S0-BBT-230

NUTRITION LABELING

Issues and Directions
for the 1990s

Committee on the Nutrition Components
of Food Labeling
Food and Nutrition Board
Institute of Medicine
National Academy of Sciences

Donna V. Porter and Robert O. Earl, Editors

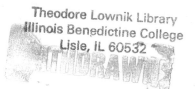

Theodore Lownik Library
Illinois Benedictine College
Lisle, IL 60532
WITHDRAWN

NATIONAL ACADEMY PRESS
Washington, D.C.   1990

363.192
I 59n

National Academy Press • 2101 Constitution Avenue, N.W. • Washington, D.C. 20418

NOTICE: The project that is the subject of this report was approved by the Governing Board of the National Research Council, whose members are drawn from the councils of the National Academy of Sciences, the National Academy of Engineering, and the Institute of Medicine. The members of the committee responsible for the report were chosen for their special competencies and with regard for appropriate balance.

This report has been reviewed by a group other than the authors according to procedures approved by a Report Review Committee consisting of members of the National Academy of Sciences, the National Academy of Engineering, and the Institute of Medicine.

The Institute of Medicine was chartered in 1970 by the National Academy of Sciences to enlist distinguished members of the appropriate professions in the examination of policy matters pertaining to the health of the public. In this, the Institute acts under both the Academy's 1863 congressional charter responsibility to be an adviser to the federal government and its own initiative in identifying issues of medical care, research, and education. Dr. Samuel O. Thier is President of the Institute of Medicine.

This study was supported by project no. 282-89-0022 from the Public Health Service, U.S. Department of Health and Human Services.

Library of Congress Cataloging-in-Publication Data

Institute of medicine (U.S.). Committee on the Nutrition
    Components of Food Labeling.
      Nutrition labeling : issues and directions for the 1990s :
    report of a study / by the Committee on the Nutrition Components
    of Food Labeling, Food and Nutrition Board, Institute of
    Medicine, National Academy of Sciences ; Donna V. Porter and
    Robert O. Earl, editors.
      p.   cm.
    Includes bibliographical references and index.
    ISBN 0-309-04326-3
    1. Food–Labeling–United States–Standards. 2. Nutrition.
    I. Porter, Donna Viola. II. Earl, Robert O. III. Title.
    [DNLM: 1. Food Labeling–standards–United States. 2. Food
    Labeling–United States–legislation. WA 33AA1 I5n]
    TX551.I56 1990
    363.19'2—cd20
    DNLM/DLC   90-13316
    for Library of Congress   CIP

Copyright © 1990 by the National Academy of Sciences

No part of this book may be reproduced by any mechanical, photographic, or electronic process, or in the form of a phonographic recording, nor may it be stored in a retrieval system, transmitted, or otherwise copied for public or private use, without written permission from the publisher, except for the purposes of official use by the U.S. Government.

Printed in the United States of America

COMMITTEE ON NUTRITION COMPONENTS OF FOOD LABELING

RICHARD A. MERRILL (*Chair*), School of Law, University of Virginia, Charlottesville, Virginia

HENRY C. McGILL, Jr. (*Vice Chair*), Department of Pathology, University of Texas Health Science Center, San Antonio, Texas

W. VIRGIL BROWN, Medlantic Research Foundation, Washington, D.C.

T. COLIN CAMPBELL, Division of Nutritional Science, Cornell University, Ithaca, New York

JOHN W. ERDMAN, Jr., Department of Food Science and Division of Nutritional Sciences, College of Agriculture, University of Illinois, Urbana, Illinois

JESSE F. GREGORY III, Food Science and Human Nutrition Department, Institute of Food and Agricultural Sciences, University of Florida, Gainesville, Florida

RICHARD L. HALL, Consultant, Baltimore, Maryland

TIMOTHY M. HAMMONDS, Research and Education, Food Marketing Institute, Washington, D.C.

ELISABET HELSING, Regional Office for Europe, World Health Organization, Copenhagen, Denmark

ALEXANDER M. SCHMIDT, Technology Advancement Center, Oakbrook, Illinois

LAURA S. SIMS, College of Human Ecology, University of Maryland, College Park, Maryland

JUDITH S. STERN, Department of Nutrition and Division of Clinical Nutrition, University of California, Davis, California

NANCY S. WELLMAN, Department of Dietetics and Nutrition, Florida International University, Miami, Florida

JOAN D. GUSSOW (*Food and Nutrition Board Liaison*), Department of Nutrition Education, Teachers College, Columbia University, New York, New York

Staff

DONNA V. PORTER, Project Director
ROBERT O. EARL, Staff Officer
JANIE B. MARSHALL, Senior Secretary

FOOD AND NUTRITION BOARD

RICHARD J. HAVEL (*Chair*), Cardiovascular Research Institute, School of Medicine, University of California, San Francisco, California

DONALD B. McCORMICK (*Vice Chair*), Department of Biochemistry, Emory University School of Medicine, Atlanta, Georgia

EDWIN L. BIERMAN, Division of Metabolism, Endocrinology, and Nutrition, School of Medicine, University of Washington, Seattle, Washington

EDWARD J. CALABRESE, Environmental Health Program, Division of Public Health, University of Massachusetts, Amherst, Massachusetts

DORIS H. CALLOWAY, Department of Nutritional Sciences, University of California, Berkeley, California

DeWITT S. GOODMAN, Institute of Human Nutrition, Columbia University, New York, New York

M.R.C. GREENWOOD, Graduate Division, University of California, Davis, California

JOAN D. GUSSOW, Department of Nutrition Education, Teachers College, Columbia University, New York, New York

JOHN E. KINSELLA, College of Agriculture and Environmental Sciences, University of California, Davis

LAURENCE N. KOLONEL, Cancer Center of Hawaii, University of Hawaii, Honolulu, Hawaii

REYNALDO MARTORELL, Food Research Institute, Stanford University, Stanford, California

WALTER MERTZ, Human Nutrition Research Center, Agricultural Research Service, U.S. Department of Agriculture, Beltsville, Maryland

MALDEN C. NESHEIM, Office of the Provost, Cornell University, Ithaca, New York

JOHN LISTON (*Ex Officio*), Division of Food Science, School of Fisheries, College of Ocean and Fishery Sciences, University of Washington, Seattle, Washington

ARNO G. MOTULSKY (*Ex Officio*), Center for Inherited Diseases, University of Washington, Seattle, Washington

ROY M. PITKIN (*Ex Officio*), Department of Obstetrics and Gynecology, School of Medicine, University of California, Los Angeles, California

Staff

CATHERINE E. WOTEKI, Director
SHIRLEY ASH, Financial Specialist
UTE S. HAYMAN, Administrative Assistant

iv

Preface

The Committee on the Nutrition Components of Food Labeling was assembled in the fall of 1989 by the Food and Nutrition Board (FNB) of the Institute of Medicine (IOM) to consider how food labels could be improved to help consumers adopt or adhere to healthy diets. The sponsors of the study, the Food and Drug Administration (FDA) of the U.S. Department of Health and Human Services (DHHS) and the Food Safety and Inspection Service (FSIS) of the U.S. Department of Agriculture (USDA), were influenced by the rapidly accumulating evidence that an individual's dietary choices can significantly affect chronic disease risk. Their support for this study reflects a shared judgment that changes in eating habits can improve the health of Americans and that food labeling, broadly defined, can materially aid wise dietary choices. The Committee agrees with both of these premises.

This Preface describes the Committee's operations and work schedule, identifies and thanks the large number of individuals and organizations that aided in the Committee's deliberations, and notes some of the limitations under which the Committee operated.

FORMATION OF THE COMMITTEE

The Committee's 14 members were convened under the auspices of the FNB and included research scientists and health professionals with experience in nutrition and health promotion as well as individuals who have experience in food formulation and food marketing and others who are familiar with the workings of the two federal agencies chiefly involved in regulating food labels, FDA and USDA. Although there were gaps in the Committee's collective experience, the members were generally aware of these limitations and took steps to augment their expertise through public hearings, workshops, and commissioned papers. Some issues are treated more cursorily than their complexity and importance warrant, but these deficiencies are, to a large extent, a consequence of the constraints, particularly of time, under which the Committee worked.

COMMITTEE PROCEDURES

From the beginning, members of the Committee appreciated that the subject of food labeling and nutrition is of intense interest to a wide range of organizations and individuals. Furthermore, it recognized that many of these organizations and individuals had information, experience, and in some instances, concrete proposals that could aid in its deliberations. Accordingly, the Committee set out to elicit a wide range of views, both through a general invitation to communicate with the Committee and by specific requests to address particular topics.

The full Committee met for 2 or more days on five different occasions, commencing in October 1989 and concluding in June 1990. In December 1989, at the second meeting, a full day was set aside to hear from organizational representatives. An announcement of the meeting was published in the *Federal Register* with a general invitation to appear, submit statements, or testify. Individual invitations were extended to 150 organizations. On December 4, 1989, 13 witnesses from 12 organizations testified at an open forum at the National Academy of Sciences (NAS) in Washington, D.C., and several other organizations and individuals submitted material to the Committee. The witnesses from these 12 organizations contributed significantly to the Committee's understanding of the issues, and the Committee wishes to identify and thank them: Sandra Bartholomey, Susan Braverman, J.B. Cordaro, Sherwin Gardner, Hilarie Hoting, Michael Jacobson, James Marsden, Allen Matthys, Elaine McLaughlin, Monica Olsen, Claire Regan, Sarah Setton, and Ann Winslow (see Appendix A).

Early in the Committee's discussions, members also realized that additional information on specific topics would be required, including issues surrounding the legal authority of FDA and USDA to adopt the type of recommendations the Committee might make, the importance of including information about specific nutrients on food labels, the utility of different types of label formats, consumer understanding and use of nutrition information, and the forces at work in the marketing of foods. The devices used to enhance understanding of these topics were through "workshops": informal conversations among Committee members and invited participants who were selected because of their experience, affiliation, or expertise.

The focus of each workshop and the invited participants, to whom we are indebted, are as follows. The workshop on label content included David Kritchevsky, Judy Marlett, Donald McCormick, Walter Mertz, Leon Prosky, and Janet Tenney. The workshop on legal issues included Edward Dunkleburger, Richard Frank, Thomas Scarlett, William Schultz, Bruce Silverglade, and Michael Taylor. The workshop on consumer understanding and use of food labels included Cheryl Achterberg, Robert Gould, James Heimbach, James Heisler, Alan Levy, and Vickie Peters. The workshop on label formats included Michael Audette, John Blair, Michael Golderman, Michael Jacobson, Pat Kuntze, Graham Moliter, Ray Schucker, and Carole Sugarman. The workshop on food marketing, label design, and promotion included Marguerite Copel, Maurice Cox, Robbi Dietrich, Harold Handley, Arthur Harckham, Doris Lennon-Thompson, Kelly Lewis, Charles Martin III, Craig Shulstad, and Robert Whermann. More detailed information about these individuals can be found in Appendix B.

The Committee appreciates the in-depth presentation on the history of food labeling regulation made by Taylor Quinn at its first meeting. It is also indebted to Robert Conley, Diane Heiman, Alvin Lorman, and Ronald Tenpas, each of whom prepared papers on relevant legal issues. Mr. Lorman's paper on the nutrition implications of FDA food standards of identity is reproduced in Appendix D.

This study is part of a larger undertaking coordinated by Michael McGinnis, deputy assistant secretary for health, and director, Office of Disease Prevention and Health Promotion (ODPHP), DHHS, that involved FDA, as well as other units of DHHS, and USDA. This effort has gone forward under the oversight of an interagency steering committee, which includes eight individuals who have provided valuable assistance to the Committee. Notable among these are Linda Meyers of ODPHP, John Vanderveen of FDA, and Ashland Clemons of FSIS.

Even before the Committee began its work, FDA and USDA had taken the first steps to prepare themselves to reform the existing requirements for food labels. The most important effort was a series of public hearings held in four cities around the United States, at which agency representatives heard from hundreds of witnesses on a series of issues, including the needed or desired changes in the nutrition contents provided in food labels. At the same time, FDA solicited public comment by publishing an announcement in the *Federal Register* (54 Fed. Reg. 32,610-32,615, Aug. 8, 1989). The regional hearings and request for public comments produced a large volume of useful information on consumer desires and food marketing practices. FDA has been generous in allowing the Committee access to all this material, and the Committee extends special thanks to agency personnel who provided assistance. The Committee also had the benefit of a study of current FDA and USDA labeling requirements prepared by Gary Kushner, under contract with ODPHP.

TIME CONSTRAINTS

Readers should be aware of an important constraint under which this report was completed. The Committee was appointed in September 1989 and met for the first time a month later; its full membership was not complete until November 1989. However, the contract between the sponsoring agencies and IOM provided for a study period of just 1 year, with a final report due by September 1990. To allow time for the National Research Council (NRC) internal review and publication processes, the Committee was required to complete its deliberations and submit a final manuscript in July 1990.

By any measure this was a short period for so complex an undertaking. The schedule was dictated, understandably, by the wishes of the sponsoring agencies rather than the complexity of the subject. This account is not intended as an excuse for the work the Committee has done or failed to do, but as background for assessing the final product.

The Committee did not attempt to produce definitive discussions of the role, content, format, and implementation of a new system of nutrition labeling for foods sold in the United States. Instead, this report attempts to advance the ongoing debate about the information that food labels should provide about nutrient content, the type of foods that should be accompanied by nutrition information, and the form in which this information should be conveyed. Many organizations and hundreds of individuals have been thinking about these subjects for many years. FDA and USDA have devoted considerable effort to studying the issues and planning for reform. In addition, many members of the U.S. Congress have displayed interest in the subject by holding hearings, drafting legislation, and pressing for its enactment.

Against this background, the Committee's report is an attempt to synthesize the scientific evidence and formulate practical proposals for improving food labels and enhancing other forms of point-of-purchase information about the nutrient content of foods. Our comparative advantage lies in the procedures and work environment of the Institute of Medicine. No member's personal well-being is dependent on the resolution of any issue discussed in the report. This is not to say that individual members lacked strong personal views or relationships that could be thought to affect their views, but members were apprised of their colleagues' affiliations and possible sources of bias, and were thus placed in a position to assess them. In addition, the Committee solicited the views of a wide range of individuals and groups with interests in the subject.

THE POLITICS OF FOOD LABELING

Although it is not appropriate in the body of this report, no serious account of the origins and progress of this study can fail to mention two developments that gained momentum in the spring and summer of 1990, some 6 months after the Committee's work had begun. Each reflected an official effort to do something about food labels promptly, and each threatened to obviate the Committee's effort.

The first development began with the announcement by DHHS Secretary Louis Sullivan in March 1990 that FDA was developing, and by mid-1990 proposed for adoption, the first in a series of revised regulations governing food labels, including information on the nutrition panel of food labels. The Committee was assured that this initiative reflected no diminution of interest in the report it had been assembled to produce and was promised that both FDA and the participants in the contemplated rulemaking would have ample opportunity to take account of the Committee's recommendations before publication of final regulations.

The second, more disconcerting development, from the perspective of the 14 individuals who volunteered their time to produce this report, has been the rapid movement of legislation that would mandate new nutrition labels on foods and that would prescribe to a substantial degree the content of those labels. No citizen who believes that more informative food labels will facilitate wiser dietary choices by Americans can be disappointed when government takes steps to accomplish this goal, and no member of the Committee believes that new legislation is, in principle, unwise. Indeed, as Chapter 8 of this report reveals, the Committee believes that legislation is desirable to confirm the authority of FDA and USDA to mandate the types of nutrition labeling that are endorsed by this report.

The Committee's concern about the legislative process has been twofold. First, investment of enormous effort and a certain pride have kindled a wish that the Committee had been able to complete work on this study before members of Congress completed theirs, desirably with an interval during which the Committee's collective recommendations could be weighed in the legislative deliberations. Second, and more important, the likelihood of legislation, combined with uncertainty about what the final product might provide, has cast a shadow over the Committee's deliberations. The Committee had no desire to disagree for disagreement's sake with the proposals pending in the Congress, but neither did it think it appropriate to express what would inevitably be seen as political positions for or against specific proposals.

The Committee's response to these external events was to ignore both of them to the extent we could. We produced the best report possible in the time available with the hope that it might be published in time to be helpful to those (FDA, USDA, and the Congress) who must make the final decisions about food labels. With respect to FDA's rulemaking initiative, the Committee assumed that the process would continue long enough to allow discussion of the recommendations before any final regulations were adopted. FDA's proposed regulations to reform food labeling were published after the Committee had completed its deliberations, and therefore, to a large extent are not addressed in this report. The same assumption could not be made about the legislative process, which appeared to be on a faster track. Even so, the Committee resisted the temptation to compare the conclusions of the study with the terms of particular legislation, none of which, until enacted, could be said to represent the judgments of Congress.

COVERAGE OF THE REPORT

As noted above, the short time frame for completing this report was the most important limitation under which the Committee functioned, and it affected the scope of the deliberations. In addition, adherence to the terms of the charge led the Committee to put aside some food labeling issues that continue to merit attention.

At its first meeting, the Committee agreed that it would not attempt to reassess, or second-guess, the conclusions about diet, nutrition, and disease that comprise the core findings of *The Surgeon General's Report on Nutrition and Health* (1988) and the NRC report, *Diet and Health: Implications for Reducing Chronic Disease Risk* (1989). The conclusions of these reports enjoy strong support within the scientific and public health communities not only in the United States but also in other countries. Moreover, the Committee's charge clearly implied that the conclusions of these reports should be taken as given and that it should focus on their implications for food labels.

The Committee reached a second self-limiting decision at the outset that was also encouraged by the sponsoring agencies. The report generally does not attempt to grapple with the phenomenon of health claims for foods. Health claims are those sorts of representations and depictions typically featured in advertising (and, thus, are beyond the jurisdiction of FDA and USDA) and on food packages, by which sellers of food have attempted to exploit the new knowledge of the relationships between diet and risk of disease. This is an area of considerable concern to the two sponsoring agencies and the Federal Trade Commission, and the commercial practices at issue have, understandably, attracted considerable interest among members of Congress. The Committee could not pretend that the subject of health claims was unrelated to its assignment—the nutrition content of food labels and other point-of-purchase labeling. The information that is allowed or required in food labels has a bearing on the types of promotional claims that should be considered legitimate. Yet, the regulatory issues presented in the latter context are more difficult, the problems of agency jurisdiction and coordination are more complex, and First Amendment limits on governmental regulation are, arguably, more potent than in the labeling context. To have grappled with the broad subject of health claims would have dramatically enlarged the Committee's work load and delayed completion of this report well beyond the established deadline.

In agreeing to exclude health claims, however, the Committee recognized that the boundary it was attempting to draw was, in some sense, an artificial one; much of the information provided in a food label can be considered a claim of some sort for that food. Thus, factual information about the level or presence of nutrients that have long-term health significance, such as fat or fiber, can be considered a type of health claim, no matter how it is presented. Moreover, the Committee was faced with the growing practice among food sellers of providing more than the basic information about the presence or levels of nutrients, a practice exemplified by labels that attempt to state or imply something about the special value of the food. Examples include such descriptors as *fat free, fiber rich,* and *low calorie.* The Committee felt obliged to examine these practices and at least attempt to suggest how FDA and USDA might deal with them. To this extent, the report crosses the boundary that the Committee initially established for itself.

It should be emphasized, however, that the Committee did not delve far into the area of health claims, nor did it attempt to identify, much less suggest definitions for, all the descriptors that have come into use to highlight the nutritional value of specific foods. Their number and variety made such an exercise imprudent. This also means that the Committee did not deal at all with terms used to describe or highlight components or features of foods that carry no obvious nutritional connotation.

Many criticisms of current food labels likewise have no nutritional implications, whatever their merits may be. For example, some critics have advocated that ingredients should be listed by percentage, others have urged that all food colors be identified by name, and still others have argued that warnings should appear on all foods that contain ingredients to which any significant number of consumers might be allergic. While sound nutrition contributes to good health, and in this sense can be considered a matter of safety, the Committee generally did not deal with criticisms of current food labels or proposals for reform that do not have an obvious bearing on the nutritional quality of foods. This report does not, however, entirely ignore the listing of ingredients on the food label. It addresses both the manner of listing and the categories of food for which the listing of ingredients is incomplete, but the discussion is confined to issues that relate to the consumer's ability to make informed choices about and among foods on the basis of their nutritional characteristics.

ACKNOWLEDGMENTS

Any undertaking of this sort accumulates debts to individuals who were not Committee members. The attempt to thank all of those who have helped the Committee complete its report would risk omitting some whose contributions were important. Therefore, expressions of appreciation are confined to the small number of individuals within IOM whose support was instrumental. Leading this list are Donna V. Porter, Project Director, and Robert O. Earl, Staff Officer.

It is no exaggeration to say that without them the report would not have been completed. We are grateful, also, to Janie B. Marshall, secretary to the project, who typed volumes, arranged travel, and assisted at meetings. Others within IOM who were very helpful in seeing this project to fruition were Catherine E. Woteki, Director of FNB; Enriqueta C. Bond, Executive Director of IOM; and Samuel O. Thier, President of IOM. Betsy S. Turvene, Michael K. Hayes, and Julie P. Phillips are to be commended for orchestrating and conducting the final manuscript editing and report preparation on a very tight schedule.

Finally, I wish to thank my 13 colleagues who comprised the Committee on the Nutrition Components of Food Labeling. They responded willingly to an unrealistic schedule, which was established after their own plans for the year were firmly fixed; they conscientiously fulfilled requests for research and writing; and they debated potentially contentious issues with tolerance and good will. In addition to producing what all Committee members hope will be an important and useful report, they made service as chairman a pleasure.

RICHARD A. MERRILL, *Chair*
Committee on the Nutrition
Components of Food Labeling

Contents

1

Summary

In 1973 the Food and Drug Administration (FDA) took the first steps to establish the current U.S. framework for the nutrition labeling of foods. For most packaged foods, FDA's regulations allowed information on nutrition content to be provided voluntarily, but prescribed a standard format. Nutrition labeling was made mandatory, however, on any food to which a nutrient was added or for which a nutrition claim was made. Not long afterward, the U.S. Department of Agriculture's (USDA) Food Safety and Inspection Service (FSIS) issued similar policy guidance for nutrition labeling on meat and poultry products. By 1990, over half of all packaged foods sold in the United States bore some type of nutrition labeling. The changes in food labels begun in the 1970s then represented a fundamental shift in regulatory philosophy and a major advance in consumer information, but from the perspective of 1990, they seem modest, incomplete, and outdated.

Criticism of the nutrition content of food labels grew intense in the 1980s. This criticism was spurred by two related developments. First, scientific investigation had convincingly demonstrated important linkages between dietary habits and the prevalence of chronic diseases, most notably cardiovascular disease, cancer, stroke, diabetes, and obesity. And at the same time, it was shown that Americans' diets were excessively abundant in such components as calories, fat, cholesterol, and sodium. The second development was a response to the first: American consumers became increasingly attentive to choices among foods. Food producers and manufacturers responded to this interest by developing foods whose composition could be promoted as reflecting this new learning about nutrition and health. Thus, in the late 1980s the expanding use of the cur-

1

rent nutrition labeling system further highlighted its inadequacies. The release of two landmark reports, *The Surgeon General's Report on Nutrition and Health* and the National Research Council (NRC) report, *Diet and Health: Implications for Reducing Chronic Disease Risk,* led to renewed efforts to reform nutrition labeling in the United States.

In 1990, the rules governing food labeling are seriously dated. Some foods subject to FDA food standards remain exempt from full ingredient labeling. No nutrition information appears on at least 40 percent of all packaged foods; nor does it accompany major segments of the food supply, including fruits, vegetables, meats, poultry, seafood, and restaurant meals. Furthermore, the information that nutrition labeling does provide is incomplete and misfocused. The current system emphasizes the presence and levels of micronutrients, disclosure of fiber and cholesterol contents is not required, and information about fat is incomplete. In addition, advertising and label claims of nutritional value or disease avoidance have proliferated with seemingly little control. It is, therefore, understandable that critics of the current system have charged that government regulation has ignored major segments of the food supply, been concerned with the wrong nutrients, and tolerated nutrition claims in advertising and labeling that are at best confusing and at worst deceptive economically and potentially harmful.

There have been earlier efforts to reform the current rules for nutrition labeling. In 1979, the U.S. Department of Health, Education, and Welfare, USDA, and the Federal Trade Commission (FTC) held hearings and considered possible changes in many areas of food labeling (44 Fed. Reg. 75,990–76,020, Dec. 31, 1979). In the past 12 years, members of the U.S. Congress have introduced legislation to overhaul FDA's and USDA's nutrition labeling regulations. Many private organizations have also put forth proposals for improved food labels generally and their nutrition content in particular.

PURPOSE AND SCOPE OF THE STUDY

In 1989 the Committee on the Nutrition Components of Food Labeling was assembled by the Food and Nutrition Board (FNB) of the Institute of Medicine to consider how food labels could be improved to help consumers adopt or adhere to healthy diets. The sponsors of the study—the Public Health Service, U.S. Department of Health and Human Services (DHHS), which includes FDA, and FSIS, USDA—were motivated by the shared judgment that changes in eating habits can improve the health of Americans and a conviction that food labeling can materially aid wise dietary choices.

The Committee was charged with addressing the following tasks: assessing the implications of the current knowledge of nutrition and health for food labeling; recommending the content and the appropriate format for food labels, taking into account the scientific data base as well as the means to communicate effectively with the public and, after examining current laws and regulations governing ingredient and nutrition labeling, proposing options for modifying current policy. The Committee was directed to use the findings of the Surgeon General's and NRC reports as the scientific basis for proposed labeling changes.

Any system of food labeling reflects assumptions about the purposes of and audience for nutrition information. The Committee believes that nutrition labeling should provide consumers with information that they can use to make choices among and between foods based on nutritional value, prevent consumer deception by providing accurate information on the product quality, and provide manufacturers with incentives to improve food products by requiring full disclosure of the ingredients and nutrient values of their products. The Committee believes that food labels must be easy to read, understandable, informative, non-deceptive, consistent across and among products, and uniform nationwide. Many consumers already use nutrition labeling, including the millions of Americans with special dietary requirements due to underlying health conditions and the many other healthy consumers who are interested in improved diets. A much larger potential audience consists of consumers who do not now use labels and who will need education before they can use labels effectively.

The Committee focused chiefly on the labels of packaged foods. However, many foods are sold without conventional labels, and some with labels are sold in conjunction with additional graphic or textual material. The Committee, therefore, considered point-of-purchase as well as conventional labels in its assessment of ways to convey nutrition information to consumers. The Committee was aware of the public interest in nutrition messages about foods conveyed in advertising. The proliferation of health claims for food products is largely a response to the scientific findings about the relationship between diet and chronic disease that precipitated the current interest in nutrition labeling reform. Since the Committee was not asked to evaluate food advertising and health claims, generally, it confined its consideration of claims to "nutrient content descriptors" on food labels and in labeling. In addition, the Committee generally did not deal with issues concerning food labels and their reform that did not have an obvious bearing on the nutritional quality of food, i.e., food safety concerns.

OVERVIEW OF THE U.S. SYSTEM FOR REGULATING FOOD LABELING

The U.S. government operates two systems for regulating food labels involving two federal agencies—USDA and FDA. Through FSIS, USDA regulates the labeling of meat and poultry products under the authority of the Federal Meat Inspection Act (FMI Act) and the Poultry Products Inspection Act (PPI Act). Operating under the Federal Food, Drug, and Cosmetic Act (FD&C Act), FDA regulates labeling of all other foods. None of these laws provide any guidance as to the information about nutrient content that must or may appear on food labels; the current rules reflect the informal judgments of FDA and USDA.

USDA and FDA regulate food labels in very different ways. USDA requires that manufacturers obtain prior approval of any label they wish to use on a meat or poultry product. USDA labeling policies are spelled out in the *FSIS Standards and Labeling Policy Book* and policy memoranda. In theory, no USDA-regulated products fail to comply, because USDA reviewers simply withhold label approval.

FDA has no legal authority to approve food labels in advance. It relies on detailed formal regulations and informal advice to describe its requirements. Manufacturers of FDA-regulated foods can use a new label and take the risk that FDA will subsequently challenge its product as being mislabeled. As a result, compliance with FDA policies depends on attentive monitoring and is resource dependent.

Although the substantive requirements of the two agencies do not differ dramatically in the area of nutrition, they do differ in some details. Moreover, there can be uncertainty as to which agency's requirements apply to a particular food. For example, the amount of meat in a pizza determines which agency has jurisdiction. A modest change in product composition can result in a change in jurisdiction.

Evolution of Nutrition Labeling of Foods

FDA's nutrition labeling regulations have undergone relatively few changes since 1973. These regulations derive their authority from the FD&C Act, which states nothing about nutrition. The Act requires that every food label must contain the name of the food, a statement of net quantity of contents, and the name and address of the manufacturer or distributor. In addition, most FDA-regulated foods must also list ingredients in descending order by weight. The Act also prohibits label statements that are false or misleading. A unique provision of the Act (section 201(n)) specifies that, in determining whether the labeling of a food is misleading, consideration should be given to whether it fails to reveal material facts about the consequences of using the product. This provision, and FDA's general power to adopt regulations to enforce the Act, formed the basis for the agency's 1973 nutrition labeling rules on packaged food labels.

It was the 1969 White House Conference on Food, Nutrition, and Health, convened to respond to reports of widespread malnutrition in America, that motivated FDA's initiative. The final report of the conference addressed the regulation of food composition and labeling, criticizing FDA's approaches to standards of identity, marketing of substitute foods, and label statements relating to nutrition and long-term health. The report stressed the need to help consumers make wise food choices by providing more nutrition information on food labels.

In response to the report, FDA initiated the adoption of regulations governing voluntary nutrition labeling for packaged foods. The regulations specified how nutrition information was to be provided if manufacturers chose to include it, and prescribed that nutrition labeling was required when a nutrient was added or a nutrition claim was made. In 1973, the goal was to enable consumers to select a diet adequate in vitamins, minerals, and protein. Thus, labels were required to provide information on the food's contribution to the desired daily consumption of these nutrients. To convey this information FDA created the U.S. Recommended Daily Allowances (U.S. RDA), which were based on the Recommended Dietary Allowances (RDA) established by FNB but reduced them to a single set of numbers applicable to healthy adults.

FDA's 1973 regulations prescribed a uniform sequence and format for disclosure of nutrition information in terms of serving size; servings per container; number of calories; amount of protein, carbohydrate, and fat (in grams per serving); and percentage of the U.S. RDA for protein, vitamin A, vitamin C, thiamin, riboflavin, niacin, calcium, and iron. A manufacturer also could list a number of other vitamins and minerals. A separate regulation allowed, but did not require, disclosure of fatty acid composition and cholesterol information, but only with an accompanying statement that such information was provided to assist individuals who were under the care of a physician. Information on the label about sodium content was required in 1984.

To convey nutrition information, FDA chose a numeric format over other alternatives. This choice seems to have been based more on informed intuition than on extensive testing of utility. FDA's scheme effectively limited the coverage of nutrition labeling. It did not have authority to require labeling on most meat and poultry products. Foods sold in restaurants and other food service operations were excluded. The agency's original plan to require nutrition labeling for fruits and vegetables, albeit with modified conditions, was withdrawn in 1975.

Although USDA has never adopted formal regulations governing nutrition labeling of meat and poultry products, it has evolved policies for such labeling that paralleled those of FDA. They are found in the *FSIS Standards and Labeling Policy Book* and policy memoranda. Policy Memorandum 039 allows a product's label to state that the food can help reduce or maintain body weight or to make a claim regarding caloric content as long as it provides nutrition information. Policy Memorandum 086, which sets forth USDA's required format for declaring nutrition information, allows either an abbreviated listing (calories, protein, carbohydrate, and fat [in grams] per serving) or the longer FDA version. USDA has also allowed provision of information about cholesterol and fatty acid content as part of either format.

The more significant differences between the two agencies concern the philosophy and manner of implementation. FDA has typically encouraged manufacturers to provide information even when it is not required, whereas

USDA has been chiefly concerned with ensuring the accuracy of whatever information appears on meat and poultry products.

Deficiencies in Current Federal
Requirements for Nutrition Labeling

Critics of current nutrition labeling cite its limited coverage, the failure to keep pace with current knowledge of the relationship between nutrition and long-term health, the amassing of information about fats and fiber, incomplete information about ingredients, misleading or undefined statements about the levels of nutrients, lack of uniformity, and inadequate consumer education efforts.

Currently, only over half of packaged foods carry nutrition information. Other foods omitted from nutrition labeling include meat, poultry, and seafood; eggs; fruits and vegetables; and foods sold in restaurants, institutional food services, vending machines, and grocery store carryout food bars. In addition, some foods subject to FDA's standards of identity (official recipes used to define the composition of standard products) still fail to list all their ingredients.

The content of current nutrition labels is incomplete given current knowledge of the relationship between diet and chronic disease. Labels are not now required to list cholesterol, saturated, monounsaturated, or polyunsaturated fatty acids, complex or simple carbohydrates, dietary fiber, and potassium, for whose inclusion there is some support. Many observers believe that labels list too many vitamins and minerals.

It is not only the nutrition information on food labels that has been criticized. Listing of ingredients by percentage has been urged. Current provision for "and/or" ingredient labeling allows manufacturers to declare a number of ingredients without specifying which ones are actually present in foods. In the case of fats and oils, it is difficult for consumers to determine the level of saturated fat in specific foods. Sugars are not currently required to be aggregated in the ingredient listing.

Confusion is reported about the meaning of both serving size and the U.S. RDAs. Nutrition information is provided as the amount per serving, but manufacturers determine the serving size, which has allowed manipulation. Serving sizes are not uniform within or between product categories. In addition, serving sizes are frequently expressed in units that consumers do not understand. The U.S. RDAs, which serve as the reference point for describing micronutrient content, have not been updated since 1972.

Finally, FDA's original choice of a numeric display rather than narrative, graphic, or symbolic presentation of nutrient information remains controversial. Some groups suggest that current dietary recommendations should also be included on labels so that consumers can compare these standards with a food's nutrient composition. There is debate, as well, over how the caloric contribution of fat can best be shown, either by calories from fat or the percentage of calories from fat.

CONTEXTUAL FACTORS INFLUENCING FOOD LABELING REFORM

Current Dietary Patterns of Americans

Since the turn of the century Americans have made extensive changes in their eating habits. More food is consumed away from home. Snacking is more common. A wider variety of foods is available year-round. Changes have occurred in the composition of foods due to improved production methods, new varieties of foods, and advances in food processing. Records maintained and surveys conducted by USDA and DHHS confirm these changes.

The primary changes in food energy sources in the past 70 years have been an increase in the percentage of energy contributed by fats, oils, sugars, and sweeteners, along with a decrease in the percentage of energy contributed by grain products. There has been no change in the amount of protein consumed, but the amount obtained from animal sources has risen. The consumption of fat and its components (certain fatty acids and cholesterol) has increased. Consumption of whole milk products and eggs has declined, whereas consumption of fats and oils, primarily salad and cooking oils, has risen. Current fat intakes are about 36 percent of total calories, compared with the frequent dietary recommendation of 30 percent of total calories from fat. Dietary fats are considered to be a current public health issue due to their association with coronary heart disease (CHD) and certain cancers. There has been a significant decrease in the proportion of carbohydrates obtained from grain products, with an increase in the consumption of sugars and sweeteners to 50 percent of total carbohydrate calories. No historical data exist on the amount of fiber available in the food supply, but current intakes are generally considerably less than the recommended minimum of 20 g/day. Americans generally consume an adequate amount of most vitamins and minerals due to new plant varieties, food fortification, and supplement use. However, there is concern about general low consumption of several micronutrients, primarily calcium and iron, and in certain population groups, vitamins A and C, folate, and zinc.

Food Marketing in the United States

A 1990 U.S. Department of Commerce document, *U.S. Industrial Outlook*, suggests that consumers demand foods with convenience, quality, variety, and healthful attributes. By 1990, an average of 12,000 new food products were being introduced annually in supermarkets, more than double the number a decade earlier. Many of these products are targeted directly at a health-conscious public and feature health and nutrition claims on their labels, and more advertising dollars are being allotted to their promotion. Sales of foods in limited-menu restaurants and foods for home use purchased in supermarkets have risen sharply, whereas those from limited-line grocery stores have fallen.

The increasing integration of the food distribution system with trade throughout the world will continue to affect the U.S. food supply. Current *Codex Alimentarius* rules and the scheduled 1992 adoption of food labeling rules by the 12 member nations of the European Community are all likely to have an impact on trade in the future, as well as the United States–Canada Free Trade Agreement. In the area of food processing, growing internationalization has occurred in food company ownership, and the pace of leveraged buyouts and takeovers has reduced funds for product research and development.

From a general marketing standpoint, it is readily apparent that nutrition "sells" food to today's consumer, and it has become an integral part of product development and marketing strategies. Manufacturers view the principal display panel of food packages as "real estate," to be reserved for sales promotion and competition with rivals, and will not willingly surrender it to government labeling requirements. Although industry can be expected to generally support labeling changes that will create a more informed consumer choice process, it will resist changes perceived to disturb consumer perception of product value, erode consumer ability to evaluate products in the context of total diet, or risk the disclosure of proprietary formulations.

Consumer Understanding of Nutrition and Use of Food Labels

No single study has adequately described how dietary patterns are developed, maintained, and changed; food choices are influenced by social, cultural, economic, psychological, and physiological factors. Familiarity is a particularly important factor in choosing foods. Education and income levels have a significant influence on food choices.

Results of the 1990 Food Marketing Institute (FMI) survey of consumer attitudes and shopping behavior indicate that over 70 percent of shoppers identified taste, nutrition, and product safety as very important factors. Those on medically restricted diets were more likely to rank nutrition first. Numerous studies have confirmed that Americans are increasingly interested in nutrition, including increasing concerns about the health risks associated with sodium, fat, and cholesterol intakes. They report eating less salt, red meat, butter, whole milk, and eggs.

Motivation is a key factor in how receptive any target audience will be to new information. Curiosity about a new claim may lead to a specific food purchase. Medical advice to limit certain food components often leads to closer attention to nutrition information. However, increased knowledge about nutrition does not guarantee dietary change by consumers. Moreover, increased concern expressed by consumers about the relationship between diet and long-term health was matched by increased food and nutrition knowledge related to dietary fats and cholesterol, except in those who are trying to avoid cholesterol. Several surveys have suggested that confusion exists over the relationship between grams and ounces; percent reductions of a food component; and the differences between fat and cholesterol, saturated and unsaturated fats, and dietary and serum cholesterol.

Although consumers may think of nutrition in terms of the positive attributes of a food, they increasingly pay attention to "negative nutrients" (e.g., calories, cholesterol, sodium, sugar, and certain chemical additives) by avoiding certain foods. Trends identified by the 1990 FMI survey indicate that consumers report that of the six food concerns listed, five related to food components that recent reports have stated need to be reduced in Americans' diets. Although consumers' stated predispositions about food components may eventually translate into food choices, no dramatic shift in dietary behavior has been observed.

Studies reveal that although consumers report that they want more nutrition information on food labels, many do not actually comprehend this information and use it in making food purchases. Research has shown that older adults are more likely to use labels to compare products or examine ingredients. The 1990 FMI survey revealed that almost one-half of respondents indicated that they read nutrition and ingredient information sometimes, whereas those on medically restricted diets are twice as likely to read labels for this information. In the 1989 FMI survey, consumers reported that labels should be easier to understand and should include more information on calories, salt and sodium, fat and saturated fats, chemicals, colorings, and dyes. Although consumers report that they understand food labels, some studies suggest that consumers often do not actually comprehend the terms and definitions used on nutrition labels, and therefore, they cannot make optimum use of them in making food purchases.

A few studies have suggested that consumers are motivated to buy foods with nutrition profiles that are more consistent with current dietary recommendations. The 1990 National Food Processors Association study reported that 51 percent of consumers were influenced "a great deal" by nutrition information at the point of purchase. The cooperative Giant Food, Inc. (Washington, D.C.), and FDA supermarket point-of-purchase program, which tracked food purchases, revealed that sales of products that were labeled with nutrition information on shelf price tags increased over sales of products that were not labeled. Several programs for meat, such as the Minnesota Heart Health and the Meat Nutri-Facts programs, have shown an increase in purchases of leaner cuts of meat, and consumers reported that nutrition information was useful in making meat selections. Other studies have suggested, however, that information programs may be more successful in improving nutrition knowledge than in changing purchasing behaviors.

Analytical Considerations Affecting Food Labeling Reform

Providing information about the nutrient content of foods on labels requires an analysis of food composition. Both FDA and USDA currently have requirements for label accuracy that reflect the current capacity of analytical chemistry. USDA permits manufacturers to provide nutrition information derived either by calculation from analyses based on official methods of the Association of Official Analytical Chemists (AOAC) or accepted references. USDA has implemented the Nutrition Label Verification (NLV) program, which includes procedures to verify labels for accuracy, although the degree of accuracy that is required imposes analytical problems on food manufacturers. FDA regulations mandate that all the required and any optional information on the nutrition information panel must be determined by direct laboratory analysis. A ± 20 percent tolerance from label values is allowed. FDA generally requires that analysis be done by AOAC-approved methods or by reliable and appropriate analytical procedures set by the Secretary of DHHS.

Acquisition of reliable food composition data is not easy. Difficulties include complexities of analytical methods and food composition, differences in the analytical capabilities of different laboratories, and the need for improved analytical methods and training of technicians. Current methods vary with respect to their applicability, convenience, expense, and the degree of analytical expertise required to perform them. Considerable improvement is needed in the validation and standardization of methods of food analysis for use in labeling as well as food composition data bases.

Soluble fiber cannot easily be measured, since it is usually calculated by determining the difference between total dietary fiber and insoluble dietary fiber, which is subject to considerable imprecision compared to a direct measurement. Thus, the method remains controversial. Measurement of total carbohydrate per serving for food labeling purposes is generally performed indirectly by determining the amount remaining after protein, ash, moisture, and fat are subtracted, resulting in potential inaccuracy and imprecision. Recent advances in the methods used to measure complex carbohydrates will allow for potentially more accurate measurement of various carbohydrate components. Total fat is currently measured routinely, and methods exist for the accurate measurement of cholesterol. Suitable methods exist for the measurement of most minerals in foods, although standardization and validation are needed. Considerable development is required to obtain reliable analytical methods for many vitamins in foods, because of natural variability, especially in plant sources.

The application of direct analytical analyses to nonpackaged foods, including meat, poultry, seafood, fruits, and vegetables, and foods sold in restaurants, is impractical. The need to expand public access to information about the nutrient content of foods suggests the desirability of using appropriate data base information as an alternative to direct analyses for these foods. The USDA National Nutrient Data Bank contains reasonably complete data on the composition of foods, although data are less complete on nutrients for which sound analytical methods are lacking. Other sources of food composition data complement USDA data, but these need to be certified by FDA and USDA to be used for nutrition labeling purposes. At best, however, data bases can indicate representative information on the composition of foods, which means that there may be large differences between data base values and the actual amounts of certain nutrients in a single sample of food.

The Committee recommends that:

- Label verification by analysis of composite samples should be made at least twice each year to ensure reasonable accuracy of nutrition labels without imposing the burden of a complete quarterly analysis.
- FDA and USDA should certify data from the National Nutrient Data Bank or other appropriate sources regarding the nutrient content of fresh foods and foods sold in restaurants.
- FDA and USDA should allow considerable flexibility in the selection of analytical methods for label verification of nutrient content.
- In proposing an alternative (nonofficial) analytical method, suitable verification must be required (e.g., recovery of samples and analysis of reference materials). In addition, appropriate quality control procedures should be used in each analysis.
- Development of additional standard reference materials for use in food analysis should be encouraged.
- Funding should be provided for the development of improved analytical methods, establishment of programs for the testing of methods through interlaboratory studies, and development of additional standard reference materials.
- Completion and expansion of the USDA National Nutrient Data Bank should be continued.

LABELING COVERAGE

Mandatory Nutrition Labeling

Although nutrition knowledge will continue to evolve, there is now sufficient consensus on diet and long-term health to serve as a basis for changes in food labeling. The Surgeon General's report and the NRC *Diet and Health* report indicate that consumers must make changes in both the dietary components and the food groups they eat, if they are to reduce their risk of chronic disease. In order to achieve the recommended dietary adjustments, consumers must be able to make informed choices in their daily selection of foods. The current lack of relevant, consistent information across the full spectrum of food products is a significant deterrent to consumers who wish to make informed choices. However, certain foods need to be either exempted from these requirements or, in the case of foods for children under age 2 with special dietary requirements, have alternative labeling requirements more suitable to that group of foods.

The Committee recommends that:

- FDA and USDA should promptly adopt regulations to institute mandatory and uniform nutrition labeling requirements for all packaged foods within their respective jurisdictions, with limited exemptions.
- Exemptions from the general requirement should only be granted in those situations in which alternatives to nutrition labeling have been fully explored and determined to be unreasonable, impractical, or too costly.
- Food designed for children under age 2 should be exempted from the general requirements; nutrition labeling of macronutrients in baby foods should be required, with the optional listing of all micronutrients, except for calcium and iron declaration.
- Nutrition labeling should be required on institutional-size packages and commodity foods or on product specification sheets.

Produce, Seafood, and Meat and Poultry

Recent dietary recommendations emphasize that Americans should reduce their consumption of fat and cholesterol by eating more fruits, vegetables, seafood, poultry, and lean meat. Nutrition information on fresh foods would aid consumers in making appropriate food choices. However, providing nutrition information about fresh foods presents some special challenges. Fresh foods are more heterogeneous than formulated foods, which are more uniform in composition and are batch tested. The variability of the nutrient content of fresh foods is due to factors such as biological variability, climate, seasonal variations, agricultural practices, and animal husbandry. The effects of storage and cooking on fresh foods further affects their nutrient composition. None of these factors are reflected in nutrient composition information provided in data bases.

For fresh foods, the use of food composition data may provide a practical alternative to laboratory analysis. Although the USDA National Nutrient Data Bank is not totally complete, the data base provides an adequate basis for use of nutrient content information in point-of-purchase labeling of most fresh foods. An alternative data bank has been developed by the Produce Marketing Association for about 30 different produce commodities. FDA and USDA currently require that nutrient information be based on analytical data of foods as actually purchased, which effectively precludes the use on the food composition data bases.

The Committee recommends that:

- Retailers should be required to provide point-of-purchase nutrition labeling information for produce, and for fresh and frozen meat, poultry, and seafood (e.g., 20 to 30 top items in each category using data base information, rather than lot-by-lot analysis). After the first 3 years, the program should be evaluated for consumer reaction, use, and understanding and modified accordingly.

- FDA and USDA should allow flexibility in the format and the nutrition information required for labeling of fresh foods.
- FDA and USDA should establish a joint committee to certify the data bases and acceptable methodologies for providing nutrient composition data for fresh foods.
- FDA and USDA should continue to improve the USDA's National Nutrient Data Bank, particularly in the area of fresh foods, in harmony with the above recommendations.

Foods Sold by Restaurants

Americans currently spend about 43 percent of their food dollar on meals eaten away from home, which is expected to total $156.4 billion in 1990. The National Restaurant Association estimates that 45.8 million Americans (about 20 percent of the population) eat in refreshment places each day. According to a 1989 National Restaurant Association survey, an increasing number of consumers are concerned about the types of foods available in restaurants.

Restaurants are paying more attention to providing foods that are consistent with current dietary recommendations. In the past 5 years, the number of restaurants reporting that they have nutrition information on their menu items available for those consumers who request it has doubled. Many restaurants have menus coded for items that are low in fat, cholesterol, salt, and calories.

Some groups have urged that restaurants provide more information on the ingredients and nutrient contents of foods served to aid consumers who are concerned about their intake of salt, fat, and sugar. Although primary attention has focused on the limited-menu segment of the restaurant industry, there is no evidence to suggest that meals served in other restaurants are necessarily more nutritious or likely to meet the recent dietary recommendations.

The nutrient composition of menu items can be computed either by the use of readily available computer software or by subscribing to programs that perform the evaluation. Nutrient content information should be based on the standardized serving sizes for foods in limited-menu restaurants. For other restaurants, normative serving sizes will need to be identified by the agencies.

Because Americans are consuming a growing number of their meals in restaurant settings where nutrition information is not routinely available, the Committee recommends that:

- All restaurants should be required to have standard menu items evaluated for their nutritional profiles and provide this information to patrons upon request.

- Restaurant menus should be required to state that "nutrient evaluation is available upon request," so that consumers can, if they desire, obtain such information.
- FDA and USDA should, through regulations, allow the use of nutrient data bases to provide nutrient evaluation of menu items.
- Food service establishments above a specified size and/or volume (limited-menu and regional/national restaurant chains) should be required to provide nutrition analysis of food items at the point of purchase. This requirement can be met by placing the information either on package wrappers and containers or at some other point-of-purchase location that allows consumers easy access and use.
- Restaurants should be encouraged to participate in programs and/or otherwise provide for appropriate symbols or descriptors on menu items that identify foods that meet criteria for low-calorie, low-fat, low-cholesterol, and/or low-sodium. Comparable definitions for symbols and descriptors should be established by FDA and USDA.
- FDA and USDA should define the categories and size of restaurant operations for which regulations based on the above recommendations are applicable.

Foods Sold by Noncommercial Food Services

In recent years, institutional food service operations have grown substantially as an increasing number of meals are being prepared, served, and consumed outside the home. Members of all age groups are eating away from home in institutional or congregate settings. Children may eat up to two meals per day at school. Long- and short-term health care facilities are feeding a growing population of elderly people. Military installations, correctional facilities, and institutions of higher education feed millions of people daily. None of these noncommercial services have strict rules on serving meals that meet current dietary recommendations. Many of their customers, however, are health conscious and/or are open to nutrition education programs.

The Committee recommends that:

- The agencies at the federal, state, and local levels that oversee or support noncommercial food services encourage voluntary nutrition labeling of meals at the point of purchase or point of selection as part of overall nutrition education efforts.

NUTRITION LABEL CONTENT

Current nutrition labeling contains information on calories, protein, fat, carbohydrate, sodium, and percentage of the U.S. RDA for protein and seven micronutrients. In light of recent dietary recommendations for changes in the consumption of certain dietary constituents, it is necessary to reexamine the nutrient information required on food labels and in labeling.

Health Relevance of Nutrient Recommendations

Calories

Despite the continued controversy over the causes of obesity, consensus exists that obesity is related to morbidity and mortality from chronic diseases. Recent dietary recommendations have emphasized the importance of maintaining a desirable weight to minimize the risk of chronic disease. An estimated 34 million Americans are overweight, and more than 80 million are trying to control their weight. In order to achieve and maintain a desirable weight, caloric intake must be in balance with energy expenditure by decreasing caloric intake and increasing energy expenditure.

Calories are the one component of the food label that most consumers understand, and its presence is useful to those who are trying to attain a desirable weight and balance their consumption of macronutrients. The principal display panel of food packages may carry a statement on calories per serving and/or a descriptive term indicating that the product has fewer calories than its counterparts in the marketplace. On the nutrition information panel, the caloric value for a single serving of the food is expressed as the number of calories per serving.

The Committee recommends that:

- FDA and USDA should continue to require the disclosure of calories expressed as kilocalories per serving on the nutrition information panel.
- If the manufacturer chooses to express nutrients as a percentage of total calories, 2,000 calories should be used and stated as the reference point for the average adult who engages in light physical activity.
- Descriptors related to caloric content of foods that are currently defined by FDA and USDA should be continued.
- FDA and USDA should define and standardize the terms *light, lite,* and *diet* and other descriptors that can be interpreted as caloric claims.

Fat and Cholesterol

Dietary fats and oils primarily provide energy and various other characteristics that relate to current health concerns. Cholesterol is another lipid component related to health concerns. The health effects of dietary fat and cholesterol range from CHD to cancer and gallbladder disease, and the high caloric density of fats has an impact on caloric intake.

The ingredient listing provides information on the sources of fat contained in foods. "And/or" labeling is currently allowed so that manufacturers can list several fats or oils that might be used in a product. In the absence of a claim, voluntary use of the nutrition information panel provides quantitative information on the amount of total fat (in grams) per serving. The principal display panel of food packages features descriptors used to highlight fat and cholesterol contents.

Current labeling requirements for fat disclosure have several limitations. "And/or" labeling fails to reveal not only the specific fats and oils used in a particular food, but also the differences in the degree of fatty acid saturation. Unless a claim is made about the fatty acid or cholesterol contents of a food or the information is provided voluntarily, the nutrition label does not contain information on the degree of saturation of fats or the cholesterol content of a food. In addition, the lack of standardized definitions for many terms used to describe fat and cholesterol contents contributes to confusion and misrepresentation.

The Committee recommends that:

- FDA and USDA should require the disclosure of total fat, saturated fat, unsaturated fat, and cholesterol contents per serving in grams (milligrams for cholesterol) on the nutrition information panel, with saturated and unsaturated fat either indented or otherwise identified as subcategories of total fat.
- FDA and USDA should require the listing of calories per serving from total fat, saturated fat, and unsaturated fat on the nutrition information panel.
- FDA and USDA should allow, as an option, the disclosure of monounsaturated and polyunsaturated fatty acid contents per serving in grams on the nutrition information panel.
- FDA and USDA should define descriptors for cholesterol content for use on the principal display panel.
- FDA and USDA should define descriptors for total fat and saturated, monounsaturated, polyunsaturated, and unsaturated fatty acid contents on the principal display panel.
- FDA and USDA should require that when a manufacturer refers to "x percent total fat" (by weight) and other similar terms on a package, it should also be required to state "x percent calories from fat" in close proximity in the same type size and type face.
- FDA and USDA regulations should continue to allow "and/or" labeling of fats and oils in the ingredient listing on the conditions that the food carries full nutrition labeling and that the stated saturated fat content listed is the

highest level that would be achieved with any mixture of the listed fats and oils.

- FDA and USDA should establish an entity to evaluate the issue of the cholesterolemic effects of stearic and other fatty acids (e.g., *trans* fatty acids) and related changes that may need to be made in redefining fatty acids for regulatory purposes.

Carbohydrates

Carbohydrates provide about 45 percent of total adult caloric intake, about half of which is provided by complex carbohydrates. Diets that exclude or are low in whole grains, fruits, and vegetables are associated with a variety of chronic health problems, including obesity, cancer, heart disease, and diabetes. The Surgeon General's and NRC's reports have recommended that Americans should increase their consumption of complex carbohydrates. Although foods high in complex carbohydrates may not contribute directly to chronic disease prevention, these foods are usually low in fat and calories and high in fiber. Health concerns about the consumption of simple carbohydrates focus on the incidence of dental caries, nutrient dilution, and potential source of excess calories.

The principal display panel of food labels may carry descriptors as well as brand names that characterize the sugar content of products but seldom provides information on carbohydrate content. In the ingredient listing, sugars are listed individually among other ingredients in the order of predominance even though they may collectively comprise the major component (by weight) of the product. The nutrition information panel lists total carbohydrate per serving (in grams). Some manufacturers voluntarily list complex carbohydrates and simple carbohydrates (sugars) separately, but this is not required.

The Committee recommends that:

- FDA and USDA should continue to require the disclosure of carbohydrate content per serving in grams on the nutrition information panel.
- FDA and USDA should allow as an option the listing of the content of complex carbohydrates (which are defined as digestible polysaccharides such as starch and glycogen), and sugars (which are defined as digestible mono- and disaccharides) per serving in grams on the nutrition information panel. The term *total carbohydrate* should be used when carbohydrate components are listed, with these subgroups indented.
- FDA and USDA should allow, as an option, the listing of calories per serving from total carbohydrate, complex carbohydrate, and sugars on the nutrition information panel.
- The ingredient listing should group all sugars together under the term *sugars* with mono- and disaccharides (including glucose [dextrose], fructose, lac-

tose, sucrose, invert sugar, and honey, as well as corn syrup, high-fructose corn syrup, and mild flavored and "stripped" concentrated fruit juices) in a parenthetical listing, in descending order by weight under this term. Sugar alcohols, such as mannitol and sorbitol, would be listed separately and would not be grouped with sugars.

- FDA and USDA should consider allowing manufacturers to use "and/or" labeling for sugars.
- FDA and USDA should define descriptors that apply to terms used for carbohydrate and sugar content on foods labels.

Dietary Fiber

For a decade, Americans have been advised to increase their consumption of dietary fiber on the basis of suggestive evidence of a possible link with the incidence of CHD, certain cancers, and diabetes, although studies of the protective role of dietary fiber per se has been inconclusive to date. Recent research suggests that soluble fiber (e.g., that found in oat bran, beans, and certain fruits) is associated with lower blood glucose and blood lipid levels. And there is some evidence that an overall increase in intake of foods that are high in insoluble fiber might decrease the risk of colon cancer. The strongest argument for an increase in consumption of dietary fiber is the important contribution it makes to normal bowel function.

FDA currently allows listing of dietary fiber on food labels, but does not require it. In addition, descriptors of fiber content are prominent on the principal display panel of some foods.

The Committee recommends that:

- FDA and USDA should require the disclosure of fiber content per serving in grams on the nutrition information panel under the term *total dietary fiber*.
- FDA and USDA should define the scope of foods from animal origin and other foods that contain little or no dietary fiber which should be exempted from this requirement.
- FDA and USDA should discourage labeling of soluble or insoluble fiber contents until methodologies approved by the agencies allow for the adequate and reproducible quantification of the soluble and insoluble fiber contents of a variety of foods.
- FDA and USDA should define descriptive terms allowed to be used for various source levels of dietary fiber on food labels.

Protein

The majority of Americans consume protein in excess of the RDA. So far there is little evidence that diets high in protein increase the risk of chronic diseases, but the hypothesis still commands continued research attention. The listing of ingredients provides information on protein sources if consumers recognize them. The nutrition information panel currently lists protein in grams per serving and as a percentage of the U.S. RDA. Protein content claims may also appear on the principal display panel.

The Committee recommends that:

- FDA and USDA should continue to require the disclosure of protein content per serving in grams on the nutrition information panel. However, protein should be moved to a position of less prominence.
- The current requirement to list protein content as a percentage of the U.S. RDA should be eliminated.
- FDA and USDA should allow, as an option, the listing of total calories per serving from protein.
- FDA and USDA should define descriptors that apply to terms used for protein content on food labels.

Sodium

For years, concern about the adverse health effects of sodium has focused on the role of sodium in causing high blood pressure, heart failure, and edema. Hypertension, which affects 60 million Americans, is a major risk factor for CHD, hypertensive heart disease, arteriosclerosis, stroke, and renal failure. Current intakes of sodium by the U.S. population are widely regarded as excessive.

The ingredient listing provides information on salt and other sodium-containing ingredients that are added to a food. FDA's original nutrition labeling regulations did not require listing of sodium content per serving, but, effective July 1986, the agency required sodium to be listed (in milligrams) whenever nutrition labeling was provided or a claim about sodium content was made. Sodium could also be declared voluntarily without triggering full nutrition labeling. These regulations also defined several descriptive terms for sodium content: *sodium free, low sodium, reduced sodium, unsalted,* and *no added salt.* USDA has adopted essentially identical guidelines.

The Committee recommends that:

- FDA and USDA should continue to require the disclosure of sodium content per serving in milligrams, regardless of source (whether natural or added), on the nutrition information panel.

- Descriptors for sodium content on the principal display panel, as currently defined by FDA and USDA, should be continued.

Potassium

Severe fluctuations in potassium levels can be life-threatening. Some studies have suggested that increased dietary potassium may lead to a reduction in blood pressure. Current FDA regulations allow, but do not require, declaration of potassium on the nutrition label. USDA's policy is identical to that of FDA.
The Committee recommends that:

- Disclosure of potassium content on the nutrition information panel should remain voluntary, unless a potassium claim is made.
- If disclosed on the label, potassium content per serving should be listed in milligrams.

Vitamins and Minerals

In the United States, dietary intakes of some vitamins and minerals are current or potential public health issues, especially in some subgroups, but the majority of Americans are at no risk of deficiency. Under FDA's nutrition labeling regulations, seven micronutrients are required to be listed as a percentage of the U.S. RDA (vitamins A and C, thiamin, riboflavin, niacin, calcium, and iron). Micronutrients would also appear in the ingredient listing when added to the product as individual ingredients. Any of these micronutrients, although most commonly calcium, iron, and vitamin C, are frequently featured on the principal display panel of foods by a descriptive term signifying their presence in a notable amount. Each of the seven vitamins and minerals, and any other voluntarily added, must be listed in the nutrition information panel as a percentage of the U.S. RDA, regardless of the label present.

Vitamin A   Vitamin A is critical for such functions as vision and the immune system. Some carotenoids without vitamin A activity may have anticancer properties. Vitamin A deficiency is generally rare among Americans, though inadequate intake is found in some children under age 5 or people with chronic fat malabsorption. Vitamin A has been accorded status as a potential public health issue.

B Vitamins   Thiamin, riboflavin, and niacin are readily available in the diets of most Americans, and the incidence of deficiency is relatively rare, except among individuals whose health is already compromised. Vitamin B_6 deficiency, which rarely occurs, is usually observed in those who are deficient in several

B-complex vitamins. Folate intakes are generally adequate. Folate and vitamin B_6 have been accorded status as potential public health issues, whereas thiamin, niacin, and riboflavin are not current public health issues.

Vitamin C   Dietary deficiency of vitamin C can eventually lead to scurvy which has been observed in the United States in infants fed diets consisting exclusively of cows' milk and in elderly individuals who are on inadequate diets. Concern about vitamin C adequacy extends to individuals with low dietary intakes, cigarette smokers, and the poor. Therefore, it has been accorded status as a potential public health issue.

Calcium   Although the mechanism is not well understood, adequate calcium intake during the formative years, when it is most efficiently absorbed, is believed to reduce the risk of osteoporosis. Calcium absorption often is impaired in elderly individuals, affected by other dietary factors and hormonal changes. Increased calcium intake has been associated with a reduction in blood pressure in some studies, although this is not yet conclusive. Because of low calcium intakes by women and its possible association with age-related osteoporosis, calcium has been accorded status as a current public health issue.

Iron   Iron's most critical role is to carry oxygen to body tissues. Inadequate intakes of dietary iron can ultimately lead to anemia. Iron deficiency is primarily observed at 6 to 48 months of age, during adolescence, and during the female reproductive period, and therefore has been accorded status as a current public health issue.

Although adequate intakes of micronutrients are important for all ages groups, intakes of a few of the seven vitamins and minerals that are currently listed on nutrition labels are current public health issues for Americans. Certain micronutrients are potential problems in specific subgroups, such as children and women of childbearing age. As a result, there seems to be little reason to continue to require all seven micronutrients to be listed, and the focus should be on those that represent clearly identified problems.

The Committee recommends that:

- FDA and USDA should continue to require disclosure of calcium and iron content per serving, but using source descriptors (i.e., *very good source of, source of,* and *contains*).
- FDA and USDA should allow, as an option, disclosure of the content of all other micronutrients for which RDAs exist.
- FDA and USDA should establish standardized definitions for the terms used to describe the micronutrient content of foods on the principal display panel and these definitions should be the same as those used on the nutrition information panel as described for calcium and iron.

PRESENTATION OF LABEL INFORMATION

Serving Size

The concept of serving is currently used as a reference unit for information about the nutrient content of foods. FDA regulations define *serving* to be the actual amount of a food likely to be consumed at a single setting or the portion of the food likely to be used as an ingredient. Nutrient information is declared in relation to the average or usual serving. Serving is also used as a tool for food and nutrient composition data bases and in dietary guidance systems that advise consumers about the number of daily servings of foods from each food group they should consume.

A number of studies have shown that a large proportion of respondents cannot accurately judge the amounts of foods and beverages they consume. There is a tendency to overestimate serving sizes, with the magnitude of the error varying with the specific food item and experience in food preparation.

There is currently wide variation in the size of servings declared on food labels, both between categories of foods and among foods in the same product category. It is frequently possible for two products with similar nutrient content to have different serving sizes. The ability of manufacturers to set serving sizes allows them to portray foods in the most favorable light to attract consumers. FDA has frequently voiced concern about the confusion in the marketplace caused by the practice of manufacturers to set serving sizes to enhance the attractiveness of a product's nutritional value. This problem is further compounded by the use of nutrient descriptors.

Several alternatives to serving size as the reference unit for nutrition information have been suggested, such as per 100 grams, and entire package. Although no reference unit is ideal, expressing nutrition information by serving seems to be preferred by consumers, health professionals, and food manufacturers.

The Committee recommends that:

- Given the alternatives available (serving size, nutrient values per package or container, 100-g portions), *serving* should continue to be the reference unit for presenting nutrition information on foods.
- Serving sizes should be expressed in common household measures, followed by the weight in grams (in parentheses) to facilitate comparisons across product categories. Serving sizes should be standardized across food categories on the basis of volume or weight measures. All serving sizes should be rounded down to the nearest whole number.
- The number of servings per package or container should continue to be specified. For a single-serving container, 50 to 150 percent of the commonly

consumed unit would be acceptable. The number of servings per container should be rounded down to the nearest in whole number.

- Consistent with the recommendation that serving sizes should be standard-ized, quantities specified by dietary guidance recommendations should serve as the main criteria for selecting the amount of food to be described as a serving. This preference for recommended amount, rather than consumed amount, has the advantage that it can be more readily applied in educational programs and will ensure consistency among serving sizes as presented in dietary guidance materials and on the food label.

- FDA and USDA should, jointly, establish serving sizes for a limited number of different food categories, (i.e., fruit juices, breads, cereals, fruits, vegetables, spreads, and salad dressings) since serving size information will be more valuable to consumers if it applies to broad categories of food. The Committee favors fewer, rather than more, categories so that nutrition information can readily be used by consumers for product comparisons and reference purposes.

- If a food manufacturer desires a serving size different from that set by the agencies, it should be permitted to petition the responsible agency to allow a deviation or to create a new subclass of foods with its own serving size.

- FDA and USDA should establish uniformity in serving size specifications within product categories and between agencies to facilitate comparisons among products, labels, point-of-purchase information, and federal and private data bases.

- Research should be conducted to determine how consumers comprehend food label information and how they interpret serving sizes declared on the food package.

U.S. Recommended Daily Allowances

The U.S. RDA reference standards were set in 1972 based on the 1968 RDA (which have since been updated several times), generally at the highest level of RDA recommended for any age or sex group in the population. The amounts of protein, vitamins A and C, thiamin, riboflavin, niacin, calcium, and iron per serving as a percentage of the U.S. RDA are currently required to be declared on the nutrition information panel. Amounts are expressed in 2 percent increments up to the 10 percent level, 5 percent increments up to the 50 percent level, and 10 percent increments above 50 percent. Nutrients present in amounts of less than the 2 percent are indicated by a zero or an asterisk, which refers to a statement at the bottom of the table indicating that the product "contains less than 2 percent of the U.S. RDA of these nutrients." When a vitamin or mineral is added to a food or a claim is made about any nutrients, the percentage of the U.S. RDA must be declared for all seven vitamins and minerals. No claim can be made that the food is a significant source of a nutrient unless a serving of the food contains 10 percent or more of the U.S. RDA of the nutrient per serving.

The Committee recommends that:

- The U.S. RDAs (or different reference term) should be updated, even if they are to play a more limited role in nutrition labeling in the future.
- FDA and USDA should require the use of the descriptors *very good source of*, *good source of*, or *contains* to characterize the content of required or optional micronutrients in foods.
- Use of the descriptive terms on the nutrition information panel would require that micronutrient meet the following or similar criteria: use of *very good source of* must provide, in a serving, more than 20 percent of the dietary standard for a given vitamin or mineral; use of *good source of* must provide, in a serving, 11 to 20 percent of the dietary standard for a given nutrient; use of *contains* must provide between 2 and 10 percent of the dietary standard for any nutrient; and a manufacturer would not be required or allowed to declare any nutrient present at less than 2 percent of the dietary standard.

Ingredient Labeling

The ingredient listing can be an important source of information about the nutrient composition of packaged foods. FDA and USDA require that ingredients be listed by their common names in their order of decreasing predominance by weight. The most significant exception to the general requirement that ingredients be disclosed is for foods covered by an FDA standard of identity for which only optional ingredients may be required to be labeled. Although FDA lacks the authority to require the labeling of mandatory ingredients, it has taken steps to amend existing standards to recharacterize most ingredients as optional. USDA requires ingredient labeling on standardized foods. The exemption of any standardized foods from mandatory ingredient labeling can no longer be justified. The Committee did not take a position on percentage ingredient labeling because it viewed the issue as having no nutritional significance, although it may have merit for other reasons.

The current format for the ingredient listing has been criticized. Ingredients typically appear as running text and often are printed entirely in capital letters separated only by commas, with no breaks or classifications and some use of parenthetical phrases to describe functions. Several useful proposals have been suggested to make this portion of the label easier to read, including required use of capital and lowercase letters, separation of major from the minor ingredients, and the use of contrasting colors. Efforts should be made to improve the readability of the ingredient listing to aid consumer understanding of the nutritional characteristics of different foods.

The Committee recommends that:

- Congress should amend the FD&C, FMI, and PPI Acts to make clear that the general requirement of full ingredient listing applies to standardized as well as nonstandardized foods.
- FDA and USDA should take steps to amend their regulations for ingredient labeling to require that the ingredients of standardized foods that are incorporated into other processed foods are declared by name on the label of the final product.
- When FDA and USDA test different basic formats for nutrition labeling, they should also seek information about consumer reactions to and use of different formats for depicting the ingredients in foods.

Food Standards of Identity

FDA has established standards of identity for nearly 300 foods, most which have existed since the 1940s and 1950s. These standards define the composition of products entitled to use the official product name. Some of these standards of identity have been criticized for impeding manufacturers' ability to offer more nutritious foods. The legal process for establishing and amending food standards of identity is extremely cumbersome, which discourages changes that would facilitate marketing of more healthful versions of products traditionally high in fat.

In theory, standards of identity need not impede the marketing of reduced-fat or low-fat substitutes for foods traditionally high in fat but critics have claimed that FDA compliance policy discourages such innovations by precluding the use of standardized names on products that contain reduced levels of fat. Although the Committee could not fully assess the criticisms of standards of identity, standards of identity certainly justify reexamination of the impact on efforts to develop more healthful versions of well-known foods.

The Committee recommends that:

- FDA's food standards should be carefully examined for their effects on the marketing of low-, lower-, and no-fat substitutes for high-fat foods.
- Congress should amend the FD&C Act to eliminate the requirement that standards be adopted and amended through formal rulemaking procedures.
- Congress should eliminate the exemption from full ingredient labeling for standardized foods.

Descriptors

Product labels have long been used for promotional as well as informational purposes, and food marketers give careful consideration to every facet of label design. Although many facets of food labels are regulated, manufacturers nonetheless have considerable choice in the information that they include and the manner in which it is displayed within the constraints of label and package size. Growing consumer interest in nutrition and specific nutritional components has led many manufacturers to feature the desirable characteristics of products. Common examples in this practice are so-called nutrient content descriptors, such as low-calorie, fat-free, no cholesterol, fiber-rich, and lite.

The proliferation of these descriptors and the growth in their usage have drawn attention from regulatory bodies, health professionals, and competitors. On the one hand, their popularity signals an encouraging interest among consumers about the links between nutrition and long-term health. On the other hand, the potential for confusion, exaggeration, and outright deception has prompted some to argue that nutrient content claims should be forbidden altogether.

The problem stems in part from failure of the current system to regulate such claims in a systematic way. Users of many content descriptors have no official definition against which to basis their claims. USDA reviews all labels individually and does not approve a label that carries an unapproved claim. FDA lacks standard definitions for most of the descriptors in common use, and at times is hampered in its efforts to prevent the use of terms in the absence of formal definitions. FDA has often relied on compliance with informal advice which depends on manufacturers' knowledge and their willingness to adhere to informal policy. Compliance with FDA's criteria is as likely to be related to the practices of competitors as to the views of agency officials. The problem is compounded when one agency has defined a descriptive term in official guidelines, but the other has not, or in the case where there are descriptors whose meanings the two agencies dispute. Without official, uniform definitions of common descriptors, food manufacturers are able to exploit consumer interest in foods that appear to be healthful. For example, the term *lite* or *light* has been used to imply fewer calories, reduced fat, lower sodium, improved texture, flavor, or color, and even the amount of breading, depending on the product. There are other practices that border on the deceptive. Although it is common to highlight desirable components of foods, rarely is there any effort to provide balanced information about other undesirable characteristics. For example, it may be literally truthful to label a food as containing no cholesterol, but even so, this may mislead consumers if it also contains substantial amounts of total fat and saturated fatty acids, particularly for unsophisticated consumers who equate cholesterol with fat. The responsible, restrained use of content descriptors may provide benefits to consumers who use them to hastily compare the main nutritional features of various foods. To promote the proper use and to aid consumer understanding of such descriptors, it is important that appropriate word definitions and criteria for their use be established. It is also important that the definitions established be the same for both agencies. Such quantitative descriptors are widely used and thus are of particular concern.

The Committee readily agreed on these elementary propositions. It found the challenge of formulating definitions for the growing variety of content descriptors in common use considerably more difficult. Each example that it undertook to evaluate seemed to present distinctive issues, and the judgments reflected in existing agency regulations and guidelines governing the use of specific terms seemed heavily influenced by precedents that cannot readily be appreciated. It quickly became clear that the Committee's work schedule would not allow the sort of in-depth study of agency policy and commercial practice that would be necessary to formulate recommendations for defining individual terms.

The Committee was also persuaded that the agencies themselves probably cannot expect to establish formal definitions for all of the terms that inventive marketers are likely to adapt or invent to describe the nutrient content of foods. The goal should be to define a core set of the terms used to describe the most important food components—fat, cholesterol, carbohydrates, fiber, and sodium. The agencies have made progress toward this goal.

The Committee was concerned that further progress would be slowed if the agencies had to treat each component—and associated set of descriptors—as presenting a unique problem. Accordingly, the Committee attempted to develop, and suggest for the agencies' consideration, a possible general framework for assigning nutrient values to such terms as *low, very low,* and *reduced.*

The Committee's suggested framework would allow the use of quantitative descriptors limited to two categories—high, low, very high, very low—with demarcations established for each descriptor. A scheme of benchmark ranges would be established for all quantitative descriptors for each nutrient based on the RDAs and other recognized dietary recommendation standards, and benchmark limits would be kept conceptually consistent for all nutrients in order to simplify the message. The use of comparative descriptors should be strictly regulated, with clear identification of the products being compared. In addition, the extent of nutrient modification should be specified and based on a modification of at least 20 percent, and descriptors should not be allowed for nutrients unless they are normally present in physiologically significant amounts (when physiologically significant amount is defined, such as 1 percent of the maximum allowance used to define the limits for very low). Synonyms of approved descriptors should not be allowed except by petitioning FDA and USDA; and descriptors that characterize other features that are not directly nutritional in nature (e.g., organic, fresh, and natural) should be controlled by narrowing the conditions for their use. Finally, the Committee believes that descriptors that imply mitigation or cure of disease or health condition should be controlled under the regulations being developed for health claims.

Comparative descriptors, such as *reduced fat*, are also widely used on many foods. Often, the compared food is not identified, and just as often the difference between the products is not described quantitatively. Use of such comparative terms should require clear identification of the product being compared and specification of the extent of modification. Descriptors that proclaim the absence of an undesired component, such as *cholesterol free*, should not be allowed on foods that do not normally contain cholesterol. And when used on foods that contain significant amounts of fat, or another undesired component, such as sodium, such claims should be accompanied by a disclosure of that fact.

Label Format Options

In 1972, when the voluntary nutrition labeling program was being developed, FDA investigated the various options that might be used to convey the nutrition information on the package and decided to use a numeric presentation. In 1982, FDA commissioned a study to develop alternative label formats, but systematic consumer testing was not undertaken. Some research has been done on the effectiveness of the current label format and various alternatives to convey nutrition information to consumers. Alternative presentations have included descriptors, graphics nutrient density with and without graphics, food equivalents calorie-based, and symbols. When any of these alternatives have been evaluated against the current format, consumers generally say they prefer the graphic format, yet they also seem to prefer nutrition information stated in absolute numbers and percentages over the alternatives.

Research on nutrition information provided at the point of purchase suggests that the form of presentation has an impact on the format judged to be most useful. Control over the individual's information input rate and ability to process data at a comfortable pace seem to reduce confusion.

In addition to the recommendations listed earlier on the mandatory and voluntary disclosure of nutrient content information, the Committee recommends that:

- Serving size should be prominently displayed on the nutrition information panel and should appear in household units.
- The amount of the serving should appear in grams or milliliters in parentheses following household units.
- Nutrient information should appear for the food as it is packaged, with the option of providing information relevant to the manner in which the food is prepared.
- Macronutrients should be listed in grams or milligrams.
- Macronutrients should be listed first, and then other food components, electrolytes, and micronutrients, or similar food components should be grouped together, except fiber and cholesterol should not appear in groupings.

- Various issues related to placement and prominence of food components on the nutrition label (e.g., increased prominence of fat components, ordering of macro- and micronutrients) should be subjected to consumer testing.
- Comparison with dietary recommendations should be optional.

Consumer Testing

Alternative label formats should be subjected to both qualitative and quantitative consumer testing prior to issuance of any final nutrition labeling requirements. However, this testing must be carefully structured to produce measurable results and, given the level of expectation for this process, carried out within a reasonable period of time. It is also assumed that before any testing procedures begin, the agencies will have determined through the comment and rulemaking process the nutrient content information to be conveyed on the label as this will affect the required nutrition information to be presented in any format tested.

The Committee recommends that:

- A brief test panel education program reviewing the current dietary recommendations and explaining the basics of the new label formats should precede label format testing.
- A formal testing procedure should include: an advisory panel to help determine the formats to be tested; an initial testing phase to include a comprehensive, qualitative review by consumers; an in-depth evaluation of the most preferred choices to assess consumer ability to use label information; and finally, large-scale surveys to determine consumer acceptance and comprehension of label information.

Educating Consumers to Use Nutrition Information on Food Labels

Two general strategies have been described for promoting dietary change. Environmental or structural interventions are strategies that encourage positive behaviors by creating opportunities for action and removing barriers so that consumers can follow health-promoting behaviors. In terms of dietary change, modification of some aspect of the food supply or improvement of consumer access to food would represent such a change. Personal or direct influence strategies are based on providing information or directing educational efforts, persuasion, and behavior modification techniques toward individuals or small groups. Techniques in these areas evolve from simple information transmission (based on the premise that knowledge of the facts will change behavior) to a variety of direct behavior modification techniques that are designed to lead directly to the development of health-promoting skills and practices.

The nutrient composition information provided on food labels should enable the public to make informed food choices. The provision of nutrition information on food labels is an amalgam of these two strategies: it is an environmental strategy because the federal government adopted an information provision policy by allowing not only nutrition information to appear, but also by setting the rules governing format, content, and placement, a personal-influence strategy for consumers to have the information to use.

Various public information campaigns aimed at promoting healthy behavior (including those for heart disease, high blood pressure, and cancer) have focused on enhancing knowledge, changing attitudes, and improving skills. Unfortunately, research suggests that improving consumer knowledge and consumer attitudes alone will not result in adoption of health-promoting practices. Consumers need information to make long-term dietary changes, but they need more than just information to achieve this goal. Educational resources will be required to effect behavioral change.

Obstacles to effecting dietary change in consumers include factors that are both cultural and psychological in nature. Most diet-related health problems develop gradually, without immediate or dramatic symptoms. Risk factor reduction and disease prevention through dietary means require an individual to make long-term and often arduous changes in food habits. However, many Americans consider themselves reasonably healthy and question whether major alterations in their dietary habits will be worthwhile in the long run.

A comprehensive national nutrition policy would ensure the availability of adequate supplies of safe and nutritious foods as well as provide consumers with the educational means for making informed food choices. A well-designed nutrition labeling program is an important component of an education program, but the provision of information is only the first stage in the behavioral change process. It cannot substitute for a comprehensive nutrition education program.

The Committee recommends that:

- Public- and private-sector initiatives should be established to help consumers understand and apply the information on the nutrition label.
- Comprehensive nutrition education programs should be developed in order to help consumers to understand the information on food labels to enable them to plan diets and make appropriate food choices.

Costs of Labeling Reform

Any reform of food labeling to provide more complete nutrition information and any expansion of the coverage of current nutrition labeling requirements will impose costs on producers, manufacturers, retailers, and ultimately, consumers regardless of who is recommending reform. It is the Committee's judgment that its recommendations for the content of nutrition labeling would require very little information that producers do not already possess. The timing of the imposition of such requirements could affect the cost of compliance. For foods that do not now bear nutrition labeling of any sort, additional costs will be incurred. The costs of analysis of these foods may not be trivial, though adequate methods and laboratory resources are available to analyze, at a reasonable cost, virtually all packaged foods for all of the nutrition components that the Committee recommends. Providing point-of-purchase nutrition information on produce and fresh meat, poultry, and seafood will impose significant new costs on retailers and consumers. The Committee is recommending that limited-menu restaurants be required to display point-of-purchase nutrient content information on their foods and that all other restaurants be required to have such information available to consumers on request. This recommendation is not likely to entail substantial additional costs, either for the limited-menu restaurant or consumers. The cost to require all other restaurants to have their menus evaluated and to offer nutrient information on request to consumers are considerably less certain. However, evaluation of the nutrition profile of menus is widely available and inexpensive, but even modest expense may prove high for small operators.

LEGISLATION AND REGULATION

The charge to the Committee to consider the implications of its recommendations for the current laws governing nutrition and ingredient labeling was interpreted as an invitation to consider whether the laws or regulations under which FDA and USDA now regulate food labels need to be changed in order to implement food labeling reform. It is the Committee's view that Congress should amend the FD&C, FMI, and PPI Acts to confirm FDA's and USDA's authority to expand the coverage and revise the content of current nutrition labeling requirements. Continuing doubt about the existence of such authority may impede actions by the agencies and result in court challenges, thus delaying implementation of needed reforms.

The Committee believes, however, that even without new legislation FDA could mandate nutrition labeling on all packaged foods. FDA's authority to prescribe the format and content of nutrition information, when it is required on food labels, appears well established as a means to prevent misleading labeling. In addition, FDA's decisions to exempt certain foods from some or all nutrition information requirements would likely be upheld.

Point-of-purchase nutrition information for produce, seafood, and foods sold in restaurants would represent a whole new area of regulation for food labeling. Most experts consulted by the Committee agreed, however, that if FDA could establish its authority to mandate nutrition labeling on foods in general, the extension of such a requirement to produce, seafood, and foods sold in restaurants would also be upheld as a matter of statutory authority. However, the practical problems associated with this expansion of nutrition labeling would be significant. FDA would have to devise an alternative to the conventional package label and would have to devise an alternative means for determining nutrient composition. FDA has frequently held the position that it has the authority to regulate the labeling of produce and foods sold in restaurants, although problems of enforcement and low priority have led it to refrain from exercising this power.

USDA's authority to expand nutrition labeling of processed meat and poultry products appears more straightforward. The FMI Act requires a label to be affixed to any meat product package, although the FMI Act does not grant general authority to USDA to require affirmative disclosures of information, nor is omission of this information classified as misleading. Section 607(c) of the FMI Act empowers USDA to prescribe the material required in nutrition labeling to avoid false or misleading statements, suggesting that nutrition information can be required on meat products whenever the Secretary of USDA concludes that it is required to prevent the label from being misleading. The same authority can be assumed under the PPI Act. USDA has ceded the authority to regulate the packaging of retail fresh and frozen meats and poultry to local agencies.

USDA's authority to prescribe nutrition labeling for meat- and poultry-containing foods sold by restaurants is more problematic. This uncertainty is of concern to the Committee, because it believes that both federal agencies should require nutrition information for foods sold at least by limited-menu restaurants.

Desirability of New Legislative Authority
for Nutrition Labeling

The foregoing discussion suggests why new legislation is, in principle, desirable. The Committee does recommend that Congress amend the FD&C, FMI, and PPI Acts to enlarge and clarify the authority of FDA and USDA, but it acknowledges that this has costs as well as advantages.

Disadvantages of New Legislation

A drawback to seeking new legislation is the possibility that such an effort may fail, causing both agencies to rethink their authority to proceed with changes in existing regulations. The second disadvantage stems from the propensity of Congress to draft legislation in such detail as to hamper administrative responses to new problems. Congress could simply require all food to bear nutrition labeling and state that FDA and USDA are to determine its content. It seems unlikely, however, that Congress will refrain from specifying the content of nutrition labeling in detail. Furthermore, new legislation could exclude important categories of foods, such as produce, seafood, meats and poultry, or foods sold in restaurants. Because the Committee is persuaded that nutrition labeling should be required for all these foods, it would consider legislation that categorically exempted or omitted them to be unsound in principle and at odds with efforts to improve the dietary habits and long-term health of Americans. An additional concern is that new legislation might encumber FDA and USDA with rulemaking procedures that would delay implementation of regulations requiring more informative nutrition labeling.

Advantages of New Legislation

An overriding advantage of new legislation is that it could lay to rest any doubt that FDA and USDA have the legal authority to mandate nutrition labeling for all packaged foods and clarify this authority to require nutrition information in connection with the sale of many foods that currently are not affected by federal labeling regulations. It would also reduce the incentives to challenge agency regulations that implement the Committee's recommendations.

New legislation could also expedite the administrative process by confirming the power of the agencies to proceed by informal rulemaking. And it could speed executive branch review by setting deadlines for proposing and promulgating initial regulations.

Successful reform of nutrition labeling requires that FDA and USDA work in tandem so that consumers can eventually make food selections in keeping with recent dietary recommendations. Legislation should mandate that the requirements of FDA and USDA be uniform and implemented on the same schedule.

Another justification for legislation is the importance of food labeling reform. The stakes involved make Congress the appropriate arena for resolving the critical issues and adjusting to the competing interests.

Design of Food Labeling Legislation

New legislation should clarify the authority of FDA and USDA to mandate nutrition labeling on all packaged foods and coverage of fruits and vegetables, fresh and frozen meats and poultry, fresh and frozen seafood, and foods sold in restaurants.

The next issue concerns what new legislation should provide regarding the content of labeling. A distinction should be drawn between those components of nutrition labeling that should be required by FDA and USDA regulations and those that should be mandated by statute. Legislation should limit itself to prescribing calories per serving, complex carbohydrates, sugars, and those components whose consumption should be restricted or curtailed (fat, saturated fat, cholesterol, and sodium). All other components to be included in nutrition labeling should be left to FDA and USDA. The Committee expects that, in addition, the agencies would agree to requiring protein, fiber, calcium, and iron.

New legislation should direct the two agencies to agree on the same reference unit for listing nutrition information, presumably a serving of food. It should also direct the agencies to adopt a uniform serving size for purposes of nutrition labeling.

The Committee believes that current legislation gives FDA and USDA adequate legal authority to adopt standard and uniform definitions of the most commonly used descriptors. However, if new legislation is enacted to resolve other questions, confirmation of the agencies' power to define commonly used nutrient descriptors would be desirable. FDA and USDA should also have the power to prohibit the use of any undefined descriptors on a food that do not conform to the definition or that are not defined by the agencies.

The Committee is reluctant to endorse any outright ban on the truthful, even if incomplete, description of nutrition components without evidence that this is the only means of preventing consumer confusion. But the agencies should have the authority to restrict the official nutrition label to designated components and relegate other components to the ingredient listing or other portions of the label. Current law appears to provide the agencies with adequate authority.

Legislation should direct FDA and USDA to identify and test different label formats and then to specify in regulations the uniform format that must be followed by all food sellers. FDA and USDA should be empowered to approve modifications of the basic format in appropriate cases, such as for foods with few mandatory components, those with very small packages, fresh foods, and foods sold in restaurants. Either agency may wish to consider other modifications for specific products, but the burden of justifying departures from the uniform format should rest on those manufacturers seeking them. Explicit confirmation of the agencies' authority to exempt certain foods from nutrition labeling would be desirable, but final decisions about which foods to exempt should remain with FDA and USDA.

A national food labeling advisory committee could periodically review the need for revision of both the format and the content of nutrition labels and labeling. Legislation should direct that regular reviews of nutrition labeling be done, prescribe deadlines for completion of these reviews, and mandate consideration of the views of the public as well as other sectors.

Allowing different formats for conveying nutrition information on food labels diminishes the utility of labels to consumers. It is essential that one format be established. A nutrition label should be prescribed by federal law, and legislation should presumptively preclude modifications or additions by state authorities or legislation to allow states to petition FDA or USDA for approval to require additional information needed by their citizens, but would disapprove of any state addition that would prevent use of the same label throughout the country.

A formal mechanism, such as a national food labeling advisory committee, including representatives from the states, should be established to provide FDA and USDA with advice on the design of nutrition labeling requirements. This could increase the willingness of the states to collaborate in enforcement efforts and would perhaps induce federal authorities to fashion their requirements to reflect the interests of the states. Establishment of such a food labeling committee would not require new legislation, but a congressional mandate would ensure creation of such a mechanism.

Finally, Congress should establish deadlines for adoption of new food labeling regulations by the agencies.

PART I

CURRENT STATE OF
NUTRITION LABELING

2

Overview

In the early 1970s the federal government took the first steps to establish the current framework for the nutrition labeling of foods used in the United States. In a series of regulations the Food and Drug Administration (FDA) expanded the information that manufacturers were required to include about the composition of foods and standardized the format in which this information was to appear. The most significant of these regulations dealt with nutrition labeling. For most packaged food products under its jurisdiction, FDA allowed information about the nutrient content of a food to be provided voluntarily. When it was provided, however, this information had to appear in a standard format. Nutrition labeling was mandatory for any food to which a nutrient was added or for which a nutrition claim was made. FDA officials encouraged manufacturers to provide nutrition information even when it was not required.

At the same time, the U.S. Department of Agriculture (USDA) proposed nutrition labeling regulations for meat and poultry products in a form very close to those of FDA. Although these regulations were not adopted, USDA issued policy guidance on nutrition labeling and encouraged manufacturers to use nutrition information on their products. By 1990 over 60 percent of the sales of FDA-regulated packaged foods sold in the United States bore nutrition labeling. Over 35 percent of the packaged foods regulated by the Food Safety and Inspection Service (FSIS) of USDA provided nutrition labeling.

The labeling reforms adopted in the early 1970s, of which nutrition labeling was a part, represented a fundamental shift in regulatory philosophy. Until that time the federal government had sought to regulate food quality chiefly through restrictions on the composition of foods, many of which were exempted from full ingredient labeling. Under the new regimen, FDA and USDA began to rely on consumer choice by allowing manufacturers to provide information on the composition and nutritional quality of the foods they purchased. Considered from the perspective of 1990, however, the changes adopted over 15 years ago seem modest. Foods subject to FDA food standards remain exempt from full ingredient labeling. Nutrition labeling was mandatory only on relatively few foods. In addition, the information that was required did not cover many important components. Thus, it is no surprise that 17 years later the food labeling regimen established in 1973 seems both incomplete and outdated.

Appreciation of the deficiencies of current labeling of the nutrient content of foods began to emerge in the 1980s. Two related developments demonstrated that food labels should be reformed. The most important development was the expanding knowledge of the relationship among diet, nutrition, and long-term health. By the 1980s the results of scientific investigation had convincingly demonstrated important linkages between the dietary habits of Americans and the prevalence of chronic diseases, most notably, cardiovascular disease, cancer, stroke, diabetes, and obesity. The central message of these findings was that, in broad terms, Americans' diets were not deficient in essential nutrients but, rather, provided excessive amounts of calories, fat, cholesterol, and sodium. Confronted with an abundant and varied food supply, Americans have found it easy to make unwise choices.

The second development can be viewed as a logical response to reports of scientific research on the relationship between nutrition and chronic disease. With the accumulating knowledge about these relationships, many Americans became increasingly attentive to choices among foods. Predictably, food producers responded to this interest by reformulating foods, creating new products, and aggressively promoting those products whose composition could be said to reflect this new learning about nutrition and health. No examples need to be cited to support the conclusion that good nutrition and disease avoidance had become central themes of food marketing in the United States by 1990.

In this environment, the current rules governing food labeling are seriously out of date. The labels of many packaged foods provide no nutrition information. No form of nutrition labeling is required for major segments of the food supply, including produce, meats, poultry, seafood, and foods served in restaurants. Advertising and label claims of nutritional value or the ability of foods to prevent disease have proliferated with seemingly little control. Moreover, the information required on those foods that do bear nutrition labeling is incomplete and misfocused. Under the current system the presence and levels of micronutrients are emphasized; disclosure of cholesterol and fiber content is not required; and information about levels, sources, and types of fat is incomplete. It is not difficult to understand why some critics charge that the federal government has ignored major segments of the food supply, been concerned with the wrong nutrients, and tolerated nutrition claims in advertising and labeling of packaged foods that are, at best, confusing and, at worst, deceptive economically and potentially harmful.

In the 15 years since FDA's regulations were adopted, concerns have been raised repeatedly about whether those requirements were too modest and should be updated in light of both the increasing use of nutrition labeling by manufacturers and growing consumer interest in the nutritional quality of their foods. Most notably, in 1978 and 1979, the U.S. Department of Health, Education, and Welfare, USDA, and the Federal Trade Commission (FTC) held hearings and examined possible changes in many areas of food labeling regulation. During the same period, bills have been introduced in the U.S. Congress to overhaul both USDA's and FDA's food labeling regulations; despite vigorous efforts to achieve consensus on needed reform, none had been enacted by the end of the 1980s. In addition, many private organizations, including health, consumer, and some producer groups, put forward improved labeling approaches.

FORMATION OF THE COMMITTEE ON THE NUTRITION COMPONENTS OF FOOD LABELING

The 1980s witnessed both the expanded use of the current nutrition labeling system and a growing consensus on the relationship between diet and chronic disease. This was exemplified by the release of two landmark reports on nutrition and health: one by the Public Health Service, *The Surgeon General's Report on Nutrition and Health* (DHHS, 1988), and the other by the National Research Council (NRC), *Diet and Health: Implications for Reducing Chronic Disease Risk* (NRC, 1989a). According to these two reports, diet plays a role in 5 of 10 leading causes of death among Americans. Health conditions that are affected by diet include heart disease (the leading cause of death), cancers (second leading cause), strokes (third leading cause), diabetes (seventh leading cause), and atherosclerosis (tenth leading cause).

The release of those two reports and the growing recognition of the need for food label reform prompted the Public Health Service (PHS) of the U.S. Department of Health and Human Services and USDA's FSIS to request, in 1989, that the Food and Nutrition Board of the Institute of Medicine conduct a study of nutrition labeling. The Board assembled the Committee on the Nutrition Components of Food Labeling, which consisted of 14 members representing the fields of analytical chemistry, dietetics, food marketing, food science, nutrition and biomedical sciences, nutrition education, and regulatory law. The Committee was charged to:

- assess the implications for nutrition labeling of current knowledge on nutrition and health,
- determine the most appropriate content and format for food labels by

taking into account the scientific data base as well as the best means to communicate the information to the public,

— examine the implications of the labeling proposals for current legislation and regulatory statutes governing ingredient and nutrition labeling, and

— propose policy options for modifying current legislative and regulatory directives (PHS contract 282-89-0022).

In responding to this charge, the Committee first reviewed the recommendations of recent reports concerned with nutrition, dietary consumption, and health as the scientific basis for reform. After examining the implications of the recommendations for nutrition labeling, it then evaluated the current information on food labels, the nutrition information that needed to be added and deleted, and the availability of valid and reliable analytical methods for use in providing information for nutrition labeling. The Committee also discussed how nutrient information should be displayed in terms of serving size, the listing of required core and optional nutrients and ingredient information, and label format. Finally, the Committee evaluated the use and appropriate definitions for quantitative and other descriptors of nutrient content.

While addressing the tasks in their charge, the Committee tried to weigh the various factors in addition to the scientific consensus that influence labeling reform, including current legal authority, existing label coverage, criticism leveled against existing food labels, current dietary consumption patterns, marketing forces, consumer understanding and use of food labels, the forces operating in the world market, the need for consumer testing of formats, the knowledge base of some consumers about the current system, and consumer education that would be needed if labels are to be changed significantly. Following the development of recommendations for food label reform, the Committee examined these options in light of the existing regulatory authority of FDA and USDA and considered the benefits and liabilities of specific legislation mandating nutrition labeling. In the process of its deliberations and final recommendations, the Committee gleaned valuable information and insights from a variety of sources, including agency officials, witnesses at a public meeting held on December 4, 1989, and invited participants at workshops on the following subjects: label content, legal authority, consumer understanding and use of labels, label formats, and the marketing aspects of label information.

RELEVANT STUDIES ON NUTRITION, DIETARY CONSUMPTION, AND HEALTH

Several studies that have examined the scientific evidence on the relationship between diet and disease formed the basis for the Committee's assessment of the kinds of information about nutrient content that food labels should provide. The Committee accepted the central findings from these reports without independently assessing their correctness. This approach was dictated by the limited time available for completing the report, but it was independently justified by the broad acceptance of these findings within the scientific community. The Committee also recognized the evolving character of the scientific understanding of the relationship between diet and chronic disease and, therefore, sought to make its recommendations in light of the changes in scientific knowledge likely to occur in the next decade.

The Surgeon General's report made a number of recommendations for change in the eating habits of Americans, including:

- reduced consumption of fat (especially saturated fat) and cholesterol;
- achievement and maintenance of a desirable body weight;
- increased consumption of complex carbohydrates and fiber;
- reduced intake of sodium;
- increased intake of calcium by women of childbearing age;
- adequate iron consumption by children, adolescents, and women of childbearing age;
- reduced amount and frequency of consumption of sugar by children; and
- addition of optimal levels of fluoride to community water systems to prevent tooth decay (DHHS, 1988).

The NRC *Diet and Health* report made more specific recommendations for the quantities of various dietary constituents that Americans should consume. The report recommended that U.S. consumers should:

- reduce total fat to 30 percent or less of calories, reduce saturated fatty acid intake to less than 10 percent of calories, and reduce intake of cholesterol to less than 300 mg daily;
- limit total daily intake of salt (sodium chloride) to 6 g or less;
- maintain protein intake at moderate levels;
- balance food intake and physical activity to maintain appropriate body weight;
- maintain adequate calcium intake; and
- maintain an optimal intake of fluoride (NRC, 1989a).

The report also described the types and amounts of foods to be consumed to achieve these recommendations.

In the fall of 1989 the tenth edition of *Recommended Dietary Allowances* (RDA) was released by the Food and Nutrition Board (NRC, 1989b). As with previous editions, the 1989 RDA updated the standards by which dietary consumption patterns were to be judged for adequacy.

Several other reports on dietary intake, disease prevention, and the food supply complete the core of the scientific data base on which the Committee relied. The earliest one was *Diet, Nutrition, and Cancer* (NRC, 1982), which offered interim dietary recommendations based on the knowledge at that time. The recommendation most relevant to the Committee's task was the suggestion that the consumption of both saturated and unsaturated fats should be reduced in the average diet of Americans. The report suggested that an appropriate and practical target was to reduce intake of total fat to 30 percent of total calories.

Designing Foods: Animal Product Options in the Marketplace was concerned with changing the food products available to consumers. The report made a number of dietary recommendations, including:

- caloric intake to match individual needs;
- no more that 30 percent of calories from fat, 10 percent from saturated fatty acids, 10 percent from polyunsaturated fatty acids, and 10 percent from monounsaturated fatty acids;
- no more than 300 mg of cholesterol per day; and
- calcium and iron in keeping with the RDAs for age and sex (NRC, 1988).

The second report on U.S. dietary consumption and nutrition status, *Nutrition Monitoring in the United States* (LSRO, FASEB, 1989), confirmed the findings of its predecessor concerning the nutritional problems and health implications for U.S. consumers. The Expert Panel on Nutrition Monitoring reported evidence of changes in eating patterns consistent with recommendations for the avoidance of too much fat, saturated fat, and cholesterol, and for the consumption of adequate amounts of starch and dietary fiber. Available data on dietary and nutritional status with respect to individual food components, however, did not indicate that there had been substantial dietary changes since the first report in 1986. According to the 1989 report, the principal nutrition-related health problems experienced by many Americans continue to be related to the overconsumption of some nutrients and food components, particularly food energy (calories), fat, saturated fatty acids, cholesterol, sodium, and alcohol. Furthermore, although the supply of nutrients is generally adequate, there is evidence of inadequate individual dietary intake or impaired nutritional status in some subgroups of the population with respect to iron; calcium; folate; zinc; and vitamins A, C, and B_6.

ROLE OF FOOD LABELS IN IMPLEMENTING
DIETARY CHANGES

The Committee believes that the reports of the Surgeon General and the NRC send a clear message that dietary changes can materially reduce the prevalence of major diseases. The Committee further believes that consumers can improve their own health and reduce their long-term risk of disease by being more careful in the food choices that they make. Better food labels can play a central role in facilitating such choices. These reports indicate that consumers need to alter their current dietary consumption patterns. The similarity and complementary nature of the recommendations of the two reports provide a strong basis on which government and the private sector can design dietary guidance, programs, and services. A host of activities can be envisioned to promote dietary change; however, food labels are only one part of the larger effort.

The Surgeon General's report outlined the activities that could lead to consumer implementation of its recommendations. The report urged that the general public be educated about dietary choices and adequate physical activity conducive to prevention and control of certain chronic diseases. The report stated that food manufacturers can improve the quality of Americans' diets by increasing the availability of palatable, easily prepared food products that will help consumers follow the dietary principles it set forth. The specific recommendations relevant to food labeling included:

- More information should be provided by manufacturers to consumers on the composition of food products, including total fat, saturated and unsaturated fatty acids, cholesterol, calories, carbohydrates, added sugars, fiber, sodium, iron, folate, and complete, explicit ingredient contents.
- Information should be straightforward, efficient, and effective.
- Health claims, if allowed, should be informative, scientific, and non-misleading.
- Health warnings on alcoholic beverage containers should warn about the hazards associated with alcohol consumption during pregnancy (DHHS, 1988).

The NRC *Diet and Health* report concluded that several sectors of society need to collaborate in the effort to implement dietary changes. Although the report did not provide specific recommendations for food labeling, it reviewed a number of issues that have implications for label reform, including serving size, macronutrient quantification, label format, food safety information, product development, and educational aspects of dietary change.

In 1973, when FDA established the current food labeling system, the seventh edition of the RDA (NRC, 1968) was the basis for establishing guidelines for the nutrition labeling of foods in the form of the U.S. Recommended Daily Allowances (U.S. RDA). The U.S. RDAs were, in general, set by taking the highest value of an RDA for a given nutrient, regardless of the age and sex group, and making it the standard for that nutrient. The tenth edition of the RDA provides a basis for changing the U.S. RDAs if they are to remain the standard for nutrition labeling, even if some other choice of name is to be used.

Designing Foods (NRC, 1988) made a number of specific recommendations for food labeling. The report recommended that regulations should not restrict truthful information at the point of purchase or on food product packaging. USDA should restrict use of the descriptors *light, lite,* or *lean* to products in the form that would be presented to the retail consumer, so that use of descriptive terminology on foods sold at the retail level should require some objective standard for the food itself. It recommended that point-of-purchase programs be developed to supplement and support information provided on the label. Finally, the report recommended that standards be set to govern serving size.

PURPOSES, CHARACTERISTICS, AND AUDIENCES OF NUTRITION LABELING

Any effort to improve the nutrition content information on food labels must begin with a set of assumptions about the purpose labels should serve and the audiences that they should be designed to inform and assist food selection. According to the agencies, the purpose of food labeling is to enable consumers to select and use products that meet their individual needs and preferences. To achieve this purpose, labeling must provide sufficient information to enable the public to identify foods and their characteristics, including ingredients and nutritional value. Effective labeling must present the information so that consumers can understand and use it in deciding what foods to buy. The agencies' guiding principles in recommending specific changes have been public health importance, the consumer's right to know, and economic protection (44 Fed. Reg. 75,992–76,020, Dec. 21, 1979).

These goals for labeling by no means exhaust the purposes of food labels. The relevant laws administered by FDA and USDA impose additional, explicit requirements for the content of food labels, which manufacturers are not free to ignore. These requirements include the name of the food, the disclosure of the quantity of contents, and the name and place of business of the manufacturer or distributor. In addition, most foods must bear a list of their ingredients. These requirements, together with demands for nutrition information, may compete with the manufacturer's own objectives for the label, which can be summarized as the desire to make the product appealing to consumers by depiction and description. Even if there were no tension among these objectives, space limitations on many food labels would necessitate compromise.

The Committee's focus was on label information about nutrient content, and it developed its own list of the purposes of nutrition labeling which formed one premise for this report. The Committee believes that nutrition labeling should:

- provide consumers with nutrition information about the food product,
- enable consumers to compare the nutritional quality of products from the same food group,
- enable consumers to choose among products from different food groups on the basis of nutritional quality,

- prevent or reduce consumer deception by providing information about the nutrient composition of the product, and
- provide incentives to improve food products by requiring manufacturers to describe fully the ingredients and nutrient value of their products.

Other characteristics of food labels can affect the extent to which any of these varied and sometimes competing informational objectives are achieved. These features include legibility, which is a function not only of type size but also of typography, background, and color; understandability of terms and illustrations; consistency among products and between agencies; and uniformity over time and across political boundaries.

The Committee discussed the audiences for which nutrition labeling is important. One very important group that nutrition labels should serve is the large number of consumers with special dietary requirements as the result of diagnosed health conditions. Members of this group have been instructed to moderate or change their diets in some way, such as to avoid salt, reduce calories, or change fat and cholesterol intake. These consumers realize that they have a health problem that can be helped by making dietary changes.

A second audience that is large, but perhaps less critical, consists of those consumers whose interest in nutrition and improved diets is largely self-generated. These consumers are already aware of dietary factors that have an impact on long-term health and wish to be provided with more useful information on the nutritional quality of food products. This group wants more and better information on food labels to enable them to select their foods wisely. For this group improved labels will serve an educative function; in truth, they are already educated and simply want better information so that they can put their knowledge to use.

A third, even larger, group consists of consumers who do not now pay attention to nutrition labels. This potentially vast audience could make use of better labels if they were educated to know why it was important to make dietary changes and how food labels can be useful in making these changes. Major educational efforts, in addition to changes in food labels, will be required to reach this new audience.

FOOD LABELS, LABELING, AND ADVERTISING

From the outset, the Committee faced a need to define its jurisdiction. Manufacturers and sellers provide information about their food products to consumers by several different means, including, but not limited to, what is thought of as the label—the printed material that is affixed to or that is part of the package. They use a wide variety of off-package textual and graphic materials displayed at the point of purchase or, more accurately, at the point of selection. In the merchandising trade these materials have a variety of titles, such as "shelf talkers" and "coupon pads." Manufacturers and sellers also rely heavily on media advertising which consumers usually encounter away from the locations at which food is sold, such as on television and in newspapers and magazines. All these potential sources of information about the nutritional content and quality of foods are, in theory, subject to federal regulation. Manufacturers and sellers use them to describe and promote the nutritional characteristics of their products.

In addition, consumers have access to several other sources of information about diet and foods, including books and articles, a growing number of health-focused newsletters, special media reports, regular health segments on television and radio, and formal and informal classes. These sources are to be distinguished, however, from information that originates with manufacturers or sellers of foods, which has special legal status, because their designers have an obvious interest in influencing consumer decisions about which foods to buy.

Federal law divides commercially inspired information into three categories for regulatory purposes. Food labels comprise the first category, and it is this category with which the Committee was chiefly concerned. Many foods are sold without conventional labels, however; and most foods that do bear labels are displayed in conjunction with additional graphic or textual material, which falls within the category of labeling as similarly defined by the laws administered by FDA and USDA. In technical terms, labeling is the broader category, for it also comprehends labels, as the Federal Food Drug and Cosmetic Act definition reveals: "The term 'labeling' means all labels and other written, printed, or graphic matters (1) upon any article or any of its containers or wrappers, or (2) accompanying such article" (21 USC § 1.3). The courts have interpreted *accompanying* expansively, which means that FDA and USDA are, in theory, empowered to regulate the contents of off-package material that describe and promote foods.

While the Committee has focused primarily on the nutritional content and format of food labels, it has also been concerned with food labeling for several reasons. The sponsoring agencies have jurisdiction over labeling, not just labels, and as the Committee's title indicates, they asked for advice regarding the nutrition components of food labeling. Furthermore, the Committee was interested in the quality of nutrition information provided in conjunction with the sale of foods that do not bear conventional labels—produce, meats and poultry, and foods provided by food service establishments, such as restaurants. Some of the Committee's recommendations contemplate action by FDA and USDA to regulate the content of labeling for such foods.

Neither FDA nor USDA has jurisdiction over manufacturer- or seller-initiated advertising, which is the province of FTC at the federal level. However, the Committee is aware that much of the public interest in nutrition and messages about foods is focused on and stimulated by advertising. The proliferation of so-called health claims for food products is, in part, a response to, as well as an effort to exploit, the scientific findings about diet and health that led to the

Committee's creation and precipitated the current congressional interest in food labeling. The Committee has not, however, studied either the content of food advertising or the manner of its regulation, and because of time constraints, there is relatively little discussion in this report about health claims. Furthermore, the study's sponsors made clear that they did not expect the Committee to address the issues surrounding health claims.

Although the Committee was content to accept this narrowed charge, it was not possible to ignore the area of health claims entirely. The growing use of so-called descriptors, which are verbal attempts to capture and highlight the distinctive nutritional value of a food, such as fat-free or low in sodium, on food labels and in labeling proved to be closely related to what is customarily regarded as nutrition labeling.

Thus, the Committee's effort to formulate advice on the nutrition components of food labeling has taken it beyond the boundaries of the food label and, in one instance, into the promotional, as distinct from the informational, facets of food labeling. This should not, however, obscure the central focus of this report: to assess the content, format, and coverage of the current FDA and USDA rules for nutrition labeling.

SUMMARY OF REPORT

The report is in two principal parts, in addition to the Summary. The remainder of Part I provides a comprehensive introduction to the work of the Committee and the nutrition labeling of food in the United States. Chapter 3 recounts the history of nutrition labeling, discusses its key features, and identifies the central themes in the growing number of proposals for reform and expansion of the system. Finally, Chapter 4 explores in considerable detail the context in which reform proposals must be evaluated, including current dietary habits of Americans, the behavior and incentives of food manufacturers and sellers, and the increasing internationalization of the food market. It concludes with a discussion of the important topic of chemical analysis of the nutrient contents of foods, both the source of the information to improve food labels and an important constraint on issues of coverage and content.

Part II sets forth the key findings and recommendations of the Committee. Chapter 5 discusses the foods to be accompanied by some form of nutrition labeling, focusing first on packaged foods and then on the important segments of the food supply that do not now bear conventional labels—produce, seafood, meat and poultry, and foods served in food service settings. Chapter 6 deals with the desired content of nutrition labeling: the nutrients that should be declared and the information about them that should be provided in a comprehensive discussion. Chapter 7 treats the important, but still poorly studied, subject of label formats: how important nutrition information should be depicted and conveyed. While the Committee offers several suggestions for the final format(s) that should be chosen by FDA and USDA, the recommendations are guarded. Chapter 7 also considers the issues of serving size, U.S. RDA, descriptors, and consumer education. Finally, Chapter 8 deals broadly with the implementation of nutrition labeling and specifically with issues of legal authority. Although it is not common for the Institute of Medicine to be asked to provide legal advice, in this instance the Committee's charge included the explicit request to consider whether FDA and/or USDA could implement the Committee's recommended reforms using their current statutory authority. And, if the Committee concluded that there might be advantages in the enactment of new legislation directing and empowering the agencies to act, the Committee was encouraged to comment on what such legislation should include. Both of these large issues are addressed.

REFERENCES

DHHS (U.S. Department of Health and Human Services). 1988. The Surgeon General's Report on Nutrition and Health. Government Printing Office, Washington, D.C. 727 pp.

LSRO, FASEB (Life Sciences Research Office, Federation of American Societies for Experimental Biology). 1989. Nutrition Monitoring in the United States: An Update Report on Nutrition Monitoring. Prepared for the U.S. Department of Agriculture and the U.S. Department of Health and Human Services. Government Printing Office, Washington, D.C. 408 pp.

NRC (National Research Council). 1968. Recommended Dietary Allowances, 7th ed. Report of the Subcommittee on the Seventh Edition of the RDAs, Food and Nutrition Board, Commission on Life Sciences. National Academy of Sciences, Washington, D.C. 101 pp.

NRC (National Research Council). 1982. Diet, Nutrition, and Cancer. Report of the Committee on Diet, Nutrition, and Cancer, Assembly of Life Sciences. National Academy Press, Washington, D.C. 478 pp.

NRC (National Research Council). 1988. Designing Foods: Animal Product Options in the Marketplace. Report of the Committee on Technological Options to Improve the Nutritional Attributes of Animal Products, Board on Agriculture. National Academy Press, Washington, D.C. 367 pp.

NRC (National Research Council). 1989a. Diet and Health: Implications for Reducing Chronic Disease Risk. Report of the Committee on Diet and Health, Food and Nutrition Board, Commission on Life Sciences. National Academy Press, Washington, D.C. 749 pp.

NRC (National Research Council). 1989b. Recommended Dietary Allowances, 10th ed. Report of the Subcommittee on the Tenth Edition of the RDAs, Food and Nutrition Board, Commission on Life Sciences. National Academy Press, Washington, D.C. 284 pp.

3

Current Food Labeling

OVERVIEW OF THE U.S. SYSTEM FOR REGULATING FOOD LABELING

The United States has no single system for regulating food labels. The federal government operates two major food labeling programs that differ in their requirements and in their modes of operation. In addition, the states may, in some circumstances, impose labeling requirements that go beyond those established by the federal government. To complicate the picture further, the authority to regulate food promotion practices that extend beyond the label, such as media advertising, lies with a third federal agency. Finally, many foods in grocery stores and supermarkets, and foods served in restaurants and institutional settings are sold without any nutrition information at all.

This complex picture can be explained in historical and political terms, and many of its features are not irrational. It may be appropriate to rely chiefly on state and local authorities to oversee restaurants and educational, medical, social, and penal institution food service operations. Similarly, consumers and producers alike might come to resent the cost and complications of a regimen that requires all produce, meat, poultry, and seafood to be packaged and sold in a form that would require conventional labeling. Other features of the splintered U.S. system for regulating food labels, however, are certainly subject to question. That, however, is not the focus of this report. The purpose of this chapter is to describe how food labels are currently regulated so that readers can better understand how food labels came to be the way they are and better assess the recommendations for reform that are made in Part II of this report.

The two federal agencies whose activities are of central interest are the Food and Drug Administration (FDA) and the U.S. Department of Agriculture (USDA). Although FDA regulates a larger share of the retail food market, it is easier to define the two agencies' responsibilities by first describing the jurisdiction of USDA. Through its Food Safety and Inspection Service (FSIS), USDA regulates the labeling of meat and poultry products pursuant to the Federal Meat Inspection Act (FMI Act, 21 USC § 601, *et seq.*) and the Poultry Products Inspection Act (PPI Act, 21 USC § 451, *et seq.*). (USDA's jurisdiction does not extend to the packaging of fresh meat and poultry at the retail level.) Operating under the Federal Food, Drug, and Cosmetic Act (FD&C Act, 21 USC § 321), FDA is responsible for regulating the labeling of virtually all other foods. It could be said that FDA has jurisdiction over the center aisles of the supermarket, while USDA regulates the side counters. This summary, however, overlooks the dairy section, the large (and growing) produce section, whose products rarely bear conventional labels, and the increasingly important seafood counter, both of which theoretically fall under FDA jurisdiction, as do the growing number of foods prepared on the supermarket premises, such as bakery products and salad bars.

The laws under which FDA and USDA operate differ in their histories, provisions, and modes of implementation. Some, but not all, of these differences have importance for this study and for the implementation of the Committee's recommendations; these are discussed in greater detail below. For the purposes of the present discussion, it suffices to note that all three laws—the FMI Act, the PPI Act, and the FD&C Act—say virtually nothing about nutrition and provide little guidance as to the information about nutrient content that USDA or FDA may require on food labels. In both systems, decisions about the information to prescribe on food labels have to a large extent reflected administrative judgments.

The laws administered by FDA and USDA disguise a more fundamental difference in their modes of operation, a difference that influences enforcement capacity and may also explain some of the reported variations in substantive policy. Although specific requirements are not obvious in the language of the FMI and PPI Acts (e.g., 21 USC § 607(d), (e)), USDA has always taken the position that a manufacturer must obtain approval in advance for any label it wishes to use on a meat or poultry product, as well as for any change it wishes to make in an approved label (Kushner et al., 1990). Research has not disclosed any challenge to this position. Indeed, many producers of USDA-regulated products probably favor the current system of prior label approval, which at least ensures certainty. In practical terms, under the USDA system no meat or poultry product bears a label that fails to meet the agency's requirements.

This label review system is a relatively small part of USDA's extensive program for regulating meat and poultry products. The FSIS work force exceeds 9,000 employees, most of whom are engaged in on-site inspection of production activities. Fewer than two dozen employees are engaged in the review and approval of labels. They process a caseload of about 130,000 requests for label approval each year (Crawford, 1990).

The USDA system displays another notable feature. Because each manufacturer must secure approval for its label, USDA has had less reason than FDA to issue formal regulations detailing its requirements. Although the agency has evolved clear policies regarding such matters as nutrition labeling, they typically cannot be found in the *Code of Federal Regulations* (CFR). Most are spelled out in the *FSIS Standards and Labeling Policy Book* and policy memoranda (USDA, 1989), which are available publicly and, therefore, are sources of guidance to applicants. Reliance on these forms of guidance has meant that USDA can, in theory, be more adaptable than FDA because it generally does not need to revise existing regulations before requiring or allowing new information on the labels of the foods it regulates. On the other hand, the failure to incorporate key policies in regulations may limit awareness of them and surely inhibits public discussion of their merits.

By contrast, FDA has never operated a system of prior approval for food labels, and any assertion of such authority now would surely be considered beyond the agency's powers. Instead, FDA has relied on publication of its labeling requirements, typically in the form of regulations, coupled with informal advice giving and periodic threats of enforcement against products whose labels fail to comply with those requirements. This mode of operation means that industry compliance with federal requirements depends on close monitoring by the agency and the ability to initiate enforcement against violative products.

Because FDA does not approve food labels, its system allows issues of labeling policy to remain unresolved, sometimes for many years. A manufacturer of meat or poultry products can always discover USDA's position on a new labeling initiative—for example, the use of a new descriptor—because it must seek approval, and the agency must provide a response. A "no" response may, in fact, mean only that USDA has not yet formulated a policy, but operationally, the answer is clear. In the FDA context, however, a manufacturer that wishes to use a new label, even one that appears to challenge the spirit of the agency's regulations, can use it and hope that the agency will not challenge its product as being mislabeled. FDA's lack of formal policy on an issue does not necessarily deter a practice unless the agency is prepared to take enforcement action. The system therefore allows FDA to ignore practices that it finds objectionable but is not prepared to challenge. It also ensures that the agency may not be aware of label changes until after they are adopted, because manufacturers are not obliged to submit copies of their labels on a regular basis.

These contrasting systems for regulating the contents of food labels might only be a curiosity if the jurisdictions of the two agencies did not overlap. The boundary between them, however, can sometimes be elusive. USDA shares jurisdiction with FDA over food labels for products containing meat and poultry, because the FD&C Act ostensibly applies to all food. The FMI and PPI Acts authorize USDA to exempt from their requirements food products that contain meat or poultry only in a relatively small proportion, and accordingly, the agency has determined that products containing less than 3 percent raw meat, 2 percent cooked meat, or 2 percent cooked poultry are subject only to FDA regulations. In addition, FDA exercises limited jurisdiction over products that remain subject to USDA's primary control. For example, no USDA-regulated product may contain a food or color additive that has not been approved by FDA (Kushner et al., 1990).

The potential overlap in jurisdictions can exaggerate the consequences of policy differences between the two agencies. A modest change in composition may cause a product to cross the jurisdictional boundary. For example, a pizza product containing cheese but little meat will fall under FDA's control, and thus escape USDA's requirement of advance label approval (GAO, 1988). For manufacturers whose product lines are under the jurisdiction of both agencies, labels for similar products may be subject to different substantive requirements as well as different approval procedures (Kushner et al., 1990).

It should be stated, however, that suggestions of serious conflict between FDA and USDA in substantive labeling requirements often appear to be unsupported on close review. The Committee found few instances in which FDA expected different information on food labels than USDA required or allowed. USDA's rules for nutrition labeling of meat and poultry products have generally tracked, although sometimes not immediately, FDA's regulations. In the Committee's judgment, the more important difference between the two systems lies in their contrasting modes for establishing and enforcing labeling requirements.

It is important to reemphasize that both FDA and USDA have jurisdiction over more than the printed label attached to a product. Under the FD&C Act, FDA's authority extends to all "labeling" for foods, a term that includes labels and other written, printed, or graphic matter on or accompanying a food. Thus, the agency presumably has the power to regulate most of the in-store point-of-purchase information that is provided about foods. The test is whether the material "accompanies" the product; virtually any material supplied by the manufacturer or displayed by the retailer near the food would qualify. USDA's authority is comparably broad, but it does not customarily require prior approval of point-of-purchase labeling for meat and poultry products.

Thus, food "labeling" encompasses a broader range of communicative devices than the printed labels affixed to products. Current FDA and USDA nutrition information requirements, however, are chiefly directed at product labels, and it is these requirements on which this report focuses. It is important, however, to understand that both agencies have the authority to challenge labels and labeling that make claims that conflict with or go beyond the content of current regulations or policies. Both agencies use statements made on off-package labeling to determine whether nutrition information is required on a product's label. In many of the contexts discussed in this report, the distinction between labels and labeling is not important. The legal authority of the two agencies to regulate labeling may prove decisive when foods are sold without conventional labels (for example, produce) or in packaging that no federal agency currently attempts to regulate (for example, foods sold by some limited-menu restaurants).

EVOLUTION OF NUTRITION LABELING FOR FOODS

FDA Nutrition Labeling Requirements

Labels on over half of all packaged foods sold in the United States currently provide some type of nutrition information. The information allowed or required on FDA-regulated foods is prescribed by regulations that the agency first adopted in 1973 (38 Fed. Reg. 2125–2132, Jan. 19, 1973). These regulations have undergone relatively few changes since they went into effect in 1975, which helps to explain the present interest in reform. Any assessment of proposed reforms, therefore, requires some understanding of FDA's original regulations and the judgments that they reflect. It is appropriate to begin this examination of current nutrition labeling policy with FDA, because its requirements antedated and influenced USDA (Kushner et al., 1990).

FDA derives its authority to regulate food labels from the FD&C Act. That law was enacted in 1938, when knowledge about nutrition was rudimentary and most links between diet and chronic disease were unsuspected. Although the FD&C Act has been amended many times, the provisions governing the labeling of conventional foods have undergone no significant change since their enactment. These provisions are written such that their broad language, coupled with the agency's explicit authority to prescribe regulations for the efficient enforcement of the Act, has allowed FDA to update the Act's requirements as processed foods have proliferated and expectations for the types of information that should appear on food labels have changed (21 USC § 371(a)).

Under section 403 of the FD&C Act (21 USC § 343), every food label must contain the name of the food, a statement of the net quantity of contents (typically net weight), and the name and address of the manufacturer or distributor. Even today, some foods are lawfully marketed with labels that bear only these three items of information, although most labels contain more. Most notably, all but a few FDA-regulated foods must also bear a list of ingredients in descending order of predominance. The exception, however, is an important one: Foods for which FDA has established a standard of identity need not list ingredients that the standard makes mandatory.

In addition to requiring these affirmative statements on food labels, the FD&C Act prohibits other statements; most significantly, it prohibits statements that are false or misleading in any particular. A related provision, section 201(n) (21 USC § 321(n)), specifies that in determining whether the labeling of a food is misleading, "there shall be taken into account . . . not only representations made or suggested . . . but also the extent to which the labeling . . . fails to reveal facts material in light of such representations. . . ." This was the U.S. Congress's way of recognizing that half-truths can often be as misleading as outright misrepresentations. Section 201(n) was originally treated as guidance for courts that adjudicated FDA charges of misbranding, but since the 1960s the agency has, on occasion, invoked this provision and its general rulemaking power to prescribe affirmative disclosures on food labels. These provisions provided the authority on which FDA relied in adopting its current requirements for nutrient information on the labels of packaged foods (38 Fed. Reg. 2125–2132, Jan. 19, 1973).

Before the 1973 regulations are discussed, FDA's early attitude toward health claims for foods and its protracted efforts to control foods offered for their vitamin and mineral contents should be mentioned. Through the late 1960s, FDA relied primarily on the FD&C Act's prohibition against misleading labeling to curb what it considered irrational fortification of foods and the sale of products that offered ingredients of no proven nutritional value. Moreover, the agency consistently objected to specific claims that a food or any component could treat or prevent disease. Agency officials took the position that any product with a label that explicitly or implicitly claimed utility in preventing or treating disease, other than nutritional deficiency, was, under the law, a "drug" and, thus, a product whose safety and effectiveness had to be proved before it could lawfully be marketed (Hutt, 1986).

Sometimes, the accumulation of knowledge about nutrition and disease seemed to challenge FDA's uniform opposition to health claims. Following the publication in 1957 of a major report by the American Heart Association recommending a reduction in dietary cholesterol and saturated fats, marketers of many foods began referring to this advice in their labeling. FDA officials viewed any reference to cholesterol or saturated fat with suspicion and they threatened to seize products whose labeling featured such references. As the evidence linking these food constituents to coronary heart disease grew stronger, however, the agency came under increasing pressure to change its position and by 1970 was no longer attempting to enforce it (Hutt, 1984).

The FD&C Act does not, in so many words, require that a label for any food provide information about nutrient content. However, Congress recognized as early as 1938 that some nutrient information might be important for certain products. In section 403(j) of the Act (21 USC § 343(j)), it authorized FDA to issue regulations prescribing the information about vitamin, mineral, and other dietary properties that must appear in the labeling of foods represented for what the law termed "special dietary use." FDA inaugurated section 403(j) in 1941 by adopting regulations governing the labeling of fortified foods, vitamin and mineral supplements, and other special dietary foods such as infant foods, hypoallergenic foods, and foods for use in weight control. The 1941 regulations specified how food components should be described if the manufacturer chose to feature them, but they did not purport to restrict the type or quantity of nutrients that could be included or limit other claims that could be made.

Over the next two decades, the types of special dietary products marketed and the claims made for them grew in number and variety. By the early 1960s, FDA officials had concluded that the 1941 regulations needed updating, and in 1966 the agency proposed a far-reaching set of changes. In addition to proposing to limit the foods that could be fortified and to restrict the nutrients that could be used in fortification, FDA proposed to curtail the number of allowable formulations of dietary supplements of vitamins and minerals. It also proposed to ban statements on vitamin and mineral supplements that Americans' diets were nutrient deficient, that common foods did not supply adequate amounts of nutrients, or that routine vitamin or mineral supplementation was prudent. The agency's most provocative proposal was to treat all products that supplied significantly more than the Recommended Dietary Allowance (RDA) of any nutrient as "drugs." The administrative hearings on these proposals lasted from 1967 to 1969, and decisions about the content of final regulations were still pending at the close of the decade.

Space does not allow, nor does the context warrant, a full account of the ensuing 5 years of litigation over the substance and legality of FDA's proposals for vitamin-mineral supplements. The final chapter of the story, however, is noteworthy. In 1976, for the first time since its passage, Congress amended the 1938 FD&C Act to *withdraw* authority from FDA, forbidding it to restrict—as unneeded or useless—the kind or amounts of vitamins and minerals that can be added to foods or sold as supplements (Merrill and Hutt, 1980).

While any summary of FDA's early food labeling policies involves over-simplification, it is nonetheless fair to describe the agency as being concerned chiefly with protecting the consumer's pocketbook by maintaining the composition of basic foods and discouraging the sale of processed substitutes. The agency started with the assumption that traditionally formulated foods and meals prepared in the home would ensure healthy diets. Furthermore, it displayed little confidence in the ability of consumers to make wise dietary choices. These policies, however, began to undergo significant change.

In 1969, President Richard Nixon convened the White House Conference on Food, Nutrition, and Health, largely in response to reports of widespread malnutrition among Americans. While this topic was the focus of the conference, the final report also addressed the regulation of food composition and labeling (WHC, 1970). The report criticized FDA's approaches to food standards of identity, the marketing of substitute foods, and label statements relating to nutrition and long-term health. While the report stressed the importance of sound nutrition, it emphasized the need to help consumers make sound nutritional choices by requiring more information on food labels. Among the conference participants were several individuals who soon after became officials of FDA, and its recommendations had an immediate impact on the agency's policies (Wodicka, 1990).

By 1973, FDA had adopted several amendments to its regulations that reflected a new emphasis on providing consumers with information needed to make informed dietary choices. Under the FD&C Act (21 USC § 343(i)) the label of a standardized food does not need to contain a list of any mandatory ingredients but must contain a list only of those optional ingredients specified by FDA. The agency urged manufacturers to list all ingredients voluntarily (21 CFR § 101.6). Then, it began (although it has not yet completed the task) to amend existing standards of identity to classify most previously mandatory ingredients as optional and to require that they be listed on the label (Hutt, 1984).

FDA's most important initiative was its adoption of regulations governing nutrition labeling for packaged foods. These regulations, the coverage and current adequacy of which are the focus of this report, did not (and still do not) require nutrition labeling of all foods within the agency's jurisdiction. Among other considerations, uncertainty about its legal authority to mandate across-the-board nutrition information led the agency to set more modest goals. The regulations specified how nutrition information was to be provided if a manufacturer chose to do so. The regulations also required that certain foods have nutrition labeling. If a nutrient were added to, or any nutrition claim was made for a food, its label had to provide nutrition information in a prescribed format.

Because these regulations established the framework for most of the nutrition information that currently appears on the labels of packaged foods, whether regulated by FDA or USDA, their examination in further detail is useful. It is important to emphasize that FDA's 1973 regulations had a different focus from those of current proposals to reform food labels. In the early 1970s, federal health officials were preoccupied about reports of undernourishment in the United States, and FDA officials wanted to ensure that consumers were provided with sufficient information to enable them to select a diet that was adequate in vitamins, minerals, and protein. At the same time they remained eager to curb excessive consumption of these nutrients. These complementary views produced agreement on a label that focused on a food's contribution to the desired daily intake of vitamins, minerals, and protein. Thus, the prescribed nutrition information panel featured those nutrients, among others, and most of them were described in terms of the percentage of the U.S. Recommended Daily Allowances (U.S. RDA) provided in a serving. The U.S. RDAs were a creation of FDA, based on the 1968 RDA established by the Food and Nutrition Board of the National Research Council (NRC, 1968) but simplified to facilitate label disclosure.

FDA's regulations prescribed a uniform sequence and format for nutrition information. The label was to set forth the following, in the indicated order: (1) serving size for the food; (2) the number of servings in the container; and per serving (3) the number of calories; (4) the amount of protein (in grams); (5) the amount of carbohydrate (in grams); (6) the amount of fat (in grams); (7) the amount of protein (expressed as a percentage of the U.S. RDA); and (8) the percentage of the U.S. RDA of each of seven micronutrients (vitamin A, vitamin C, thiamin, riboflavin, niacin, calcium, and iron). The regulations also allowed a manufacturer to list any of a dozen other vitamins and minerals, in terms of the percentage of the U.S. RDA in a serving (21 CFR § 101.9(c)).

The explanation accompanying the regulations did not always spell out the agency's reasons for the choices it had made. Contemporary statements by FDA officials indicated little more than that the list of required nutrients was consistent with the opinions of professional nutritionists consulted by the agency (Stokes, 1972). Among the major constituents, only protein was to be described in terms of recommended intake, and it seems clear that FDA officials were not concerned about excessive protein consumption but, rather, about deceptive claims for protein content. The agency required that protein be listed, by percentage of the U.S. RDA, "unless the product contained no substantial amount of protein." In that case, protein could be omitted (21 CFR § 101.9(c)(7)(ii)).

FDA's regulations required the disclosure of total fat content but not fatty acid composition. A separate regulation that addressed this subject allowed manufacturers to include information about fatty acid composition, with certain conditions (21 CFR § 101.25). If the fatty acid composition was listed, the regulations specified that it was to be described in terms of polyunsaturated, saturated, and percent calories from fat. Furthermore, reflecting FDA's long-standing opposition to label claims about saturated fats and coronary heart disease, the regulations provided that if fatty acid composition was listed, the label also had to include the following statement: "Information on fatty acid content is provided for individuals who, on the advice of a physician, wish to modify their total dietary intake of fatty acids" (Dunning, 1973). The agency adopted the same position regarding cholesterol. Stating cholesterol content was optional, but if it were included the manufacturer had to add a similar statement that the purpose was to assist individuals who were under a physician's care (21 CFR § 101.25).

Sodium was treated somewhat differently. Under the 1973 regulations, listing of sodium (in milligrams per serving) was optional, but it could also be listed in the absence of full nutrition labeling (21 CFR § 101.9(c)(8)(i)). The objective was to encourage the provision of sodium information without subjecting manufacturers to the expense of determining the amounts of other nutrients in a food. However, rules adopted in 1984 required sodium to be declared when nutrition information was provided.

FDA's 1973 regulations reflected important decisions regarding the format of nutrition labels. First, the agency specified that nutrition information, when provided, was to appear on the information panel or principal display panel of the package (21 CFR § 101.2). Another regulation had previously fixed the location of these label components (21 CFR § 101.1). The goal was to make sure that nutrition information appeared in the same location on similar foods and in roughly the same position on all foods, so that it would be "more easily found and read by consumers under normal conditions of purchase and use" (37 Fed. Reg. 6493–6497, Mar. 30, 1972).

Second, for the presentation of nutrition information, FDA chose a numeric format over verbal and pictorial alternatives. This choice was based in large part on studies the agency had commissioned by the Consumer Research Institute (CRI) (Johnson, 1973; Wells, 1972). The agency apparently had already decided that the U.S. RDAs should provide the framework for describing nutrient content; it asked CRI to test three approaches for communicating this information. One format, the one that was chosen, presented the information numerically as a percentage of the U.S. RDA. One of the two rejected, the so-called verbal format, described the content of individual nutrients as fair, good, and excellent. In the other, the pictorial format, the proportion of the U.S. RDA provided by a serving was expressed by small circles, stars, or smiling faces. According to an FDA official, all three formats were understood by uneducated, low-income consumers as well as by educated consumers, although the former group had greater difficulties with the verbal design. Consumers found the pictorial format least desirable; many thought it condescending (Johnson, 1973). See Figure 3-1 for an example of a nutrition information panel based on current FDA regulations.

FDA's original nutrition labeling regulations embodied several decisions that ensured that its system would not be comprehensive. Because of its understanding with USDA, FDA could not make its regulations applicable to meat and poultry products. Foods sold by restaurants and other food service institutions

```
                    2% LOWFAT MILK
              Nutrition Information Per Serving
    SERVING SIZE .........................      ONE CUP
    SERVINGS PER CONTAINER ..    8
    CALORIES ...............................  120
    PROTEIN ...............................      8   GRAMS
    CARBOHYDRATE .....................     11   GRAMS
    FAT .......................................      5   GRAMS
    SODIUM..................................  130   mg

                   Percentage of U.S.
          Recommended Daily Allowances (U.S. RDA)
    PROTEIN ..........    20   RIBOFLAVIN .....   25
    VITAMIN A ........   10   NIACIN.............      *
    VITAMIN C ........     4   CALCIUM.........   30
    THIAMINE..........    6   IRON ................      *
    *CONTAINS LESS THAN 2% OF THE U.S. RDA FOR THESE NUTRIENTS
```

FIGURE 3-1   Sample nutrition information panel for 2% low-fat milk (½ gallon) under current FDA regulations (minimum requirements).

were also excluded, chiefly, but not solely, because of problems of enforcement (DHEW/USDA/FTC, 1979). The agency originally contemplated labeling for fresh fruits and vegetables, albeit with modifications, but it eventually exempted them from the regulations, ostensibly on the grounds of infeasibility (38 Fed. Reg. 32,786–32,787, Nov. 28, 1973). FDA never finalized a later proposal to extend nutrition labeling to produce (40 Fed. Reg. 8214–8217, Feb. 26, 1975).

In sum, FDA's 1973 nutrition labeling regulations applied only to retail packaged foods other than meat and poultry products. Even for these retail packaged foods, the agency's requirements were not universally binding. By their terms, the regulations required nutrition labeling on a packaged food only if the manufacturer of a food added a nutrient or made a nutrition claim for the product.

The decision to make nutrition labeling essentially voluntary was carefully considered. Although it was not spelled out in the preamble, almost surely one of FDA's reasons for this was uncertainty about its legal authority to require affirmative disclosure of nutrient information on foods for which no nutritional claim, implicit or express, was made (Wodicka, 1990). The agency's chief source of power in the FD&C Act, in addition to its general power to adopt regulations for the efficient enforcement of the Act, was the section 403(a) prohibition against misleading labeling, coupled with section 201(n), which, arguably, is activated by what manufacturers chose to say about their products. FDA had other reservations as well, however, as its preamble in the *Federal Register* explained:

> The Commissioner has concluded that insufficient information is known about the nutrient content and variability of some foods, and that the analytical methodology and capacity of some food manufacturers, processors, and distributors is inadequate to permit adoption of a requirement at this time that all foods bear nutrition labeling. Experience under this new regulation is required before expansion to all foods on a mandatory basis can be considered (38 Fed. Reg. 2125–2132, Jan. 19, 1973).

Although changed in some details, FDA's current nutrition labeling regulations still make nutrition labeling mandatory only for foods to which a nutrient has been added or for which a nutrition claim has been made.

USDA Nutrition Labeling Requirements

Soon after FDA issued its final nutrition labeling regulations, USDA proposed a similar set of requirements for meat and poultry products (Mussman, 1974). However, the department never completed this rulemaking. Its system of prior label approval allows it to effect compliance with departmental policies without issuing regulations, and apparently, USDA officials concluded that it was preferable to set forth its policies in a less formal fashion. USDA's current nutrition labeling requirements can be found in the *FSIS Standards and Labeling Policy Book* and policy memoranda.

The first FSIS policy relating to nutrition labeling dates from 1982, but the agency had previously approved numerous labels containing nutrition information before then. Policy Memorandum 039 provides that a label may state that a meat or poultry product can help reduce or maintain body weight or may make a claim regarding caloric content (USDA, 1982). Either type of claim obligates the producer to provide nutrition information in an abbreviation of the FDA required format. The memorandum reflects a judgment, similar in substance to FDA's but presumably not considered necessary to establish USDA's legal authority, that consumers should be provided full information in order to assess the utility of products for which specific nutrition claims are made.

Policy Memorandum 086 sets forth USDA's required format for providing nutrition information (USDA, 1985). FDA regulations allow the information to be provided on the principal display or information panel of the label. Use of FDA's comprehensive format is authorized, but it is not required. Instead, the manufacturer of a meat or poultry product may list only calories and the amounts of protein, carbohydrate, and fat stated as grams per serving. This abbreviated format focuses on major nutritional components, ignoring vitamins, minerals, and notably, sodium.

USDA has also adopted an informal policy toward cholesterol and fatty acid labeling similar to FDA's historical policy. Information about cholesterol and/or fatty acid content may be included with nutrition information when it is provided in the FDA format or in the abbreviated USDA format. USDA does not require a manufacturer that makes a cholesterol claim or that provides cholesterol information to provide information about fatty acid content as well.

The most significant differences between USDA's nutrition labeling requirements and FDA's current regulations do not relate to content or format. Rather, they reflect, on the one hand, the possible different outlooks and, on the other, the previously discussed important different modes of implementation. While FDA officials have frequently encouraged manufacturers to provide nutrition information even when it is not required, USDA has been chiefly concerned with ensuring the accuracy of whatever information appears on meat and poultry products. The need to obtain FSIS approval may have discouraged some producers from volunteering nutrition information, because FSIS demands that producers submit data to support statements about nutrient content (as well as other statements). This may mean that nutrient levels described on USDA-approved labels are better verified than those on labels for foods regulated by FDA, which has no general authority to require submission of supporting data.

USDA's more cautious approach to nutrition labeling for meat and poultry products does not appear to reflect doubt about its authority to require such information—even on meat and poultry products for which no nutrition claim is made. While neither the FMI Act nor the PMI Act uses the word *nutrition* and both say relatively little about the type of information USDA may require on labels, the universal acceptance of USDA's prior approval system, coupled with the broad language of these statutes, would appear to put any such doubts to rest.

DEFICIENCIES IN CURRENT
REQUIREMENTS FOR FOOD LABELS

For 15 years, nutrition labeling has been used to provide consumers with information to make more informed food choices, primarily to avoid certain nutrient inadequacies. Critics of the current system stress the need to provide information to help consumers manage their total dietary pattern in line with current dietary recommendations (ADA, 1990; AIN/ASCN, 1990; CNCFL, 1989; CSPI, 1989; DHEW/USDA/FTC, 1979; DHHS, 1988; FDA, 1978, 1989a,b; FNLG, 1989; GAO, 1988; ORC, 1990; U.S. Congress, 1989a,b). Their criticisms of current food labels fall into several categories:

- Nutrition labeling should be mandatory; currently, it is not required on all packaged foods and is not used in conjunction with the sale of other important classes of foods.
- Nutrition panel information is not uniform across all food products.
- Current nutrition labeling as well as efforts to make labeling changes should be accompanied by a consumer education program.
- Nutrition panel information includes some nutrients that should not or do not need to be listed, while other information is omitted.
- Ingredient labeling is incomplete and misleading.
- Current format is too confusing and complex.
- Label disclosures of nutrient contents are misleading and are not based on established standard definitions.

Foods Not Currently Covered or Exempted from
Nutrition Labeling Regulations

Recent estimates are that about 60 percent of packaged products regulated by FDA have nutrition labeling; for USDA, more than 35 percent of regulated packaged products carry nutrition labeling. This means that almost half of all packaged foods do not bear nutrition labeling. Moreover, nutrition information is not required on or in conjunction with the sale of fresh and frozen meats, poultry, eggs, and seafood; fruits and vegetables; foods prepared and sold for immediate consumption by restaurants, carryout food bars, and many supermarkets; and most foods served in institutional settings.

Many consumer and health and nutrition organizations have called for mandatory nutrition labeling of all foods under FDA and USDA jurisdiction, either based on current law or mandated by new legislation. These groups also argue that FDA and USDA requirements for such labeling should be uniform.

Industry groups have expressed concern over the potential for a multiplicity of food labeling rules by the states and have argued that food labels throughout the United States should bear uniform information that is subject to supervision and enforcement by FDA and USDA. However, many proponents of nutrition labeling changes have opposed preemption of state labeling laws and expressed concern that efforts to achieve uniformity could extend beyond nutrition and ingredient information on food labels into areas such as food safety.

Virtually all groups urge that legislative or regulatory reforms of food labels should include a comprehensive consumer education component developed and funded jointly by the public and private sectors.

Deficiencies in Information About Nutrient Content

There is considerable public health interest in several food components that are currently not required on the standard nutrition information panel, including cholesterol; saturated, monounsaturated, and polyunsaturated fatty acids; complex carbohydrates; fiber; and potassium. Although current rules allow voluntary declaration of some of these food components, none of this information is now mandatory.

Fat and Cholesterol

Current FDA and USDA regulations permit the voluntary inclusion of fatty acid and cholesterol contents, in addition to total fat content, as part of nutrition labeling (21 CFR § 101.25; USDA, 1985). The rules allow a food label to include information on fatty acid content if the food contains 10 percent or more fat on a dry weight basis and not less than 2 percent of fat in an average serving. If any claim about fatty acid and/or cholesterol content is made for a product, full nutrition information becomes mandatory. In addition, current regulations on fat content require an accompanying statement, for example, "Information on fat [and/or cholesterol, where applicable] content is provided for individuals who, on the advice of a physician, are modifying their dietary intake of fat [and/or cholesterol, where applicable]." However, FDA has not enforced the requirement for several years and the disclosure now rarely appears on food labels.

Health professional and consumer groups have called for more comprehensive information about fat and cholesterol to be included on food labels. Suggestions for expanded fat information include mandatory disclosure of saturated, monounsaturated, and polyunsaturated fatty acids, and cholesterol. Some also urge that each fat component be disclosed by weight (in grams), number of calories, and/or percentage of total calories.

Carbohydrates

Both FDA and USDA require the disclosure of total carbohydrates when nutrition information is provided (21 CFR § 101.9(c)(5); USDA, 1985). Various consumer groups have called for more complete information on complex and simple carbohydrates (starches and sugars, respectively). These groups are concerned that high levels of sugar consumption contribute to dental caries, nutrient dilution, and, potentially, excess calories. Quantitative declaration of carbohydrate components has been urged as consumers have become increasingly concerned about the quantity of sugars they are consuming.

Numerous critics have argued that the amount of sugar and other sweeteners should be declared by weight, or by both percentage and weight, either on the nutrition panel or ingredient listing. Many industry groups, however, have questioned whether current analytical techniques are adequate to support mandatory disclosure of total carbohydrates, simple carbohydrates (sugars), and complex carbohydrates.

Fiber

Over the past several years, breakfast cereal manufacturers and other segments of the food industry have included fiber content declarations on their food labels as a result of consumer interest. Although not required, FDA policy currently states that if fiber content is reported, it must be expressed as dietary fiber and declared in grams. Consumer and health advocates support the mandatory declaration of fiber content on the nutrition information panel.

Sodium and Potassium

Sodium content (in milligrams) is a required component of the nutrition information panel when it is used voluntarily or a claim is made on the label. However, sodium content can be declared on a food label without providing full nutrition information labeling (21 CFR § 101.9(c)(8)(i)). In the absence of a claim, listing of the sodium content remains voluntary under USDA Policy Memorandum 049C (USDA, 1984). FDA applies similar rules to potassium; however, declaration is voluntary (21 CFR § 101.9(c)(8)(ii)).

For more than a decade, consumer, professional, and industry groups, as well as legislators, have supported mandatory labeling of the sodium and, sometimes, potassium contents on all foods. Recommendations from these groups vary as to whether the total and/or added sodium or salt should be declared on the nutrition information panel and whether it should be declared by weight or percent.

Other Nutrients

Micronutrients of current public health concern (e.g., folate, zinc, and vitamin B_6) have been proposed by various groups to be required components of the nutrition information panel. Most groups seem to agree, however, that federal agencies should have regulatory discretion to add or subtract nutrients from the required label information as knowledge of dietary patterns and the relationship of nutrition to long-term health change.

Incomplete Ingredient Information

When the 1938 FD&C Act first mandated the listing of ingredients on most packaged foods, the requirement was viewed primarily as a means of providing consumers with basic information about the value of foods. While the listing of ingredients does not provide direct information about a product's nutrient composition, it does provide information about the components used to make the food and about ingredients that consumers may wish to avoid, such as certain fats. Current interest in the ingredient listing has focused on the health implications of specific ingredients and consumers' ability to identify and avoid certain food constituents.

Current FDA and USDA regulations generally require that, except for for standardized foods, if a food is formulated from two or more ingredients, the ingredients must be listed on the label in descending order of predominance by weight (21 CFR § 101.4; 9 CFR § 317.2). Each ingredient is to be listed by its common or usual name, except for spices, flavors, and colors, which generally may be listed in categorical groupings (21 CFR § 101.22).

Percent Ingredient Labeling

Many groups have proposed that the ingredient panel disclose the percentage of each ingredient in a food product. Current FDA and USDA regulations do not require percent ingredient labeling. The possibilities for listing percentages of ingredients range from listing the major ingredients to listing all of them. Manufacturers have resisted this proposal, arguing that it would reveal proprietary formulations.

"And/Or" Ingredient Labeling

Current FDA regulations allow the use of "and/or" ingredient labeling for the declaration of leavening agents, yeast nutrients, dough conditioners, firming agents, and fats and oils (21 CFR 101.4(b)(14). "And/or" labeling allows the manufacturer the flexibility to switch among interchangeable ingredients without revising food labels, when price, availability, or both vary. Particular attention has focused on the implications of this practice regarding the fat composition of foods.

Continued use of "and/or" labeling for fats and oils is opposed by groups which believe that consumers should be able to avoid certain fats and oils with high levels of saturated fatty acids. Many groups argue that "and/or" labeling could continue to be allowed for fats and oils only if nutrition information labeling is mandatory for total fat and saturated and unsaturated fatty acids.

Some consumer groups have proposed extension of the use of "and/or" labeling to nutritive carbohydrate sweeteners, which would have the effect of aggregating all sugars under a single entry in the ingredient list. These groups have expressed concern about the quantity of sugars in Americans' diets and claim that many ingredients being used in foods would not be identified as sweeteners by consumers. By grouping these ingredients together on the label, they argue, consumers would realize that, in addition to sugar, other ingredients (e.g., corn syrup, honey, or molasses) are being used to sweeten a given product.

Confusing and Complex Disclosures

Several critics argue that a number of items currently required or allowed on food labels create confusion and are difficult for the average consumer to grasp, including the concept and sizes of servings and the U.S. RDA.

Serving Size

A critical element of the nutrition information panel is the serving size of the food, for "serving" provides the reference unit for declaring nutrient content. While both agencies require that serving size be declared when nutrition information is provided, neither FDA nor USDA has established serving sizes for any class of foods; they allow manufacturers to set the serving size. FDA regulations define serving size as that reasonable quantity of food consumed as part of a meal (21 CFR § 101.9(b)(1)).

There are notable disparities in serving sizes among foods. Some manufacturers have clearly manipulated serving sizes to promote perceived or real benefits from the nutrition information panel (e.g., calories per serving). Some serving sizes appear to be altogether unrealistic. For example, a 12-fluid-ounce (355-ml) can of a carbonated beverage lists two servings per container at 6 fluid ounces (177 ml) each when most individuals would consume the entire contents at one time. Critics also point to the lack of uniformity within product categories. Different serving sizes within product categories make comparisons between similar foods difficult. Concerned about these practices, FDA proposed a procedure for standardizing serving sizes in 1974 (39 Fed. Reg. 20,887–20,888, June 14, 1974), but it never finalized the rule. Professional and consumer organizations have recommended that FDA and USDA standardize the serving sizes used in nutrition labeling to make comparisons among products easier and to prevent misleading manipulation.

Consumer groups and some food manufacturers believe that many consumers are unfamiliar with serving sizes expressed in grams and milligrams; they are more familiar with food measurements in household units, such as teaspoons and cups.

It has also been argued that all foods that require additional ingredients for the usual forms of preparation should be required to provide serving size and nutrition information for the food in the form that is consumed, not just in the form that is packaged. For example, since milk is routinely added to breakfast cereal, the nutrition information panel should be required to provide nutrient information for both the dry cereal and the cereal as consumed.

U.S. Recommended Daily Allowances

Amounts of protein, vitamins, and minerals per serving are currently required to be expressed as a percentage of the U.S. RDA. FDA developed the U.S. RDAs in the early 1970s for use in nutrition labeling by taking the highest level of the NRC 1968 RDAs (NRC, 1968) for each nutrient and making it the standard for expressing nutrient levels (21 CFR 101.9(c)(7). RDAs were updated in 1974, 1980, and 1989, the current 10th edition (NRC, 1974, 1980, 1989). The U.S. RDAs, however, have not been updated since 1972.

Most professional and consumer groups have recommended that the U.S. RDA system at least be updated to reflect the 1989 RDAs. Some have also urged adoption of the quantitative nutrient intake recommendations from recent reports as standards for expressing amounts of macronutrients. Many groups have also expressed concern about consumers' understanding of the U.S. RDA. Some evidence suggests that consumers have difficulty understanding and using percentages. It appears that many consumers do not understand that the U.S. RDA percentages for different nutrients on food labels cannot collectively be added up to reach a total of 100 percent for their U.S. RDA for the day. Other critics question whether the concept of the U.S. RDA is sound in principle. They suggest that there should be a different system for presenting nutrition information to consumers and, at the very least, some better way to educate consumers about the nutrition information on food packages.

Nutrition Label Format

Although there seems to be widespread support for changing the content of nutrition labeling, opinions diverge on the best format for depicting nutrition information on food labels. Current research provides little guidance about the best nutrition label format for consumers. Advocates of label change, however, have proposed a variety of untested new label formats. Other label expression issues include weight versus percentages, "and/or" labeling, and the listing of the ingredients discussed above.

Critics of the current numeric labeling system have urged federal agencies to use market research techniques, including focus groups, to determine consumers' ability to use different presentations of nutrition information on food labels. They argue that education, media, and marketing experts should be included in the development and analysis of new potential label formats. A variety of groups have also supported the need for strong efforts to educate consumers about the use of a new label once a new label format is developed and approved for implementation.

Nutrition Information Panel

The expression of fat content by weight (grams or household measures), as calories from fat, or as a percentage of total calories has been widely discussed. Although many supporters of additional fat information do not support use of the percentage of calories from fat, they acknowledge that it may be useful when comparing similar foods.

Numeric Displays

The current label format presents nutrition information as numbers in columns. Many critics believe that the current format is confusing, complicated, and difficult for consumers to understand. When FDA established nutrition labeling regulations in 1973, it prescribed text and numbers rather than text alone or text with graphics because results of the limited amount of consumer research available suggested that consumers preferred numbers to indicate the amounts of nutrients in a food.

The nutrient content of a food can be expressed as absolute amounts, such as grams and milligrams, or as a percentage of a daily intake standard. Currently, only protein, vitamins, and minerals are expressed in terms of a daily intake standard. Some have suggested that other food components such as fat, carbohydrates, and fiber should be expressed in a similar fashion.

Descriptive (Adjectival) Display

Descriptors are already widely used to describe the nutrient content of foods on the principal display panel, and some argue that their use should be expanded to describe nutrient content on the nutrition panel. It is argued, for example, that terms such as *excellent, good,* and *fair,* or *high, medium,* and *low* are more easily understood by most consumers than are the metric weights (grams and milligrams) currently used. Others note, however, the difficulty of defining such terms and point to the lack of consistency in their use among agencies. Some also argue that descriptive terms alone may not provide sufficiently precise information on the nutrient content of a food, and numeric ranges would need to be defined for the use of each term.

Graphic Display

There have been several innovative suggestions for the use of visual representations to convey nutritional value. Pie charts have been proposed to present information on the protein, fat, and carbohydrate contents of a food, with the information being presented either on a weight basis or as a percentage of calories. Critics of such approaches note that vitamins and minerals cannot be presented in this manner since they make no caloric contribution to the food.

The bar graph is another graphic option that has been proposed to express nutritional values as a percentage of a daily intake standard. It has been noted, however, that bar graphs confront problems in expressing nutrient values that exceed 100 percent of the standard (e.g., over 100 percent of the U.S. RDA), and some worry that consumers would perceive that only long bars are good.

Symbolic Display

Another approach to providing consumers with nutrient information is the use of symbols. Various types of symbols (colors) have been suggested, including the use of stoplight colors (e.g., red is bad or high, yellow is caution or moderate, and green is good or low) and icons for low-fat, low-cholesterol, low-sodium, high-fiber, and low-sugar. Symbols of this type currently appear on some restaurant menus.

Groupings and Sequences

Some commentors have suggested the grouping of nutrients in positive and negative clusters. Protein, fiber, vitamins, and minerals would appear in a group, possibly at the top of the label, whereas fat, cholesterol, sugar, and sodium would be clustered, perhaps, at the bottom of the label. Another variation would be to provide groupings according to nutrient type; that is, all carbohydrates, all fats, and all micronutrients would appear in separate blocks on the nutrition panel.

Typography and Color

The type sizes of words on labels are frequently criticized as being too small and, therefore, illegible to many consumers. Individuals with sight problems, especially the elderly, are thought to find labels difficult to use. Better use of color has also been recommended to make information more readily distinguishable. Some industry representatives argue, however, that the use of multiple colors on labels may add significant costs and present additional comprehension problems.

Nutrient Content Claims

The growing practice of labeling packaged foods with descriptors that characterize a food's nutrient content has led FDA and USDA to establish or propose definitions for certain descriptive terms, such as *low calorie* (21 CFR § 105.66), *sodium free, low sodium* (21 CFR § 101.13), *no cholesterol*, and *low cholesterol* (55 Fed. Reg. 29,456–29,473, July 19, 1990). Other widely used terms, however, such as *natural, organic*, and *fresh*, have never been defined by either agency or have been defined by only one. As a result, some descriptors are used to refer to several different product characteristics, creating confusion among consumers. For example, the term *lite* has been used by various manufacturers to describe color, taste, texture, fat, sugar, calories, salt or sodium, weight, and even breading. Furthermore, other descriptors are used in different ways to describe the same nutrient.

Most groups urge that regulations be established to define terms such as *high, reduced, low, no, lite*, and others as they are needed. Most groups have requested formal definitions of descriptors for all nutrients that appear on the nutrition information label. There is disagreement whether certain claims should be allowed only when a food meets other characteristics (e.g., not allowing a no-cholesterol claim when a food is high in saturated fat).

REFERENCES

ADA (American Dietetic Association). 1990. Position of The American Dietetic Association: Nutrition and health information on food labels. J. Am. Diet. Assoc. 90:583–585.

AIN/ASCN (American Institute of Nutrition and the American Society for Clinical Nutrition). 1990. Position Statement on Food Labeling. Nutrition Notes January:7–9.

CNCFL (Committee on the Nutrition Components of Food Labeling). 1989. Information presented at a public meeting of the Committee on the Nutrition Components of Food Labeling, Food and Nutrition Board, Institute of Medicine, December 4, 1989. Unpublished.

Crowford, L.M. 1990. Testimony before the Subcommittee on Rural Development, Agriculture, and Related Agencies, Committee on Appropriations, U.S. House of Representatives, Washington, D.C., March 5, 1990.

CSPI (Center for Science in the Public Interest). 1989. Food Labeling Chaos: The Case for Reform. CPSI, Washington, D.C. 37 pp.

DHEW/USDA/FTC (U.S. Department of Health, Education, and Welfare; U.S. Department of Agriculture; and Federal Trade Commission). 1979. Food Labeling Background Papers. Government Printing Office, Washington, D.C. 124 pp.

DHHS (U.S. Department of Health and Human Services). 1988. The Surgeon General's Report on Nutrition and Health. Government Printing Office, Washington, D.C. 727 pp.

Dunning, H.N. 1973. Integration with other labeling concerns. Food, Drug, Cosmetic Law J. 28:118–122.

FDA (U.S. Food and Drug Administration). 1978. FDA Food Labeling Consumer Survey. Government Printing Office, Washington, D.C. 188 pp.

FDA (U.S. Food and Drug Administration). 1989a. Summary of regional hearings on food labeling (Chicago, San Antonio, Seattle, Atlanta). Unpublished FDA staff document.

FDA (U.S. Food and Drug Administration). 1989b. Comments received from the FDA Advanced Notice of Proposed Rulemaking on Food Labeling, Docket No. 89N–0226. Dockets Management Branch, FDA, Washington, D.C.

FNLG (Food and Nutrition Labeling Group). 1989. Joint Statement on Nutrition Labeling. FNLG Coordinating Committee (American Association of Retired Persons, American Cancer Society, The American Dietetic Association, American Heart Association, Center for Science in the Public Interest, and Public Voice for Food and Health Policy) and 18 other professional nutrition and health organizations. FNLG, Washington, D.C. 2 pp.

GAO (U.S. General Accounting Office). 1988. Food Marketing: Frozen Pizza Cheese— Representative of Broader Food Labeling Issues. Report to the Chairman, Subcommittee on Oversight and Investigations, Committee on Energy and Commerce, U.S. House of Representatives. Government Printing Office, Washington, D.C. 47 pp.

Hutt, P.B. 1989. Regulating the misbranding of food. Food Technol. 43(9):228.

Hutt, P.B. 1986. Government regulation of health claims in food labeling and advertising. Food, Drug, Cosmetic Law J. 41:3–73.

Johnson, O.C. 1973. Nutrition labeling—a foremost concern. Food, Drug, Cosmetic Law J. 28:108–117.

Kushner, G.J., R.S. Silverman, S.B. Steinborn, and R.A. Johnson. 1990. A Guide to Federal Food Labeling Requirements. Draft prepared for the U.S. Department of Agriculture and the U.S. Department of Health and Human Services. Government Printing Office, Washington, D.C. 37 pp.

Merrill, R.A., and P.B. Hutt. 1980. Food and Drug Law: Cases and Materials. The Foundation Press, Mineola, N.Y. 959 pp.

Mussman, H.C. 1974. USDA nutrition labeling regulations and the growth of voluntary nutrition labeling on meat. Food, Drug, Cosmetic Law J. 29:425–428.

NRC (National Research Council). 1968. Recommended Dietary Allowances, 7th ed. Report of the Subcommittee on the Seventh Edition of the RDAs, Food and Nutrition Board, Assembly of Life Sciences. National Academy of Sciences, Washington, D.C. 101 pp.

NRC (National Research Council). 1974. Recommended Dietary Allowances, 8th ed. Report of the Committee on Dietary Allowances, Committee on the Interpretation of the Recommended Dietary Allowances, Food and Nutrition Board, Assembly of Life Sciences. National Academy of Sciences, Washington, D.C. 128 pp.

NRC (National Research Council). 1980. Recommended Dietary Allowances, 9th ed. Report of the Committee on Dietary Allowances, Food and Nutrition Board, Assembly of Life Sciences. National Academy of Sciences, Washington, D.C. 185 pp.

NRC (National Research Council). 1989. Recommended Dietary Allowances, 10th ed. Report of the Subcommittee on the Tenth Edition of the RDAs, Food and Nutrition Board, Commission on Life Sciences. National Academy Press, Washington, D.C. 284 pp.

ORC (Opinion Research Corporation). 1990. Food Labeling and Nutrition: What Americans Want. Survey conducted for the National Food Processors Association. ORC, Washington, D.C. 178 pp.

Stokes, R.C. 1972. The Consumer Research Institute's Nutrition Labeling Research Program. Food, Drug, Cosmetic Law J. 27:249–262.

U.S. Congress. 1989a. Hearing before the Subcommittee on Health and the Environment, Committee on Energy and Commerce, U.S. House of Representatives, Washington, D.C., Aug. 3, 1989. 261 pp.

U.S. Congress. 1989b. Hearing before the Committee on Labor and Human Resources, U.S. Senate, Washington, D.C., Nov. 13, 1989. Unpublished.

USDA (U.S. Department of Agriculture). 1982. FSIS Policy Memorandum 039. Food Safety and Inspection Service, Washington, D.C.

USDA (U.S. Department of Agriculture). 1984. FSIS Policy Memorandum 049C. Food Safety and Inspection Service, Washington, D.C.

USDA (U.S. Department of Agriculture). 1985. FSIS Policy Memorandum 086. Food Safety and Inspection Service, Washington, D.C.

USDA (U.S. Department of Agriculture). 1989. FSIS Standards and Labeling Policy Book. Food Safety and Inspection Service, Washington, D.C.

Wells, B.H. 1972. The Consumer Research Institute's nutrient labeling research. Food, Drug, Cosmetic Law J. 27:40–44.

WHC (White House Conference on Food, Nutrition, and Health). 1970. Final Report. Government Printing Office, Washington, D.C. 341 pp.

Wodicka, V.O. 1990. The 1970s: The decade of regulations. Food, Drug, Cosmetic Law J. 45:59–67.

4

Contextual Factors Affecting
Food Labeling Reform

A number of external factors have an influence on food labeling reform. Although an exhaustive discussion of all these factors is not possible in this report, a brief review is necessary in order to convey the milieu in which proposals for changes in food labeling will be evaluated. The factors that are considered in this chapter include current dietary patterns, food marketing in the United States, consumer understanding of nutrition and use of food labels, and analytical considerations that affect food labeling information.

CURRENT DIETARY PATTERNS OF AMERICANS

Since the turn of the century, Americans have made extensive changes in their eating habits. More food is purchased for consumption away from home. Snacking is more common. A wider variety of foods is available year-round. Changes in the composition of foods have occurred due to improved methods of cultivation and animal husbandry, the introduction of new varieties of plants and animals bred for either nutritional or other features, and advances in food processing that permit the formulation of foods with desirable characteristics. The data on which a discussion of these changes is based come primarily from records maintained and surveys conducted by the U.S. Department of Agriculture (USDA) and the U.S. Department of Health and Human Services (DHHS). Most of the trend data discussed here are based on the U.S. Food Supply Series and the Nationwide Food Consumption Survey (NFCS) conducted by USDA and the National Health and Nutrition Examination Survey (NHANES) conducted by DHHS.

Sources of Data and Issues of Interpretation

Major changes have occurred in what and where Americans eat; however, care needs to be taken in the interpretation of the available data. The data that are collected represent four different levels: national food supply, use of food in households, individual food intakes, and nutritional and health outcomes that are influenced by diet. A variety of methods is used to collect the data, and the collective evaluation of such data needs to be sensitive to these different methods.

Systematic collection of data on the U.S. food supply began in 1909, when USDA initiated tracking the availability of foods in the U.S. marketplace. USDA has been able to calculate annually the approximate amount of food available per individual by dividing the total amount of foodstuffs available by the civilian population of the United States at a given time. The total amount of foodstuffs is calculated as [(food produced + beginning inventories + food imported) − (food exported + food purchased by the military + year-end inventories + food having nonfood uses)]. Through the use of food composition tables, a rough estimate can then be made of the nutritive value of foods available for consumption by Americans. Refinements of these types of calculations have led to the development of estimates of the per capita availability of 25 nutrients in approximately 350 foods as they "disappear" into the U.S. food distribution system.

Data on food availability represent quantities that are larger than those actually eaten, because the amounts do not account for the losses that occur during processing, marketing, and home use. Calculations of the nutritive value of the food supply overlook some sources of nutrients such as alcoholic beverages (which provide calories, but few nutrients) and vitamin and mineral supplements (which provide micronutrients, but essentially no calories). Because the per capita availability of food and nutrients is based on the total U.S. population in any given year, comparisons over time do not take into account the changing demographic structure of the U.S. population. With these caveats in mind, and recognizing that food supply data do not provide information on the actual foods that are eaten, they are still useful for reflecting changes in the overall patterns of the foods and nutrients available over time.

At the second and third levels, data are collected by using household-based surveys (i.e., use of food in households and individual food intakes). At approximately 10-year intervals since 1936, USDA has conducted its NFCS. The first four surveys collected data only on the use of foods in households. In 1965, data on the consumption of food by individuals were added to the information collected. Surveys were conducted in 1965–1966, 1977–1978, and 1987–1988. Beginning in 1985, USDA began the Continuing Survey of Food Intakes of Individuals (CSFII), which is performed annually except in years when the more comprehensive NFCS is conducted.

DHHS conducts a variety of surveys and surveillance activities that provide information on food intakes and the nutritional and health status of the U.S. population and subgroups of the population. The Total Diet Study, which has been conducted annually since 1961 by the Food and Drug Administration (FDA), estimates intakes of certain essential minerals as well as the extent of contamination of foodstuffs by industrial chemicals and pesticides. The Ten-State Nutrition Survey was conducted from 1968 to 1970 to examine the diets and nutritional status of the poor. The first National Health and Nutrition Examination Survey, NHANES I, which was conducted between 1971 and 1974, collects an ambitious set of data, including not only the dietary intakes of individuals but also health and medical histories, physical examinations, and laboratory data. Particular attention is paid to nutrition-related diseases. NHANES II was conducted from 1976 to 1980, the Hispanic HANES (HHANES) was carried out from 1982 to 1984, and NHANES III began in 1988.

In 1977, the U.S. Congress directed that a comprehensive, coordinated nutrition monitoring system be created. The National Nutrition Monitoring System (NNMS) was begun as a collaborative program between USDA and DHHS. NNMS is meant to coordinate the survey activities of these two federal departments and to issue joint survey reports through the Interagency Committee on Nutrition Monitoring. Reports issued in 1986 and 1989; these reports compared data from the 1977–1978 NFCS, 1985–1986 CSFII, NHANES II, HHANES, and USDA's historical data series (DHHS/USDA, 1986; LSRO, FASEB, 1989).

Data from the surveys mentioned above and historical data series can be useful in assessing major shifts in eating habits and the resulting nutritional status of Americans; however, the nature of the information requires that these conclusions must be reached with consideration of the limitations of the sources. All of the information, whether derived from food supply data or dietary surveys, is dependent on the quality of estimates and assumptions that permit the calculation of nutrient intakes. Dietary intake surveys of individuals often use a technique called the 24-hour dietary recall, relying on the respondent to accurately recall and describe the foods consumed during the preceding day or in the past 24 hours. Much of the data concerning the per capita disappearance of food consists of gross estimates of the amount of food produced; no adjustments are made for discarded, wasted, and spoiled foods. In addition, the data represent the average amount of food and nutrients available to the population, regardless of differences in age, sex, race, and economic status. However, major shifts in eating habits and the resulting nutritional status of Americans can be discerned from the available data.

More detail on changes in food consumption over the years than is offered here are provided in the National Research Council (NRC) report, *Diet and Health: Implications for Reducing Chronic Disease Risk* (NRC, 1989) and the

Expert Panel on National Nutrition Monitoring report, *Nutrition Monitoring in the United States* (LSRO, FASEB, 1989).

Food Energy

The daily food energy content (or calories, as it is expressed on food labels) of the food supply is substantially higher (3,500 calories in 1985) than intakes recorded in surveys. The primary changes in food sources of energy in the past 70 years have been from an increase in the percentage of energy contributed by fats, oils, sugars, and sweeteners, along with a decrease in the percentage contributed by grain products. Of the percentage of calories obtained from macronutrients from 1909 to 1985, protein contributed about 11 percent, fats increased from 32 to 43 percent, and carbohydrates fell from 57 to 46 percent (NRC, 1989). In 1985, the major sources of food energy in the food supply were fats and oils (20 percent); grains (19.9 percent); meat, poultry, and fish (19 percent); and sugars and sweeteners (17.8 percent) (LSRO, FASEB, 1989).

Data from the 1985–1986 CSFII indicate that children aged 1 to 5 have mean energy intakes that fall within the range for their age groups, with little difference observed between blacks and whites or among those from families with different income levels. The reported mean intakes by women, however, fall below the recommended range. In addition, intakes are lower in older (40 to 49 years) than in younger (20 to 29 years) women, lower in blacks than in whites, and lower in women below the poverty level than in those above the poverty level (LSRO, FASEB, 1989).

Despite the low caloric intakes reported, more than a quarter of American adults are overweight. Data from NHANES I, NHANES II, and HHANES reveal that women are more likely than men to be overweight (LSRO, FASEB, 1989). A comparison of NHANES I and health survey data from 1960 to 1962 reveals that the average weight gain was a 3-pound increase for women and a 6-pound increase for men (NRC, 1989).

Data from national surveys reveal that reported caloric intakes have decreased over time, while the prevalence of overweight individuals has remained the same or increased slightly. Whether an individual's weight changes or is maintained depends on the balance between caloric intake and physical activity, body size, body composition, and metabolic efficiency. The paradox of the reported low caloric intakes in conjunction with the high prevalence of overweight individuals in the United States has yet to be fully explained. A number of reasons have been suggested, including underreporting of caloric intake, heredity, decreased physical activity, and metabolic mechanisms. However, JNMEC considered it probable that low levels of physical activity have a significant relationship to the high prevalence of overweight individuals observed in the United States (DHHS/USDA, 1986). Concern exists that recommendations to reduce caloric intake further without a concomitant increase in nutrient density may compromise nutritional status.

Food energy is considered a current public health issue due to the relationship of total caloric intake to both its association with body weight and the implications for overall nutrient intakes and chronic diseases (LSRO, FASEB, 1989).

Fats and Cholesterol

The per capita amount of fat available in the food supply, the food sources, and the types of fat have changed considerably during the twentieth century. The amount of fat available per capita has increased to the current level of 169 g/day. The types of fat have also changed. Since 1909, the per capita amount of saturated fatty acids has remained constant at approximately 60 g/day, but the amount of monounsaturated fatty acids has gradually increased to the current level of 68 g/day, and since the mid-1960s the amount of polyunsaturated fatty acids has doubled to 33 g/day (LSRO, FASEB, 1989). Cholesterol in the food supply increased from 500 mg/day in 1909 to a peak of 570 mg/day in 1947. It subsequently fell to 480 mg/day in 1977, where it has remained. The decline in the availability of cholesterol is primarily due to the reduced use of eggs, from a peak of 49 pounds per person per year in 1951 to 32 pounds per person per year in 1985 (NRC, 1989).

Sources of dietary fats in the food supply have also changed. The proportion of total fats from meat, poultry, and fish has changed little, amounting to about 31.4 percent in 1985. Fat from whole milk has declined steadily, from 10.4 percent in the late 1940s to 3 percent in 1985, while a significant increase has occurred in the amount from fats and oils, increasing from 38 to 47 percent during the same period. The proportion of saturated fatty acids from meat, poultry, and fish has changed little since 1909, although there has been an increase in poultry consumption (LSRO, FASEB, 1989). Since the mid-1960s, a shift in dairy product consumption has occurred, with about a 50 percent decrease in whole milk consumption, a doubling of low-fat milk consumption, and a 173 percent increase in the consumption of cheeses (NRC, 1989). Within the fats and oils group, the proportion of saturated fatty acids obtained from animal sources has declined, while the amount obtained from vegetable sources has increased, due to the use of salad and cooking oils, which has increased from 2 to 25 pounds per capita since 1909 (NRC, 1989). In 1985, meat, poultry, and fish, fats and oils, and dairy products contributed almost all of the saturated fatty acids to the food supply. The proportion of polyunsaturated fatty acids from meat, poultry, and fish has decreased, while the amount from fats and oils has more than doubled in the past 70 years. In 1985, the food groups contributing most of the cholesterol were meat, poultry, and fish (43 percent), dairy products (13 percent), and eggs (39 percent) (LSRO, FASEB, 1989).

The most recent data on dietary fat intakes are derived from the 4-day dietary intakes from the 1985–1986 CSFII. Women aged 20 to 49 and children aged 1 to 5 consumed 37 percent and 35 percent of total calories from fat, respectively. Only about 10 percent of women surveyed had fat intakes below 30 percent of total calories. Fat intakes by women in this survey were higher among whites than among blacks and were higher for those in higher socioeconomic groups. However, race and economic status have been shown to have little to do with the percentage of calories from fat. Saturated fatty acids comprised an estimated 13 percent and 14 percent of calories in the diets of women and children, respectively. Monounsaturated fatty acids accounted for 13 percent of calories in both groups. Polyunsaturated fatty acids provided 6 percent of calories for children and 7 percent for women. Mean cholesterol intakes were 277 mg/day and 228 mg/day by women and children, respectively. More than 25 percent of women had mean cholesterol intakes in excess of 300 mg/day. Estimated intakes by men have remained high, at 423 to 466 mg/day (LSRO, FASEB, 1989).

Comparison of 1-day data from the 1985–1986 CSFII and the 1977–1978 NFCS reveals similar intakes of total fat by children and adult males, whereas for females aged 20 to 49 there appeared to be a decrease of about 10 percent between the surveys. The data can be considered to suggest that only women's fat intakes have actually changed. However, from 1977 to 1985 the percentage of total calories from fat has declined for children (37 to 35 percent) and adult males and females (42 to 37 percent). This change may be the result of an increase in carbohydrate consumption (LSRO, FASEB, 1989).

Data on mean serum cholesterol levels from national surveys have been compared (NRC, 1989). For adult men and women aged 20 to 74, the mean serum cholesterol levels have decreased 3 to 4 percent since the early 1960s, and the declines are statistically significant for both men and women, for all whites, but not for blacks (LSRO, FASEB, 1989). According to the definition of the National Cholesterol Education Program, 36 percent of all adults aged 20 to 74 are candidates for medical advice and intervention for high blood cholesterol levels (Sempos et al., 1989).

In view of the continuing indications of the high per capita availability and higher than recommended intakes of dietary fats and cholesterol, dietary fats are considered to be a current public health issue due to their association with heart disease, certain cancers, and obesity. As a result, the high consumption of total fat, saturated fatty acids, and cholesterol has a high priority in public health monitoring (LSRO, FASEB, 1989).

Carbohydrates

The per capita amount of carbohydrates in the food supply declined from the turn of the century until the mid-1960s. In the past 70 years there has been a significant decrease in the proportion of carbohydrates obtained from grain products and an increase in the proportion obtained from sugars and sweeteners; in particular, high-fructose corn syrup has replaced sucrose in many products since the 1960s. In 1909, the proportion of carbohydrates in the food supply was about two-thirds from complex carbohydrates and one-third from sugar. In 1985, sugars and sweeteners contributed 39.6 percent of the carbohydrates in the food supply, while grain products, fruits, and vegetables provided most of the remainder (35.8 percent, 6.6 percent, and 9.2 percent, respectively) (LSRO, FASEB, 1989).

Four-day data from the 1985–1986 CSFII showed that the carbohydrate intake for women aged 20 to 49 was 175 g/day, providing 46 percent of calories; and the intake for children aged 1 to 5 was 184 g/day, providing 52 percent of calories (LSRO, FASEB, 1989). The 1977–1978 NFCS found that carbohydrate intake averaged 47 percent of calories for children aged 1 to 8 and 46 percent of calories for females and 45 percent of calories for males aged 9 to 18. Based on 1-day estimates, the general trend during the past two decades seems to indicate an increase in the mean percentage of calories obtained from carbohydrates in most age groups (NRC, 1989).

Dietary Fiber

Data on the amount of fiber in the food supply are not available. Dietary fiber sources include whole grains, fruits, and vegetables. Oat bran, beans, and dried fruits provide soluble fiber, while wheat bran is a source of insoluble fiber.

Four-day estimated mean intakes of dietary fiber from the 1985–1986 CSFII were 11 g/day for women aged 20 to 49 and 10 g/day for children aged 1 to 5. Only 5 percent of the women surveyed had dietary fiber intakes of 20 g or more per day, as currently recommended by the National Cancer Institute (NCI). One analysis indicated that vegetables, grains, and fruits supplied 50 percent, 30 percent, and 12 percent, respectively, of the dietary fiber consumed by women. One-day intake data from the 1985–1986 CSFII indicate that, on average, the dietary fiber intake by men aged 19 to 50 was 17 g/day, a level higher than the dietary fiber intake by women (LSRO, FASEB, 1989).

Dietary fiber is considered a potential public health issue worthy of further study due to its possible role in reducing the risk of certain chronic diseases (LSRO, FASEB, 1989).

Protein

Since early in the twentieth century, the food supply has provided approximately 11 percent of calories as protein, or the equivalent of about 100 g of protein per person per day (NRC, 1989). Over the years the source of protein has changed from plant sources to increased levels from animal sources. During the period from 1909 to 1913, approximately 52 percent of protein came from animal sources; by 1982, the amount had increased to 68 percent as a result of the increased use of meat, poultry, fish, and dairy products, with a concomitant decrease in the use of eggs, flour, cereal products, and potatoes (NRC, 1989).

The amount of protein available per capita is considerably higher than the 1980 Recommended Dietary Allowances (RDA) for protein, which is 56 g/day for men over age 15 who weigh 70 kg and 44 g/day for women in the same age group who weigh 55 kg (LSRO, FASEB, 1989). According to the 1977–1978 NFCS, the average protein intake was 74.3 g/day for all respondents, with race, economic status, region, urbanization, and season having little influence on dietary protein levels (NRC, 1989). Protein contributed an average of 17 percent of total calories in the diets of males and females. In 1985, meat, poultry, and fish supplied 43.4 percent, dairy products supplied 20.6 percent, and grain products supplied 19 percent from the food supply (LSRO, FASEB, 1989).

Sodium and Potassium

Data on the amount of sodium in the food supply are not available. The daily per capita amount of potassium has been declining since 1909, to a level of 3,460 mg in 1985. Dietary sources of sodium include meat, dairy products, some vegetables, and sodium-containing compounds added to foods during processing, preparation, or at the table. The major sources of potassium in the food supply are vegetables; dairy products; meat, poultry, and fish; and fruits.

Four-day data from the 1985–1986 CSFII provide estimates of individual sodium intakes. The mean intake by women aged 20 to 49 was 2,372 mg/day (excluding salt added at the table), with many exceeding the upper limit of estimated safe and adequate intakes. Intakes were slightly higher in whites, those above the poverty level, and those with higher education levels. The mean sodium intake by children aged 1 to 5 was 2,036 mg/day. Estimates from NHANES II and 1985–1986 CSFII data (1-day) reported mean intakes in excess of 3,300 mg/day by males aged 12 to 49. Sodium intake is considered a public health issue due to its relationship to hypertension.

Four-day data from the 1985–1986 CSFII indicated that the mean potassium intake by women aged 20 to 49 was 2,073 mg/day, with at least 25 percent of women having intakes below the lower limit of the safe and adequate range. Intakes were higher by white women, those above the poverty level, and those with higher education levels. For children aged 1 to 5, mean intakes were almost all above the lower limit of safe and adequate intakes, and some intakes exceeded the upper limit. In 1980, only 4.5 percent of the adult U.S. population obtained potassium in the form of supplements, and only a few exceeded the upper limit of the safe and adequate level.

Vitamins

Vitamin A and Carotenes   From 1909 to 1985 there was an increase in the daily per capita amount of vitamin A available in the U.S. food supply, and since 1965 there has been an increase in carotenes. Both nutrients reached a peak in 1985, at 1,610 retinol equivalents (RE) for vitamin A and 660 RE for carotene. The increases in availability were primarily the result of the development of new varieties of deep yellow vegetables with higher carotene contents and the fortification of margarine and other dairy products. Vegetables have accounted for three-fourths of carotenes in the U.S. food supply, particularly dark green and yellow varieties. Vitamin A is also supplied by meat, poultry, and fish, as well as dairy products (LSRO, FASEB, 1989).

Individual dietary intake data from the 1985–1986 CSFII indicate that the mean intake of vitamin A by women is 832 RE, although considerable individual variation was observed. Data from HHANES suggest that poor young children may be at risk for low serum vitamin A levels (LSRO, FASEB, 1989).

A survey of dietary supplement use found that 25 percent of the U.S. adult population obtained vitamin A from supplementary sources (LSRO, FASEB, 1989).

Although the availability and intakes of vitamin A are generally adequate, it is considered a potential public health issue due to the low serum levels found in certain groups (LSRO, FASEB, 1989).

Thiamin   Key sources of thiamin in the food supply include grain products (42.3 percent); meat, poultry, and fish (25.7 percent); vegetables (10.9 percent); and dairy products (8 percent). About 2.2 mg of thiamin per capita per day is available in the U.S food supply, which is 40 percent higher than that in the pre-World War II era, when the level was 1.6 mg per capita per day. The introduction of enrichment of flour with thiamin is primarily responsible for the increase (LSRO, FASEB, 1989).

Women aged 20 to 49 in the 1985–1986 CSFII (4-day) had a mean intake level slightly above the 1980 RDA. Only 5 percent of women had intakes that were below 50 percent of the RDA. Mean thiamin intakes by children aged 1 to 5 were above the RDA among all races and were highest among black children. Data from the 1977–1978 NFCS and the 1985–1986 CSFII (1-day) indicate that mean intake levels increased 9.3 percent for children aged 1 to 5, 18 percent for men aged 20 to 49, and 10.8 percent for women aged 20 to 49 (LSRO, FASEB, 1989).

In 1980, supplements containing thiamin were ingested by 30 percent of the population, with the median intake being about five times the 1980 RDA (LSRO, FASEB, 1989).

Riboflavin Riboflavin is currently available in the food supply at about 2.3 to 2.4 mg per capita per day, which is about 30 percent higher than that prior to World War II, when the level was 1.8 mg per capita per day. The amount available has remained unchanged since World War II, when enrichment of flour with riboflavin was implemented (LSRO, FASEB, 1989). Primary sources of riboflavin in the food supply include dairy products (34.7 percent); grain products (24 percent); and meat, poultry, and fish (24.3 percent).

The mean intake of riboflavin by women aged 20 to 49 in the 1985–1986 CSFII (4-day) was 12.5 percent above the 1980 RDA, with only 5 percent having intakes below 50 percent of the 1980 RDA. Mean riboflavin intakes by children aged 1 to 5 were at least 60 percent above the 1980 RDA, with 95 percent of children having intakes of at least 0.9 mg/day. Comparison of intakes from the 1977–1978 NFCS and 1985–1986 CSFII shows that the mean intake levels of riboflavin increased by 4.3 percent for children aged 1 to 5, 8.1 percent for men aged 20 to 49, and 8.3 percent for women aged 20 to 49 (LSRO, FASEB, 1989).

In 1980, supplements with riboflavin were taken by 30 percent of the adult population, with the median intake being about four times the 1980 RDA (LSRO, FASEB, 1989).

Niacin The daily per capita amount of preformed niacin available in the food supply was 26 mg in 1985, which has increased since the 1940s, when enrichment of flour with niacin was instituted. Major sources of niacin in the food supply include meat, poultry, and fish (46 percent) and grain products (30 percent) (LSRO, FASEB, 1989).

Four-day data from the 1985–1986 CSFII reveal that mean intakes of preformed niacin in all age groups of women and in children aged 1 to 5 are well above the 1980 RDA. Tryptophan conversion to niacin is not included in these values but would undoubtedly contribute to even higher niacin intake levels. There does not seem to be any real difference in niacin intake by age, race, or degree of urbanization. Comparison of data on niacin intakes from 1971 to 1986 showed a slight increase over time (LSRO, FASEB, 1989).

Supplements containing niacin are used by 30 percent of the adult population, and the median intake of niacin from these products is 190 times the 1980 RDA (LSRO, FASEB, 1989).

Vitamin B_6 The daily per capita amount of vitamin B_6 available in the food supply has changed little since early in the twentieth century, but the food sources have changed. The contributions from meat, poultry, and fish have increased dramatically, whereas the amounts from potatoes and grains have decreased. In 1985, the daily per capita amount in the food supply was 2.1 mg; the major sources were meat, poultry, and fish (41.1 percent); vegetables (21.9 percent); dairy products (10.7 percent); and fruits (10.6 percent).

Intakes by children aged 1 to 5 exceeded the 1980 RDA, as determined in the 1985–1986 CSFII. The mean intake by women was well below the 1980 RDA (approximately half) and varied by age.

Thirty percent of the adult U.S. population consumed supplements containing vitamin B_6, at a median level of 1.4 times the 1980 RDA (LSRO, FASEB, 1989).

Due to the low intakes by a substantial number of individuals, vitamin B_6 is considered a potential public health issue (LSRO, FASEB, 1989).

Vitamin C   The daily per capita amount of vitamin C in the food supply has fluctuated since the turn of the century, but it has not changed consistently. In 1985, 115 mg of vitamin C per capita per day was available, an amount well in excess of the 1980 RDA. Major food sources of vitamin C have changed; contributions from citrus fruits have increased whereas those from potatoes and vegetables other than dark green and deep yellow types have decreased. In 1985, the food groups that contributed the major shares of vitamin C to the food supply were vegetables (47.9 percent) and fruits (42.7 percent), especially citrus fruits (27.7 percent).

Four-day data from the 1985–1986 CSFII revealed that mean intakes of dietary vitamin C in women aged 20 to 49 and children aged 1 to 5 were well above the 1980 RDA. A comparison of intakes of vitamin C during the period from 1971 to 1986 showed an increase, although results are not consistent over all surveys. Greater changes may be observed in the future with the introduction of higher levels of vitamin C fortification in a variety of foods and beverages (LSRO, FASEB, 1989).

In 1980, 35 percent of the adult U.S. population consumed vitamin C in supplements, and the median amount consumed was three times the 1980 RDA.

Vitamin C is considered to be a potential public health issue due to low intakes in groups with low socioeconomic status; however, recent vitamin C fortification may have affected intakes by this group (LSRO, FASEB, 1989).

Folate   The daily per capita amount of folate has not changed substantially since the early 1900s which was nearly 300 µg in 1985. The contributions from meat, poultry, and fish, and fruit have increased, whereas the contribution from grain products has decreased. In 1985, the major sources of folate in the food supply were from vegetables (24.8 percent), legumes, nuts, and soybeans (19.5 percent), grain products (12.7 percent), meat, poultry, and fish (12.6 percent), and fruits (12.4 percent) (LSRO, FASEB, 1989).

Mean dietary folate consumption from the 1985–1986 CSFII (4-day) was estimated to be below the 1980 RDA by over 95 percent of women aged 20 to 49 and over 50 percent of children aged 3 to 5. In contrast, 90 percent of children aged 1 to 2 had folate intakes that were above the 1980 RDA (LSRO, FASEB, 1989).

The serum and red blood cell folate levels measured in NHANES II are difficult to reconcile with the dietary data. The interpretive criteria for the blood levels are not certain, and the prevalence of low levels of serum and red blood cell folate are low (LSRO, FASEB, 1984). However, women aged 20 to 44 appear to be at greater risk of folate deficiency than are other population subgroups (LSRO, FASEB, 1989).

Supplemental folate was consumed by 20 percent of the adult U.S. population at a median level of two times the 1980 RDA (LSRO, FASEB, 1989).

Folate is considered to be a potential public health issue due to the lower than recommended intakes by some groups (LSRO, FASEB, 1989).

Minerals

Calcium The daily per capita amount of calcium in the food supply was greater than 900 mg in 1985, indicating that, overall, the food supply contains an adequate amount for most of the population. Dairy products are the primary source, providing 76.8 percent in 1985 (LSRO, FASEB, 1989).

Four-day data from the 1985–1986 CSFII indicate that the mean intakes by women aged 20 to 49 continue to be below the 1980 RDA, causing concern about osteoporosis. For children aged 1 to 5, the mean intake of calcium was 804 mg/day; the median intake was 769 mg/day, indicating that over half of the group had intakes below the 1980 RDA (LSRO, FASEB, 1989).

In a comparison of data from NHANES I and NHANES II with data from CSFII, some tentative conclusions can be drawn about trends in calcium intakes since 1971. For men aged 20 to 49, mean calcium intakes ranged from 750 to about 1,100 mg/day, with little change over time having been observed, suggesting that their calcium intakes are adequate. For women aged 20 to 49, mean calcium intakes have ranged from 530 to 690 mg/day, which is well below the 1980 RDA. For children aged 1 to 5, mean calcium intakes ranged from 750 to 920 mg/day. In general, calcium intakes seem to have remained fairly constant over the 15-year period (LSRO, FASEB, 1989).

Data on dietary supplement use indicate that 13.5 percent of the population and 34.9 percent of supplement users consumed calcium supplements. The median level of supplemental calcium was 16 percent of the 1980 RDA, indicating that calcium supplements are consumed at relatively low doses. Major promotion and use of calcium supplements and calcium-fortified foods as a means of preventing osteoporosis have occurred since the 1980 survey (LSRO, FASEB, 1989).

Calcium is considered to be a current public health issue due to the low calcium intakes by vulnerable groups, especially women. The influence of the recent calcium promotion may have an impact on the overall calcium status of vulnerable groups (LSRO, FASEB, 1989).

Iron   The amount of iron in the food supply increased during the 1940s due to the introduction of iron enrichment of flour. Recent increases have resulted in a level of 17 mg/day in 1985. The iron supplied by various food groups in 1985 included 41 percent from grain products, 23.8 percent from meat, poultry, and fish, and 12.6 percent from vegetables (LSRO, FASEB, 1989).

Estimates of mean iron intake from NHANES I and II, the 1977–1978 NFCS, and 1-day 1985–1986 CSFII data reveal remarkably close values, with a range of 9.2 to 10.8 mg/day by women of childbearing age. The mean intakes are less than 60 percent of the 1980 RDA for this group. Four-day 1985–1986 CSFII data show that over 95 percent of women aged 20 to 49 and over 90 percent of infants aged 1 to 2 have iron intakes below their age-specific 1980 RDAs. Iron intakes are below the 1980 RDA for 50 percent of children aged 3 to 5.

Despite the low levels of iron intake with respect to the 1980 RDA, the prevalence of iron deficiency in the population is relatively low. Data from NHANES II and HHANES indicate that the prevalence of iron deficiency ranges from 2.4 to 14 percent in women of childbearing age. There are several explanations for the discrepancies with dietary intake data. The 1980 RDA for iron may be overly generous and, therefore, not attainable by most women who eat otherwise nutritionally adequate diets. Also, iron intake is not directly related to iron status, since absorption of iron increases substantially when body iron stores are low (LSRO, FASEB, 1989).

Supplemental iron (taken alone or in a multinutrient form) was consumed by about 22 percent of the U.S. population in 1980. Supplemental iron was consumed by 56 percent of all supplement users, and the median level consumed was 1.2 times the 1980 RDA (LSRO, FASEB, 1989).

Iron is considered to be a current public health issue, due to the extent of low intakes by vulnerable groups such as women of childbearing age (LSRO, FASEB, 1989).

Zinc   The per capita amount of zinc in the food supply has remained essentially unchanged at about 12 mg/day since 1909, despite fluctuations over the years (NRC, 1989). In 1985, primary sources included meats, poultry, and fish (48.7 percent); dairy products (19 percent); and grain products (12.6 percent). A large decline has occurred in the percentage of zinc obtained from grain products (LSRO, FASEB, 1989).

Four-day data from the 1985–1986 CSFII indicate that the mean dietary intake of zinc by women aged 20 to 49 is about half the 1980 RDA, with a large percentage of intakes falling well below that level. Zinc intakes were lower for blacks, those below the poverty level, and those with lower education levels. Mean intakes by men were higher and closer to the 1980 RDA. For children aged 1 to 5, mean intakes were close to the 1980 RDA (LSRO, FASEB, 1989).

An estimated 13.5 percent of the adult population used supplements containing zinc in 1980, and the median intake by users was 50 percent of the 1980 RDA (LSRO, FASEB, 1989).

Zinc is considered a potential public health issue due to the low dietary intakes by some groups, particularly women (LSRO, FASEB, 1989).

Conclusions from Survey Data

The foregoing discussion of the per capita availability of food and nutrients, levels of dietary intake, and prevalence of impaired nutritional status leads to several conclusions. The supply of food is abundant and the nutrient levels in the food supply are generally adequate. The principal nutrition-related health problems experienced by Americans are related to overconsumption of food energy, fat, saturated fatty acids, cholesterol, and sodium. Despite the abundant food supply, some subgroups in the population may not have sufficient food for a variety of reasons. There is evidence of inadequate individual dietary intake of specific nutrients or impaired nutritional status in some subgroups of the population. Iron deficiency continues to be the most common single nutrient deficiency observed among women of childbearing age and young children. Low calcium intakes by females from childhood through early adulthood may contribute to less than optimal bone mass that can predispose them to osteoporosis later in life. The survey evidence is less conclusive for vitamin A, vitamin C, folate, zinc, and vitamin B_6 than it is for iron or calcium. Dietary surveys indicate that intakes are low with respect to recommended nutrient levels in specific subgroups of the population. However, there is limited information from these surveys or other studies to suggest that health problems exist in the general population that would justify nutrition labeling of all these micronutrients.

Factors Influencing Future Dietary Changes

Several major changes in Americans' life-styles have had major impacts on eating habits. Perhaps the most significant change is in the number of meals eaten away from home. Approximately one-third of all food is now eaten away from home as packed lunches (9 percent), meals at restaurants (20 percent) and limited-menu restaurants (13 percent), and meals at schools (16 percent) and workplaces (20 percent). Another 16 percent of meals are eaten at someone else's home. In general, the nutrient densities of meals eaten away from home are somewhat less than those of typical meals eaten at home (NRC, 1989).

Americans snack more; it has been estimated that as many as 20 percent of calories now come from snacking. The number of Americans who snack increased from 60 percent in 1977 to 80 percent in 1985. Fewer young people eat breakfast, more people are dieting, and more vitamin and mineral supplements are being consumed. In 1977, only 35 percent of Americans took food supplements; that figure grew to between 45 and 60 percent among all age groups by 1985 (LSRO, FASEB, 1989; NRC, 1989).

Other factors affecting dietary habits include many of those mentioned above: income (and related factors such as employment and household size), availability of food assistance programs, education, and number of meals eaten at home. In addition, race, ethnicity, geographic origin, and health status also help to determine eating habits.

It can be assumed that even more changes in food consumption patterns will occur in the near future, reflecting changes in the U.S. population as well as the food supply. As the demographics of U.S. society shift to an older, but more ethnically heterogeneous composition, shifts in demand for different types of foods are expected. A higher proportion of the population with higher levels of education may portend more concern with health and nutrition. As households become smaller and as an even greater proportion of families are headed by single parents or two working parents, there may be an even greater demand for easy-to-prepare meals. Biotechnology has enormous potential to improve the composition of the U.S. food supply. Considering the aggregate effects of these and other unforeseen changes, it is anticipated that Americans' diets will continue to experience dynamic changes.

FOOD MARKETING IN THE UNITED STATES

The introductory language of the U.S. Department of Commerce's *1990 U.S. Industrial Outlook* report illustrates the changing nature of today's food industry. The section on food, beverages, and tobacco, "Food Chain in Transition," opens with the following paragraph:

> Growing numbers of consumers are demanding foods with convenience, quality, variety and healthful attributes. Today, 70 percent of U.S. households own microwave ovens; some industry researchers estimate 15 minutes is the maximum most Americans are willing to spend preparing an ordinary meal. Demographics are changing. Only 28 percent of American families now have one spouse at home and one at work. The remainder have either two wage earners or a single parent. Dual-income families often purchase more convenience type products. Travel, ethnic restaurants, and television have encouraged many consumers to experiment with new varieties of food. Hence, many retailers now offer numerous types of

exotic foods. Concerned with health, many consumers want high fiber products genuinely free of fat and cholesterol (DOC, 1990, p. 34-1).

It is clear that the U.S. food industry is faced with a rapidly changing marketplace. As the industry has searched for profitable marketing niches in this changing environment, the number of new products introduced annually has exploded. Until 1981, an average of 2,500 grocery products were introduced each year. By 1990, the number has grown steadily to an annual average of 12,000 items (Friedman, 1990). Many of these products are targeted directly at a more health-conscious public and, as a result, feature health and nutrition claims on the label. In addition, the decade of the 1980s produced a variety of structural changes that complicate labeling issues. This section explores the relevant structural issues pertaining to major sectors of the food processing and distribution systems, including the growing integration of the food system into the world community of trade and issues that have an impact on marketing, promotion, and labeling decisions.

World Trade

No consideration of food labeling issues should ignore the growing integration of the U.S. food distribution system with trade throughout the world. The United States is the world's largest exporter of agricultural products, generating an agricultural trade surplus every year since 1959. However, U.S. competitiveness declined during the 1980s as the European Community shifted from being the world's largest importer of grains to one of the largest exporters.

In 1988, the United States exported $35 billion of agricultural products, while agricultural product imports hit a record $21 billion. Imports can be classified into two general categories: (1) noncompetitive imports of products that cannot be produced at all, or at least not profitably, in the United States; and (2) competitive imports that compete directly with U.S. products. During the 1980s, competitive imports doubled, with meats becoming the largest single U.S. food product import, surpassing coffee in 1988 for the first time in 16 years (USDA, 1989b). While most agricultural trade is still in commodities rather than processed food products, the share of processed products is growing in the import market. It is also clear that more and more imports compete directly with products that are also produced in the United States. The volume of international trade is an important issue not only for U.S. consumers but for the balance of U.S. trade as well. Labeling changes must be sensitive to their international trade implications.

Food Processing

The food processing sector is huge and incredibly diverse. The industry is divided into 48 separate SIC (standard industry classification) codes. During

1989, food product shipments totaled over $345 billion (DOC, 1990). A full survey of this sector is beyond the scope of this report. However, a few general observations that bear on label revisions can be made.

First, the growing internationalization of the food industry is evident in the ownership of food processing companies. From a balance of U.S. investment abroad of $8.2 billion versus foreign investment in the United States of $8.3 billion in 1984, there has been a shift over the past 5 years toward more foreign ownership in the United States. In 1988, U.S. investment in food product industries overseas totaled $13 billion versus $16.4 billion of direct foreign investment in the United States. The Netherlands accounted for the largest share of direct foreign investment, followed by the United Kingdom. The largest non-European Community investor was Canada, followed by Japan (DOC, 1990).

Second, the pace of leveraged buyouts and takeover activities during the 1980s has had a direct impact on the food processing industry. For a variety of reasons, the food processing industry was a major target of hostile takeovers during the decade. Increased corporate debt to fund takeovers or to defend against a hostile raid diverted cash flows to cover interest payments. As a result, food processors have much less capital investment flexibility for product research and development in the 1990s than they did in the 1980s. Food processing or labeling changes will take longer to implement during the 1990s.

Third, as consumers have become more interested in health and nutrition, more funding has been allocated toward the promotion of health-oriented products. It is estimated, for example, that one-third of the $3.6 billion spent on food advertising in 1988 contained some type of health or nutrition message (DOC, 1990). This trend is a vivid demonstration of the fact that, in the 1990s, nutrition "sells."

Food Retailing

U.S. shoppers spent $410 billion on food in 1988, $155 billion of it on food consumed away from home and $255 billion of it on food consumed at home (USDA, 1989b). This amount represents 11.8 percent of disposable personal income after taxes in 1988 versus 15.3 percent in 1965.

The growth of sales in limited-menu (fast-food) restaurants represents the most significant shift in recent times in expenditures for food eaten away from home. In 1987, one-third of all food eaten away from home was purchased in limited-menu restaurants versus only 10 percent in 1963. Restaurants, lunchrooms, and cafeterias represented almost half of this market in 1963 but declined to 40 percent in 1987 (USDA, 1989b). Since foods sold in restaurants and noncommercial settings are an increasing part of American diets, this sector is very important in any program aimed at dietary improvement.

There was a significant shift in sales at supermarkets for food consumed at home in the 1980s. Supermarket sales grew from about 45 percent of the market for food consumed at home in 1963 to just over 73 percent in 1989. Sales at limited-line grocery stores declined from 30 percent in 1963 to just under 19 percent in 1989. Over this same period, convenience store sales grew from almost zero to just under 8 percent (Sansolo, 1990). Not all large supermarkets are operated by large businesses. There are approximately 147,000 grocery stores in the United States. Chains operate 17,300 units, representing 50.1 percent of total food sales; independent businesspeople operate 72,700 units, representing 42.2 percent of total food sales; and convenience stores number 57,000, representing 7.7 percent of total food sales. In-store information programs would, therefore, have an impact on a large number of small businesses.

In addition, the major costs associated with food products incurred after they leave the farm differ between food consumed at home and that consumed away from home. The differences are greatest for processing (31 percent compared with 16 percent) and retailing (23 percent compared with 60 percent) (USDA, 1989a). Therefore, the issue of cost is a consideration in food labeling reform. Since processing and retailing costs already make up the majority of the retail cost of food, increases in costs related to food label changes for either or both of these sectors should be expected to have an impact on the prices consumers pay for foods. Reforms should be evaluated to ensure that consumers perceive the benefits of increased label information as a trade-off for any price increases that they may experience for individual foods. A more complete discussion of the costs of food labeling reform appears in Chapter 7.

General Marketing Considerations

The limited scope of this section permits only a cursory examination of food marketing and labeling considerations. As was made clear during the Committee's marketing workshop, because nutrition concerns help to sell products to today's consumers, the health and nutrition groups within food manufacturer organizations are becoming an increasingly integral part of product development and marketing teams. Prior to this shift, almost all decisions in this area were subordinated to the brand management team. As a result, health, nutrition, and labeling considerations are becoming an important part of the marketing strategy for a growing number of food products.

This is an encouraging development in one very important respect. The marketing motivation provides a powerful incentive to develop new nutritious and healthful products. Therefore, even though this motivation may lead to aggressive, and at times even overzealous, claims on the label and in advertising, the incentive to satisfy consumer demand for more healthful products is an important asset if it is channeled in the proper direction.

It was also clear during the Committee's marketing workshop that consumer feedback is a powerful motivating tool for including nutrition labeling and creating more healthful products. Feedback takes many forms, including consumer purchase data, focus group responses, taste panels, complaints, and requests for additional product information through the mail or the use of toll-free telephone numbers. In short, consumer choice forms the basis for a powerful feedback mechanism that helps food product manufacturers to know whether they are in tune with today's consumers and, through trial and error, shapes the nature of product development. The cornerstone of consumer feedback is informed consumer choice. Improved label information will not only help consumers make more appropriate immediate decisions, but it also improves the direction and quality of future product development decisions.

The views within the industry as to how much importance to place on health and nutrition issues differ, depending on the nature of the product. There are many products that the industry views as indulgence or reward foods for which they feel the consumer has little or no expectation that they will make a nutritional contribution to their diets. There are other products that the industry feels make such a minimal nutrition contribution that the consumer has little interest in detailed information (spices or condiments, for example).

The views of different elements of the industry also differ with regard to where the information is placed on the label. The principal display panel is viewed as a commercial vehicle, with its primary purposes being sales promotion and competition with rivals. Manufacturers guard this product "real estate" with a fervor not applied to other areas on the package. Design, color, visual impact, balance of presentation, and overall image of the product are the driving forces for the principal display panel. Detail and elaboration are generally left to the back or side panels. This possessive attitude helps to explain why label regulations that have an impact on the principal display panel are much more likely to meet with strenuous opposition than are any other kinds of labeling proposals.

The product design, development, and marketing process is complicated, and thus, it is useful to place these aspects in perspective. The dominant view within the industry is that all positive attributes of a product, no matter how carefully they are developed, are lost if the product will not sell. For the product to sell, it must taste good and be attractively packaged, priced right, and convenient for the consumer to use in the way it was intended. The industry will generally support label changes that create a more informed consumer choice process. It will, however, strongly resist changes viewed as being so costly as to disturb the consumer perception of product value, so directive in tone that they erode the ability of the consumer to think in terms of a total dietary context (i.e., creating a good food/bad food image for single products), or run the risk of disclosing proprietary formulations.

CONSUMER UNDERSTANDING OF NUTRITION AND USE OF FOOD LABELS

The U.S. food supply is diverse and abundant. Consequently, consumers can choose from over 20,000 items in most supermarkets. As Timmer and Nesheim point out, "To the consumer who has the *motivation, knowledge,* and *financial means,* the American food system offers a diet as healthy, safe, and appetizing as any in history" (1979, p. 155).

Factors Influencing Food Consumption Behavior

Despite comprehensive study, no single factor or set of factors has yet been found to adequately describe how dietary patterns are developed, maintained, and changed (Hochbaum, 1981). Factors that influence consumers' food choices are many and varied, including internal as well as external factors (Sims, 1981). External influences include social, cultural, and economic factors. Dramatic examples of the influence of culture, geography, and food availability on eating habits and chronic disease prevalence can be cited. Internal factors include individual physiological and psychological factors, as well as acquired preferences and knowledge about foods. In addition, interpersonal or social factors are also important; family and group situations dominate many food acquisition, preparation, and consumption situations (Glanz and Mullis, 1988).

Assuming that foods are available and can be purchased at a reasonable cost, familiarity is one factor that perhaps exercises influence over all others. Sociocultural forces dominate the associations made with foods that have been familiar and consumed since childhood. Psychological factors also influence food choices; many individuals go out of their way to find comfort foods (such as chocolate or ice cream) when they are bored or lonely.

Motivations, particularly those related to health, play a strong role in influencing food choice decisions. Only the most foolhardy do not try to comply with advice from a physician or other health professional that a change in diet must be undertaken in order to ameliorate symptoms or cure a medical condition. Others have been persuaded that if they make certain dietary changes now, these changes will help to promote health and prevent disease in the future.

Education and income are moderating factors that influence how amenable certain individuals are to making dietary changes. Those with more education are more knowledgeable about nutrition, and many individuals make food choices consistent with this knowledge. In addition, those with higher incomes can be expected to have more flexibility when it comes to choosing from among the foods available for purchase.

The latest survey of consumer attitudes and shopping behavior conducted by the Food Marketing Institute (FMI, 1990) asked respondents to rate the importance of various factors in food selection. Over 70 percent of the consumers interviewed identified taste, nutrition, and product safety (in that order) as "very important" factors when they purchase food. Those on medically restricted diets were significantly more likely to rate nutrition considerations as highly important, as were women and those over age 50. Nutrition is, therefore, perceived as being extremely important by consumers, but only as one part of a complex decisionmaking process, when purchasing food (FMI, 1990). Price was deemed very important by two-thirds of the consumers in the 1990 FMI survey. FMI believes that economics has remained important to consumers over the past 10 years but that the dominant themes have now shifted to nutrition, product safety, and convenience.

Consumers' Knowledge of Nutrition

Knowledge of food and nutrition is undoubtedly one factor that influences food choices and dietary behavior. Fanelli and Abernathy (1986) reported that for older adults, the reading of food labels was significantly related to their level of nutrition knowledge.

It had long been thought that if nutrition knowledge were increased, improvements in food choices and eating habits would follow. Research in this area has shown this to be a misleading, if not false, assumption (Hochbaum, 1981). Surveys, however, continue to assess the nutrition knowledge of target groups on the assumption that at least minimal understanding of basic nutrition must be present for an individual to make decisions that result in nutritionally sound food choices.

Numerous surveys have confirmed that Americans are increasingly aware of and display interest in nutrition (Sloan, 1987). Five of the six concerns listed by more than 10 percent of the sample in the FMI survey were dietary components that both the Surgeon General's (1988) and NRC (1989) reports recommended should be consumed at low levels or reduced in the diet. The sixth concern was vitamins and minerals, which moved from number 2 in rank in 1983 to number 6 in 1990 (FMI, 1990).

Despite such promising claims about increased consumer nutrition knowledge, it cannot be assumed that increased awareness leads to enhanced nutrition knowledge, which in turn leads to improved dietary behavior. The results of the 1988 FDA Health and Diet Survey are an example of this point (Levy and Stephenson, 1990). Despite the public's increased awareness about dietary fats and cholesterol as risk factors for heart disease in recent years, the results of the 1988 Survey showed no increase in food and nutrition knowledge related to dietary fats and cholesterol between 1983 and 1988. Only 3 of 11 questions asked in the 1988 Survey were answered correctly by more than 50 percent of the respondents.

However, consumer concerns about food components do seem to translate directly into their reported food choices. A number of FDA surveys have shown that Americans are increasingly aware of health risks from sodium, fats, and cholesterol and that they report eating less salt, red meat, butter, whole milk, and eggs as a result (Heimbach, 1985, 1986). Putnam and Weimer (1981) reported that roughly two-thirds of surveyed households claimed to have made at least one change in food consumption, almost always to avoid a negative nutrient. Of the 10 most frequently mentioned reasons for changes in eating habits, nine were related to reducing the intake of negative food components.

Although awareness of the relationship between diet and risk of disease seems to be at an all-time high, actual dietary behavior has not shifted dramatically. Despite consumer reports of awareness, nutrition is only one factor, and usually not the most important one, that influences food choice. The 1988 Prevention Index Survey, which is conducted annually by Harris & Associates, concluded: "Almost no change has taken place in the last five years in the structure of the American diet as it relates to preventing illness" (CNI, 1988, p. 1). Likewise, after examining dietary changes of women between 1977 and 1985, the CSFII conducted by USDA reported that although consumption of red meat had declined substantially, the overall fat intake by these groups had not declined because women had correspondingly increased their intake of salad dressings, table spreads, and rich desserts (Harris and Welsh, 1989).

Sources of Nutrition Information

As consumers have developed a more intense interest in diet and disease, they clamor for more information in an easier-to-understand form. Nutrition advice seems to dominate the airwaves and the printed page. Not only has the amount of information about diet and disease proliferated, but the sources and settings in which such information is offered have increased as well. Nutrition education programs are found in schools, community groups, fitness centers, and the workplace, as well as in various community sites such as supermarkets, restaurants, shopping malls, museums, and libraries (ADA, 1990).

Surveys have confirmed that doctors are still regarded by consumers as the best source of nutrition information, although media sources are assuming increasing importance (Rahn, 1980; Woolcott, 1983). Consumers who responded to a recent Gallup survey overwhelmingly cited the media as the source they used to get information about food and nutrition: television, magazines, and newspapers were named as the chief sources of nutrition information by 68 percent of the respondents (IFIC/ADA, 1990). Consumers who participated in focus-group discussions conducted by the Institute of Food Technologists (IFT) also cited mass media, including print (newspaper and magazine articles, books), television, and radio, as the major sources of information about foods and nutrition, although a number of the participants expressed concern about the reliability of the information they received (Snider et al., 1990).

A recent survey on the reading habits of Americans (Robinson, 1990) has shown that, since 1965, the amount of time people spend reading has fallen by more than 30 percent, primarily as a result of a decline in newspaper reading. Today, television is the dominant mode of receiving information for most consumers. The survey of reading habits confirmed that people who are older and well educated spend the most time reading.

These findings have particular relevance for a study of nutrition labels. Venkatesan and fellow researchers (1977, 1986) concluded that the medium used for the presentation of nutrition information (television, advertisements, or labels) influenced the formats that consumers perceived to be the most useful. Television viewers appeared to find a variety of presentation formats equally useful, whereas readers of print media preferred detailed information as opposed to graphic or summary presentations.

Thus, in order to provide nutrition information to a communication-saturated, time-starved public, the message must be simple, short, and practical (Shepherd, 1990). The issue then becomes how to best present the nutrition information on food labels to measure up against these criteria.

Impact of Nutrition Information on Food Purchase Decisions

Format of Information

Given the level of interest in nutrition expressed by consumers but the high level of confusion over the interpretation of some of the currently available information, it is useful to examine whether point-of-purchase information makes a difference in food choices when presented in a format relevant to current dietary recommendations. Although the number of research reports is limited, several studies have demonstrated that consumers can be motivated to buy foods more consistent with current dietary recommendations by providing point-of-purchase information (Glascoff et al., 1986; Hixson et al., 1988; Light et al., 1989; Mullis et al., 1987).

In a survey conducted for the National Food Processors Association (NFPA) (ORC, 1990), consumers were asked whether ingredient and nutrition information influenced their actual purchase decisions. Fifty-one percent stated that it influenced their purchases "a great deal," while another 32 percent said their purchases were influenced "somewhat." By category, nutrition information had the most influence on the purchase of cereal (35 percent), canned products (26 percent), and prepared foods (13 percent). Nutrition information was reported to have the least influence on the purchase of snack foods (15 percent), produce (12 percent), and dairy products (9 percent) (ORC, 1990).

One study that supported the contention that supermarket operators are willing to undertake informational programs at their own expense because they believe that consumers find them useful was a cooperative effort between Giant Food, Inc., of Washington, D.C., and FDA (Levy et al., 1985). This program, called Special Diet Alert (SDA), consisted of shelf tags next to the product price information that identified products that were low in or had reduced levels of sodium, calories, fat, or cholesterol, all of which were accompanied by special media campaigns and other printed material. Consumer purchases of SDA and non-SDA products were tracked through computer-assisted checkout (scanner) data in two market areas. Results over a 2-year period showed that sales of SDA-identified products increased, on the average, 4 to 8 percent more in the Washington test market than they did in the Baltimore (control) market. Undoubtedly, some segments of the population (e.g., those with medical conditions) are very interested in this type of information, whereas others are not.

Glanz and Mullis (1988) reviewed more than 20 reports of nutrition information programs in supermarkets, restaurants, and cafeterias and on vending machines, and concluded that point-of-purchase information programs in supermarkets were more successful in improving nutrition knowledge and attitudes than they were in changing consumer purchasing behaviors. In studies that documented significant changes toward the purchase of more nutritious foods, an emphasis on brand name choices appears to have been influential. Glanz et al. (1989) believe that the conclusions of the review neither support nor discredit the value of programs for improving diets; rather, they believe that the findings reflect weaknesses in the design of some interventions as well as identify shortcomings in research designs and measures. Thus, while the idea of providing nutrition information at the point of purchase in grocery stores and restaurants is appealing and well liked by consumers, research to date has not conclusively demonstrated that such programs are directly responsible for changing consumer behavior in making more healthful food choices.

Information Processing and Behavioral Change

Consumers learn based on the way in which they process the information they receive. McGuire (1969) pointed out that whether acquisition of a certain piece of information leads to some desired behavior depends, in part, on whether the information has been appropriately processed by the receiver. Thus, an educational program may deliver a nutrition message to individuals or groups, but whether it produces the desired effect depends on how the recipient of that information processes or internalizes it to make decisions or guide behavior.

A change in food choices and purchases may be the ultimate effect of information programs such as food labeling, but there must be prior cognitive changes (Mazis and Staelin, 1982). Thus, in order to judge the effectiveness of nutrition labels on food products, more reliance must be placed on an analysis of how such information is processed by individuals rather than on surveys based on consumer reports of how frequently they read the food label or how well they understand the label content (Olson and Sims, 1980) (Figure 4-1). An information processing perspective allows an examination of the conditions under which information and persuasive messages may lead to behavioral changes.

Social scientists believe that individuals pass through a series of steps in acquiring, processing, and using information that eventually leads to the adoption of new behavior (McGuire, 1976), a conceptualization of sequential impact that has been referred to as a "hierarchy of effects" (Russo et al., 1986). For the purposes of this discussion, the framework suggested by Mazis and Staelin (1982, p. 3) is used:

Exposure: data come into contact with one or more of the consumer's five senses.
Attention: the consumer selects certain stimuli out of the environment for further processing.
Comprehension: the consumer understands and assigns meaning to the message conveyed.
Retention and Retrieval: information is stored in memory for later use when a decision is made.
Decisionmaking: the consumer sorts out and synthesizes information stored in memory or available at the point of sale.

This framework is useful in discussing how nutrition information on food labels can ultimately affect consumer choices. Each factor in the framework and the effects it may exert in terms of consumer use of nutrition labels are discussed below.

Exposure   Consumers must come into contact with the information on the label before it can have any effect on their food choice decisions. Mazis and Staelin (1982) identified several roadblocks that can prevent consumers from ever being exposed to nutrition information: destruction or removal of the information, information unavailability, inappropriate timing of the message, or targeting problems. Therefore, nutrition information on the food label must be appropriate to consumer needs. For those who have been advised to follow a medically prescribed diet or who have hypersensitivities to certain food components, specific information identifying particular food components and ingredients must be placed on the label. Likewise, for those who wish to compare the nutrients in foods among various product categories, the information must be presented in a readily identifiable format.

The issue of coverage of food products with nutrition labeling also relates to the notion of exposure. If only about half of packaged foods and far fewer fresh products carry nutrition information in the grocery store, and few restaurants or other sites offer nutrition information, nutrition labeling on only a limited number of products cannot be expected to have much of an impact on food choices.

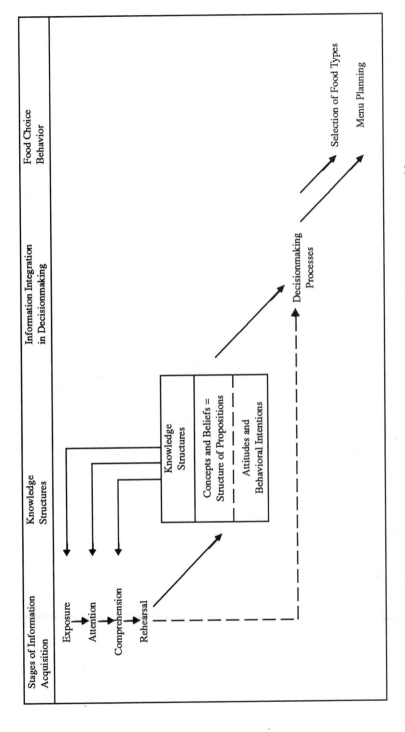

FIGURE 4-1 A model of information processing stages showing the central importance of knowledge structure stored in memory.
SOURCE: Olson, J., and L.S. Sims. 1980. Assessing nutrition knowledge from an information processing perspective. J. Nutr. Ed. 12(3):157–161.

Frequency and Prevalence of Label Reading   When queried, consumers indicate that nutrition knowledge and the availability of nutrition information on the label are important. Several studies have confirmed that most consumers are aware of and want nutrition information (Heimbach and Stokes, 1979), and some studies suggest that consumers would be willing to pay extra for it (Daly, 1976; Lenahan et al., 1972).

The survey recently conducted for NFPA, *Food Labeling and Nutrition: What Americans Want*, revealed that,

> **Most shoppers read food labels.**   About eight in ten consumers report that they usually read product labels for general information, nutrition information or the list of ingredients the first time they purchase a specific product. Four in ten shoppers always read this information on their first purchase. On subsequent purchases, only one in five always reads labels, while about six in ten consumers say that they read the labels at least sometimes for this information. Women, older shoppers, and those with more formal education are among the most frequent label readers, as are consumers who are on restricted diets (ORC, 1990, p. iii).

Approximately one-third of the consumers in the FMI survey responded that they read labels for nutrition information "pretty much every time" when they buy packaged foods, with another 45 percent reading them "sometimes." The proportion of consumers who read labels for ingredient information was almost identical to the proportion who read them for nutrition information. Those on medically restricted diets were twice as likely to read labels for ingredients and nutrition information (FMI, 1990).

Consumers are significantly more likely to read labels the first time they purchase a product than they are on subsequent purchases. Ingredient information is read by 53 percent of first-time consumers, and nutrition information is read by 49 percent of consumers the first time they purchase a product, in contrast to 36 percent for ingredients and 36 percent for nutrition information by repeat purchasers. Only about 5 percent of consumers say they never read labels for nutrition or ingredient information, which is true for first-time as well as repeat purchasers of a product (FMI, 1990). One-half of those consumers who responded to the FMI survey said they felt that the current labels provided "no more than some" of the desired information. Those on medically restricted diets were the most likely to judge nutrition labels as being inadequate.

The desired changes in the label by those who need additional nutrition information were probed in the 1989 FMI survey. These changes included the need to make the label easier to understand (25 percent) and for information about calories (24 percent), salt/sodium (21 percent), fat/saturated fat (18 percent), and chemicals, colorings, and dyes (10 percent) (FMI, 1989).

Attention   Information is of little use unless consumers consciously decide to pay attention to it. Because consumers are exposed to so much information simultaneously, they have neither the time nor the inclination to pay attention to all of it. It is at the attention stage that consumers sort out and actively examine stimuli (e.g., a warning or a nutrient claim) for the purpose of further processing the information, while they ignore or filter out other messages.

Attention is affected by internal as well as external factors. Consumers pay attention to the information that they feel is consistent and pertinent to their own personal needs, values, and goals (internal factors) and tend to be attracted to messages that are distinctive, have sufficient intensity, and are not subject to distraction from competing messages (external factors). Shepherd et al. (1989) examined the content and graphic design features of nutrition labels (i.e., external factors) that consumers considered to be the most appealing and useful; the features that consistently drew the most favorable reactions were bright, "food-like" colors and organizational cues (such as indexing and clustering of related information).

Motivation, an important internal factor, also plays an important role in determining how receptive the target audience is to new information. For example, consumers who are attracted by a new claim on the principal display panel of the food label may be curious enough to check out the actual information on the back of the label. This curiosity may not actually lead to the purchase of that food item, a behavioral indicator of label reading. However, consumers who have been advised by a physician to limit the amount of a certain food component (e.g., calories, sodium, fat, sugar, or cholesterol) may closely inspect the nutrition information that is provided on a label in order to choose the most desirable product. For example, at least one high-fiber breakfast cereal benefited from unprecedented shifts in market share because consumers were influenced by an advertising campaign that indicated the possible benefits of consuming a high-fiber, low-fat diet for preventing some types of cancer (Levy and Stokes, 1987).

Consumers pay attention to information that is presented in a style that they prefer. Although some studies have suggested that consumers prefer a graphic presentation of numeric information, other research points to consumer preferences for absolute numbers and percentages listed on the label (Geiger et al., 1990; Sims and Shepherd, 1985). The study by Geiger et al. attributes these results to a manifestation of the respondents' preference for more information. This conclusion confirmed the results of a study by Scammon (1978) in which consumers felt more satisfied and less confused with their purchase decisions when more information was presented.

Consumer preference for more detailed information on food labels was substantiated by the findings from the recent NFPA survey which asked consumers to rank six pairs of label formats according to their usefulness in making food purchase decisions (ORC, 1990). Consumers reported that they wanted more information to be included on product labels, particularly information on key nutrients and daily dietary recommendations. They also expressed an interest in acquiring more detailed product information, such as the breakdown of fat and carbohydrate contents compared with current dietary recommendations, and they wanted complete nutrition information, including data on micronutrients. Consumers preferred a label that provided nutrition information on key ingredients and nutrients (even if they were not present in that product) to a label that provided nutrition information only for those nutrients contained in the product. Consumers preferred having quantities presented in grams and milligrams over grams alone, and they also wanted quantities expressed numerically, to the point of specificity that included decimals. Consumers expressed some interest in having sugars grouped on the ingredient label for better identification.

Although presentation in a numeric format may require more information processing than graphic formats would, Bettman (1979) concluded that as long as consumers have control over the information input rate and can process the data at a comfortable pace (as when they are reading a nutrition label), presentation of larger amounts of data is unlikely to result in confusion during the decisionmaking process. After testing printed label format alternatives, Hammonds (1978) found that consumers preferred numeric data, which allowed them to make choices for themselves, over graphic representations, which consumers perceived as "leading the label reader toward a particular choice." Likewise, Muller (1985) concluded that consumers preferred numeric ratings for individual nutrients in order to determine for themselves which brands were more nutritious.

The work of McCullough and Best (1980) confirmed that the appropriate information load may be determined individually. They used the marketing research technique of conjoint analysis to measure consumer perceptions of the usefulness of various nutrition label configurations, which were portrayed as five different information type levels and three different information load levels. The results identified three groups of label readers: (1) predominantly blue-collar workers, who preferred less information and retaining the current nutrition labeling format; (2) white-collar workers, who strongly preferred increased amounts of information; and (3) another group of white-collar workers, who preferred more information in more complex forms. The investigators concluded that it is impossible to develop a single suitable label format, because changes made in label information for one group appeared to be disadvantageous for another group.

Comprehension   Studies that have examined consumer reactions to and use of nutrition information on food labels reveal a startling dichotomy. Although consumer interest in nutrition information appears to be high at present, a less positive conclusion can be drawn about the actual level of consumer comprehension of nutrition information. Some surveys report that consumers say they understand food labels, but other studies suggest that consumers often do not actually comprehend the data on current nutrition labels and, therefore, do not make optimal use of this information in their food purchase decisionmaking (DHEW/USDA/FTC, 1979; Heimbach, 1982; Jacoby et al., 1977).

Conflicting results appear from studies that have been conducted to assess consumer comprehension of food label information. The survey conducted for NFPA presented a rather optimistic view:

> **The vast majority of shoppers understand food label information.** Reported lack of attention given to labels is more a result of low interest than confusion or lack of understanding. Consistent with previous research, only about one in ten shoppers claims to have a serious lack of understanding about ingredient and nutrition information. Use of chemical and technical terms causes the most confusion (ORC, 1990, p. iv).

A less positive conclusion about the level of consumer comprehension of food label information emerges from results of other studies that have examined this issue. In the 1979 Food Labeling Background Papers, the following statement on consumer acceptability of food label information appears:

> In the Consumer Food Labeling Survey, 23 percent of the 64 percent of those consumers who use the nutrition label responded that at least some aspects of the label are confusing. Terminology was stated to be confusing by 79 percent of the people, the use of the metric system by 27 percent, "big words" by 16 percent, and U.S. RDAs and the use of percentages by 15 percent; the fact that they do not know what to do with the information was stated by 8 percent. In the food labeling hearings and written comments, 189 commenters stated that nutrition labels are confusing, with the single most often cited source of confusion being U.S. RDAs (90). Sixty comments did not specify the confusing aspects of the label (DHEW/USDA/FTC, 1979, p. 41).

Daly (1976) found that even though consumers expressed positive attitudes about the importance of nutrition labeling, comprehension of the terms used on the label was low. After summarizing the data from six studies, Jacoby et al. (1977) suggested that although a high percentage of consumers indicated that they were aware of and reported that they used the nutrition information provided on food labels, only a small percentage were able to define nutrition terms and accurately assess their total dietary intakes. Those investigators concluded that many consumers simply do not comprehend nutrition information as currently provided on package labels (Jacoby et al., 1981).

The following caveat must apply in interpreting the findings from surveys that report that a large number of respondents say they understand food label information. Undoubtedly, in some cases consumers respond with the answer they believe the questioner wants to hear. When asked a direct question about their level of understanding, a consumer who does not wish to appear to be misinformed or unintelligent will usually respond affirmatively. Or, they may say that they "think" that they understand the information, until they are probed on specifics or asked to apply the information to make food purchase decisions.

During this comprehension stage, consumers begin to actively transform and assign meaning to the information they read. In order for information to pass successfully through this stage, it must be understandable, and it must be presented in a context that allows it to be encoded into memory. Consumers do not understand many of the terms now used on food labels, for example, scientific terms for nutrients or food components or the metric units used to indicate nutrient compositions (Achterberg, 1990). In addition, the concept of serving size has no consistent meaning, either for food manufacturers or consumers. These problems do not allow for adequate consumer comprehension of food label information.

Levy and Stephenson (1990), after studying consumers' nutrition knowledge about dietary fats and cholesterol, confirmed that respondents had a number of common misconceptions, particularly about sources of cholesterol and the caloric value of saturated versus other fats. More than half of the respondents in that study did not know the meaning of hydrogenated, and most had not heard of monounsaturated fatty acids or oils. The only subgroup of respondents who had improved their scores over the 5-year evaluation period were those who had been told they had high blood cholesterol or others who were consciously trying to reduce their blood cholesterol through dietary means.

Examination of consumer comprehension of the key nutrition concepts, terms, and numeric expressions used on food labels may help to explain the major causes for poor understanding of the information presented. One survey found that only 36 percent of the sample knew that ingredients are listed in decreasing order by amount (Lecos, 1988). Only 6 percent knew the relationship of grams to ounces. Only 44 percent could correctly calculate the reduction in milligrams when the amount of salt was reduced by one-third.

A sample of Pennsylvania adults expressed the most confusion about fats and cholesterol in two areas: the difference between saturated and unsaturated fatty acids, and the difference between fat and cholesterol (Achterberg et al., 1990). Related to the misconception about saturated versus unsaturated fatty acids was the fact that respondents did not know what the fat was saturated with. Those consumers also had difficulty differentiating between the concepts of fat and cholesterol (probably because the terms are so often used together) and between the notion of dietary cholesterol and serum cholesterol.

The process that transforms data into usable information is referred to as *encoding*. The consumer may transform information as it is presented into what is actually intended. The use of inconsistent terminology may result in confusion. Consumers need to be able to reorganize the information in their own minds so that it becomes meaningful. When ideas must be communicated to consumers and no frame of reference exists (e.g., the term *high-fat*), the label could show relevant range data or reorganize information into groupings that help to facilitate memory processes.

A continuing issue concerns the importance of the format in which nutrition information is presented. Russo et al. have conceptualized the "costs" faced by consumers who want to base their brand choice on nutrition information. They concluded that "currently [consumers] must collect the nutrition information from many different product labels, comprehend it, and then determine how to aggregate the different nutrients to identify the most nutritious brand" (Russo et al., 1986, p. 49). At least three types of "effort costs" are involved: collection, comprehension, and computation of information. It appears that consumers conduct an informal cost-benefit analysis and use information only when they perceive that benefits exceed the costs. For those consumers who actually do such an analysis, it is likely to be done subconsciously. Even if the information per se is free (as it is for nutrition information on food labels), consumer efforts to process the information is still a cost to them. Therefore, an important tactic for making information provision programs more successful is to decrease the effort required by consumers to process the information. Russo et al. (1986) view effort reduction as changing the information environment to adapt to people and suggest that "it may be more effective to change the shopping environment [i.e., the food label] to adapt to people than to change people to adapt to an effortful environment" (p. 68).

The initial research conducted in the early 1970s to determine nutrition label format examined only numeric, percentage, pie chart, and verbal presentations (Asam and Bucklin, 1973; Babcock and Murphy, 1973; Lenahan et al., 1972). The study by Lenahan et al. (1972) on consumer reactions to nutrition compared nutrient content in terms of (1) units as a percentage of the RDA, in which a unit represented 10 percent of the RDA, (2) adjectives (e.g., excellent, very good, and fair), and (3) percentage of the RDA. Consumers reported preferring the percentage of RDA format over the other two options.

Babcock and Murphy (1973) tested a food equivalent labeling system against the proposed RDA format. This system used a pie chart that graphically related a food's nutritional value to that of a reference food based on a nutrient-to-calorie ratio. Testing of the RDA label in comparison with the food equivalent pie chart label showed that the RDA label increased sales by 55 percent, while sales increased 63 percent with the food equivalent labels. They concluded that the use of a reference food utilizing a pie chart was more effective than the FDA-proposed label format in conveying nutrition information to consumers.

In 1979, FDA reported on the written comments it had received on the type of nutrition label that consumers felt would be most useful:

> 84 [of the 494 received] supported the present system. The most popular was a pictorial or graphic display, with 151 comments. Other proposed alternatives included using words to describe the "quality" of nutrition (64), nutrition scores (44), nutrient density (43), and a food group system (24) (DHEW/USDA/FTC, 1979, p. 41).

Because formats with such alternatives as graphic presentations were not included in the original consumer testing, it is important to examine those studies that have modified the label format in an effort to aid consumers in processing the nutrition information the label presents. While the concept of a nutrient density label has been recommended (Hall, 1977), this format has not been extensively evaluated. Hansen et al. (1985) strongly recommended a graphic format for the nutrition label because it rapidly conveyed important information and encouraged comparisons between brands.

Mohr et al. (1980) suggested that a graphic nutrient density label was more effective in aiding consumer nutrition decisions than the traditional label format was. A replication of this study by Rudd (1986), who added a graphic label, reaffirmed the findings of Mohr et al., and also demonstrated that a simple graphic label format produced the same effect as that of the graphic nutrient density format. Rudd (1989) recently found that the addition of a calorie-based identification statement to the graphic nutrient density label had an impact on consumer perceptions of nutrient quality.

Geiger et al. (1990) reported the results of a study of consumer perceptions of label usefulness in purchase decisions by using the marketing research technique of adaptive conjoint analysis. Results indicated that for food purchase decisions, consumers preferred the graphic format over the others; consumers in that study also expressed a preference for the most nutrition information load, presentation of numbers and percentages, and a rearranged order of nutrition information (placing those nutrients to be consumed in smaller amounts at the bottom of the label).

One technique used to assess the level of information processing is cognitive response analysis. Leung-Chung et al. (1985) studied homemakers' cognitive responses to nutrition information presented in a conventional versus a graphic format. Each verbalized thought was categorized according to whether it contained nutrition or nonnutrition content references and whether the thought content was semantic (i.e., the respondent made inferences about the nutritional quality of the product, a product attribute, or label characteristics) or sensory (i.e., the respondent repeated verbatim a statement or comparisons exactly as they were presented on the label). Results showed that the graphic label elicited a greater number of semantic responses containing nutrition content than did the conventional label. Consequently, it was concluded that a food label that presented information in a graphic format, as opposed to the conventional numeric format, enhanced the processing of nutrition information in a meaningful way.

Retention and Retrieval   In order for information to be useful to the consumer, it must be retained in memory, activated, and retrieved for use in decisionmaking. Food labels must be designed that will be acted upon by both short- and long-term memory. Because short-term memory has very limited storage capacity, the aim must be to keep the label information as simple and relevant as possible. Information processing through long-term memory can be facilitated by providing appropriate cues for retrieval. Therefore, informational cues presented on the label must be congruent with the manner in which the same information is likely to be stored in memory. Venkatesan and fellow researchers (1977, 1986) concluded that in a presentation format experiment, the majority of consumers preferred a standardized listing of nutrient contents over a summary score or an index of nutritional quality.

Decisionmaking   When faced with making a decision, most consumers do not attempt to consider all the relevant factors. Instead, they construct simplifying rules that allow them to reach a satisfactory decision. Mazis and Staelin (1982) described a number of general principles that should be followed in helping consumers make appropriate decisions. The first principle is concreteness. A decisionmaker tends to use only the information that is explicitly provided and uses it only in the form in which it is displayed. Information is more likely to be used if it is in a form that is directly compatible with the question the consumer is trying to answer, for example, "Is this product high in fat?" or "What is the sodium content of this product?" Also, if the information is poorly organized, consumers will not engage in an extended acquisition effort; thus, attention to the design of an appropriate label format is essential for facilitating consumer comprehension of label information. Another principle is anchoring and adjustment. People ease the strain of integrating information by first using a natural starting point (an anchor) and then adjusting to accommodate additional information. Those informational approaches designed to encourage more comparison shopping must contend with this process, which helps to explain why it is difficult for consumers to learn or try something new or unfamiliar.

Most people seem to think of nutrition in terms of positive attributes, that is, the components of food necessary for good health. However, consumers have recently increased their attention to certain food components that can be referred to as negative nutrients (e.g., calories, cholesterol, sodium, sugar, and various chemical additives) in an effort to avoid these items altogether or choose foods that contain lower amounts of these items (Russo et al., 1986).

Consumers think that knowledge of both positive and negative nutrients is important. When it comes to making food choices, however, they are more concerned with avoiding the negative nutrients (Heimbach, 1987; Heimbach and Stokes, 1979) than they are with choosing foods for their beneficial effects. Heimbach (1982) reported on a survey of consumers in which they were asked to rate the importance of 38 food components, 29 positive and 9 negative. All 9 negative food components were ranked in the top 12 most important components. Indeed, it has been shown that consumers read food labels more to avoid particular food constituents (such as fat, cholesterol, sugar, and sodium) than to seek out positive attributes (Heimbach, 1987).

Asam and Bucklin (1973) varied brand, price, nutrition information, and store location to determine the effect of nutrition labeling on consumer purchase preferences. The investigators concluded that nutrition labels that used vague descriptors to indicate nutrient content did not affect consumer choice patterns. In addition, detailed nutrition labels that showed average values were used by some consumers and appeared to affect the perception of product quality, while promotional campaigns lessened the effect of nutrition labels.

Some studies have suggested that nutrition information on food labels helps consumers decide which brand of a product they should buy. In one study to determine the impact of full disclosure on labeling sales of the leading store brands and private-label brands, consumers purchased foods in a simulated supermarket environment (Yankelovich, Inc., 1971). The results indicated that the dominant brand in each product category held its market share when full disclosure nutrition labeling appeared on a secondary brand, thus suggesting that full disclosure had its strongest effect on the purchase of secondary brands, as long as the brand was not a private label.

While consumers appear to use nutrition information on food labels to make comparisons of the same food sold under different brand names, it is disappointing to note that consumers rarely used such information to choose from among general groups of foods to achieve more balanced diets (Rudd and Glanz, 1990). Fanelli and Abernathy (1986) found that 40 percent of the older adults in their survey reported that they never read food labels to compare products or to examine ingredients.

Summary of Consumer Understanding

The field of nutrition is clearly more complex than it was 15 years ago, when the use of nutrition labels became effective; likewise, the amount of nutrition information to which consumers are exposed has expanded exponentially. It is the responsibility of regulatory agencies to require that food manufacturers present nutrition information on food labels in a format that consumers can readily understand and use.

Several factors currently contribute to consumer confusion. About 40 percent of all food labels do not carry the nutrition information panel and were not designed to be directly relevant to today's dietary recommendations, particularly with respect to consumption of macronutrients, such as fat and cholesterol. In addition, current regulations allow confusion to continue in terminology (e.g., light, low, reduced, and diet) and definitions (e.g., serving sizes). These problems can largely be resolved by a new, well-designed, mandatory nutrition labeling system.

ANALYTICAL CONSIDERATIONS AFFECTING FOOD LABELING REFORM

Overview of Analytical Issues

The compositions of all food products vary as a result of factors that are not readily controlled or predicted. As with all biological materials, some degree of variability occurs with respect to the composition of foods. Substantial variation in the composition of plant-derived foods occurs as a result of various factors, including soil and climatic variables; maturity of plants at the time of harvesting; conditions of postharvest storage and handling; and conditions of processing, subsequent storage, and handling by consumers (Nagy and Wardowski, 1988; Salunkhe and Desai, 1988). In addition, genetics and diet affect the composition of animal-derived foods (Froning, 1988; Ockerman, 1988; Renner, 1988). The composition of seafood is also subject to wide variability (Krzynowek, 1988).

Of the various food components, vitamins and minerals are generally subject to the greatest natural variability. For example, as much as 100 percent variation in the folate concentration has been reported among samples of certain vegetable products (Mullin et al., 1982), and extensive variation in ascorbic acid and vitamin A activities also have been reported in vegetables (Klein and Perry, 1982). Even greater variability in the levels of trace minerals (e.g., selenium) can occur as a function of geographic variation and soil type.

For the purpose of nutrition labeling, the precision of analytical methods must be considered in light of the variability of food composition. For example, the natural nutrient composition of some plant-derived foods varies so greatly among samples that determination is difficult or impossible even when the least amount of precision is required. In this case, current nutrition labeling regulations that specify that the actual nutrient content must be within 20 percent of the label claim appear to be overly stringent. The net effect of such regulations is that the stated nutrient values must be set sufficiently low that, within analytical variability, nutrient content of all samples of a product fall within the 20 percent tolerance range. In contrast, the composition of many formulated foods is much more constant, and application of the 20 percent limit is consistent with the need for accuracy and precision but may not be within the accuracy and precision of certain analytical methods. The nutritional significance of minor inaccuracies of label data is probably minimal.

A major purpose of analyzing the composition of foods is to provide information concerning the quantities of the various nutrients and other food components as they relate to nutritional status and health. Consumers and health professionals use such information, along with estimates of food intake, for the assessment of dietary adequacy. In the food industry, analytical data are used to monitor processing and manufacturing procedures and as a basis for the data provided in nutrition labeling. Regulatory agencies use analytical data to monitor label claims and to enforce the law against products for which false or exaggerated claims are made. In each situation, the adequacy of methods of food analysis and the accuracy of the results are critical considerations. Continuous improvements are needed in the methodology of food analysis in all applications (i.e., for manufacturing quality control, and regulatory and research purposes).

It should be recognized that frequently there are differences in the bioavailabilities of nutrients; that is, there is often variation in the extent of intestinal absorption and/or metabolic utilization of various nutrients. Thus, analytical data describing food composition ideally should be interpreted with respect to the bioavailability of each nutrient. This is a particularly significant consideration for such nutrients as iron, calcium, zinc, folate, niacin, and vitamin B_6. However, current knowledge of vitamin bioavailability, particularly with respect to folate and vitamin B_6, precludes *a priori* estimation. Similar uncertainty exists in the case of many minerals, especially iron.

This discussion covers issues concerning the analytical basis of food labeling data and verification of data provided on labels, the adequacy of food composition data bases, and the status of analytical methods for the generation of food composition data.

Current Analytical Basis of Food Labeling Information

The authority to regulate nutrition labeling is divided between USDA (meat and poultry) and FDA (all other foods). These agencies differ substantially with respect to their procedures and verification requirements, although the nutrition information provided is similar (Frattali et al., 1988; Kessler, 1989; Kushner et al., 1990).

Summary of USDA Requirements

USDA permits food processors and manufacturers to provide full nutrition labeling in the format and style specified by FDA (Houston, 1985; USDA, 1989c). In addition, USDA also permits an abbreviated format that provides only the content of calories, protein, carbohydrate, and fat per specified serving. Important features of the USDA labeling regulations are that the agency must approve a label prior to its use and that data must be provided to verify the continuing accuracy of nutrition information on the label.

The information provided on the label must be accurate, whether determined by calculation from accepted references (e.g., the USDA data base) or from analyses by validated laboratory procedures, such as the *Official Methods of Analysis* of the Association of Official Analytical Chemists (AOAC, 1989) or the USDA *Chemistry Laboratory Guidebook* (USDA, 1979). In the past, the agency had established a partial quality control (PQC) program to ensure label accuracy through formulation control with periodic laboratory analyses, laboratory analyses only, or a combination of formulation control and laboratory analyses (Houston, 1985). The PQC program was allowed to be waived if there was an adequate data base for a manufactured product (Houston, 1985). In the interest of accuracy and efficiency, the PQC program was phased out and in its place, USDA initiated Nutrition Label Verification (NLV) procedures to verify that labeling is "reasonably accurate."

The quantity of supporting data and the degree of precision required on nutrition labels under the NLV program of the Food Safety and Inspection Service (FSIS) may impose analytical problems for many food processors (USDA, 1988). The NLV program requires either quarterly (level I) or annual (level II) submission of analytical data on a randomly selected composite sample of the finished product. The label claim must be no less than 80 percent of the analytical values for protein, vitamins, and minerals and no more than 120 percent of the analytical data for calories, fat, cholesterol, fatty acids, sodium, and carbohydrate. It is stated in Policy Memorandum 085B (USDA, 1988) that "because some variability in analytical values can be expected, even though compositing tends to minimize this to a large extent, some over-declaration of calories, carbohydrates, etc., and some under-declaration of protein, vitamins, and minerals is acceptable . . . . However, the over or under-declaration should be selected so as not to be excessive." USDA generally requires a label change, even when the difference in value is within the 80/120 rule, if a year's worth of data show another number is more accurate.

The degree of leeway allowed is not specified. For products that are out of compliance, the manufacturer or processor must resolve the problem (e.g., reformulate) and perform additional analyses for each nutrient in question. Analytical data from at least 10 consecutive production lots of the revised, corrected formula must be submitted to indicate that the product is within the permitted tolerances (USDA, 1988).

Summary of FDA Requirements

In 21 CFR § 101.9, FDA specifies the procedures for nutrition labeling of foods, whether the information is provided voluntarily or is required when the product is formulated with the addition of any nutrient or any nutrition claim is made. Labels provide information on the composition of the products in the form in which they are packaged. There may be a declaration of nutrient content of the product as consumed after typical (specified) preparation (e.g., breakfast cereal with milk).

The nutrition information required on food labels is reviewed in Chapter 3. Although FDA differs from USDA in that it does not require prior approval of nutrition labeling information, the agency may challenge a label to ensure compliance (21 CFR § 101.9(e)). If, on analysis, values of nutrient contents declared on the label are not within the defined deviations, the food may be declared misbranded. For foods containing added vitamins, minerals, and proteins, the content of a nutrient in a composite sample must be at least equal to the value for that nutrient indicated on the label. In contrast, for naturally occurring nutrients, the nutrient content must be at least equal to 80 percent of the value declared for that nutrient on the label. A provision is made for analytical imprecision, in that no regulatory action will be made for nutrient values less than 80 percent of the label claim by a factor less than the variability generally recognized for the analytical method employed. Furthermore, the regulations specify that reasonable excesses in vitamins, minerals, and protein are acceptable and consistent with good manufacturing practices; reasonable deficiencies of fat, calories, and sodium are similarly allowable. The main specification concerning the accuracy of label claims for calories, fat, carbohydrate, and sodium is that the product will be declared misbranded if the content of each of these components is more than 20 percent in excess of the value indicated on the label.

Also included in section 101.9(e) are specifications concerning the methods to be used for ensuring compliance with FDA nutrition labeling regulations. A sampling protocol is specified for taking a composite sample. The composite is to be analyzed by official methods of AOAC or, if no AOAC method is available, by reliable and appropriate analytical procedures. The regulations also indicate that alternative (i.e., non-AOAC) methods of analysis may be submitted to FDA for determination of their acceptability. The criteria used to evaluate the acceptability of an alternative method are not indicated, however. Alternative methods may be used by the industry provided that they have been validated (e.g., shown to be equivalent to AOAC official methods) such that they will be acceptable in the event of a regulatory challenge (Victor Frattali, Center for Food Safety and Applied Nutrition, FDA, personal communication, 1989).

FDA goes through several steps to enforce compliance with regulations. If labeling information is not comparable to the information obtained by FDA laboratory analysis, within established limits, FDA first issues a warning letter to the manufacturer. If the violation continues, the agency can seize a product, although seizure of a product for nutrition label misbranding is very rare.

Requirements for AOAC or Other Official Methods

USDA and FDA rely primarily on official methods of AOAC in the implementation and regulation of nutrition labeling. Furthermore, the analytical basis of all areas of food and drug regulation is the validation process developed by AOAC (Hutt, 1985). In this context, an official method is one that has been subjected to an interlaboratory collaborative study to demonstrate its accuracy and precision under the conditions of its intended use. Methods that exhibit suitable performance in such an evaluation are given official final action by

AOAC for inclusion in the *Official Methods of Analysis* (AOAC, 1989). These methods are published at approximately 5-year intervals. It is important to recognize that the AOAC official methods are often not the methods of choice in terms of speed, simplicity, and suitability for automation; and with the time required to set up, conduct, and evaluate an interlaboratory study, they often do not represent the most current technologies. Thus, the need exists for flexibility in the selection of analytical methods for verification of food label data by the food industry and the regulatory agencies. In practice, the regulatory agencies apparently allow considerable latitude in the selection of the methods of analysis required for nutrition labeling. The criteria that they use for the selection of alternative (i.e., non-AOAC) methods have not been clearly stated.

Designation of a method as official by AOAC requires that the method perform satisfactorily in interlaboratory collaborative studies under the conditions of intended use. In an important change of policy, the Official Methods Board of AOAC recently took a highly restrictive view of applications of official methods. In a memorandum to James Tanner of FDA (May 19, 1990), AOAC indicated that: "The Official Methods Board recommends that collaborative study results apply only to those commodities for which the method was approved. Extension of the method to other commodities should be subjected to a mini-collaborative study."

The implications of this policy are far-reaching and detrimental to the regulatory agencies that rely on official methods in regulating labeling compliance. For example, if an official method for measurement of a certain food component was subjected to collaborative evaluation with respect to an analysis of the nutrient composition of broccoli, it would not be considered applicable to other foods unless the results of further collaborative study were approved by AOAC. Although the scientific rationale is justified, from a regulatory viewpoint this policy effectively removes AOAC official method status from most analytical methods used in the regulation of compliance in nutrition labeling.

This problem is particularly acute in specialized aspects of mandatory nutrition labeling, such as specified for infant formula (21 CFR § 107.70). The legal status of the AOAC methods used to monitor compliance of infant formulas, which were not subjected to an AOAC collaborative study for that application, is seriously in question.

Selection and Validation of Methods of Food Analysis

Among the problems associated with the acquisition of reliable data for food composition are (1) difficulties in the proper implementation of often complex methods of analysis; (2) the complexity of food composition, which makes selection of an appropriate analytical method of primary importance; (3) differences in analytical capabilities of different laboratories, such that different methods might, by necessity, be used to achieve the same measurement; and (4) the need for improvement of analytical methods as well as better training of technicians (Stewart, 1988, 1989). These factors apply equally to the generation of data for food labeling, the expansion of food composition data bases, and all aspects of food regulation.

The current methods of food analysis leave much to be desired. Methods vary with respect to the suitability for various types of food composition, the convenience and expense, and the degree of analytical expertise required to perform tests (Beecher and Vanderslice, 1984). As proposed by Stewart (1981), the result of an analytical test should be within 10 percent of the actual value when the nutrient of interest is present at nutritionally significant concentrations. Many methods of food analysis are not fully adequate when their accuracy and precision are critically evaluated (Beecher and Vanderslice, 1984). Precision within a 10 to 15 percent relative standard deviation has been considered to be adequate for all nutrients, except those that are present at nutritionally low concentrations (Beecher and Vanderslice, 1984; Stewart, 1981). Many methods of nutrient analysis fail to meet these criteria of accuracy and precision, particularly when they are evaluated on an interlaboratory basis. Methods of quality control for nutrient analysis should be strictly specified, but are lacking for nearly all current methods, including the official methods of AOAC and similar organizations.

Considerable improvement is needed in the validation and standardization of methods of food analysis for use in nutrition labeling and in the generation of food composition data (Stewart, 1985). In addition to the evaluation of the accuracy and precision of a method at the time of development, validation of each set of analytical data should also be provided (Stewart, 1989). Particular emphasis should be placed on the validation of each analysis through proper use of standard laboratories, standard instruments, certified analysts, certified algorithms, internal standards, pooled samples, standard reference materials, and audit trails (Stewart, 1989). The National Institute of Standards and Technology has developed several biological materials for use as standard reference materials in the determination of various inorganic and a few organic elements in foods (Alvarez, 1984). Unfortunately, similar reference materials do not exist for many organic food components. It should be noted, however, that the American Association of Cereal Chemists does provide certified bran products suitable for use in fiber analysis and the American Oil Chemists' Society has developed standards for fatty acids and cholesterol. However, further development and implementation of appropriate reference materials is needed.

Analytical Issues Related to Expansion of Nutrition Labeling

Problems with Nutrients Proposed for Inclusion on Nutrition Labels

Dietary Fiber Of all the methods for analyzing food components subject to nutrition labeling, those for measurement of dietary fiber have undergone the greatest transition in recent years but remain the most controversial. Because of its heterogeneous nature, dietary fiber is difficult to measure by either chemical or gravimetric methods.

Selective hydrolysis and chemical analysis of dietary fiber components (e.g., the Southgate method) provide important qualitative and quantitative information (Lanza and Butrum, 1986). However, the lengthy sample preparation time and the multiple chromatographic analyses required for each sample render such methods unsuitable for routine use in food labeling.

A gravimetric approach for the measurement of total dietary fiber has received official final action by AOAC (Prosky et al., 1985). This method is not well suited for rapid, repetitive analysis due to its labor-intensive nature, which minimizes automation, although there are currently no suitable alternatives. Previous methods of gravimetric analysis (e.g., crude fiber and neutral detergent fiber methods) underestimated total dietary fiber as a result of losses of soluble fiber components. Although the AOAC method provides generally acceptable results, evidence of some inaccuracy has been reported. For example, Marlett and Navis (1988) observed that the AOAC method overestimated total dietary fiber by 14 percent and 18 percent in chemical analyses of fiber components in samples of apples and a total diet composite, respectively.

In view of the physiological properties of certain water-soluble forms of dietary fiber for the reduction of serum cholesterol, there is interest in extending food labeling to include total, soluble, and insoluble categories of dietary fiber. In this regard, the AOAC method was modified to permit measurement of the soluble and insoluble fiber components (Prosky et al., 1985, 1988). In an interlaboratory study of the modified method, generally acceptable results were obtained for most foods that were examined, although the need for further refinement of the fractionation procedure was evident. Currently, there is no simple gravimetric method that is acceptable for measurement of soluble dietary fiber in foods. Because soluble fiber ordinarily makes up a small proportion of total dietary fiber, calculation of soluble fiber by difference (i.e., total dietary fiber minus insoluble fiber) probably would be subject to excessive imprecision.

Carbohydrates For the purpose of nutrition labeling, the measurement of total carbohydrates in foods is ordinarily performed indirectly. Total nutritionally available carbohydrates are calculated as total sample weight minus analytical values for protein, fat, moisture, ash, and total dietary fiber. These values are also used in the calculation of caloric content of protein, carbohydrate, and fat on the basis of 4, 4, and 9 kcal/g, respectively. At present there are no convenient methods for the direct measurement of total available carbohydrates. It should be noted that this indirect method for determining total available carbohydrates is subject to potential inaccuracy and imprecision. Large variations have been reported between measured values for available carbohydrates (sugars and starch) and indirectly calculated total carbohydrates based on handbook values for proximate composition (Li et al., 1988).

Recent improvements in liquid chromatographic and gas chromatographic methods of sugar analysis have provided means for convenient qualitative and quantitative analyses of sugars in foods. Similar methods are available for the measurement of starch and derived oligosaccharides by measuring the amount of glucose released during specific enzymatic hydrolysis. Thus, the potential exists for more accurate, precise, and direct measurements of total carbohydrates, specific sugars, and starches. Problems in the enzymatic hydrolysis of starches in foods that have been subjected to extensive browning (Maillard or caramelization) have been noted, although this would not preclude accurate measurement in most cases.

Fats and Cholesterol   The Surgeon General's report (DHHS, 1988) recommended that total fat, saturated and unsaturated fatty acids, and cholesterol contents be listed in nutrition labeling. Although this is clearly justified on a nutritional basis, it will inevitably cause substantial increases in the analytical loads of all laboratories that perform these analyses. The measurement of total fat is a technically simple but cumbersome procedure, although it is routinely performed for all foods with nutrition labels.

Extension of nutrition labeling policy to require data on the fatty acid content in foods represents a major analytical difficulty. In this regard, a nonchromatographic spectrophotometric method is available for measurement of total polyunsaturated (*cis,cis*-methylene-interrupted-polyunsaturated) fatty acids (AOAC, 1989, method 28.082). The method is limited in that it does not identify the fatty acids present. In addition, it was designed for analysis of vegetable oils and requires extensive sample preparation if it is applied to complex samples (e.g., plant and animal tissues and multicomponent foods). Gas chromatographic determination of the individual fatty acids may be performed by using a traditional packed-column method (AOAC, 1989, method 28.060) or by a capillary-column procedure (Slover and Lanza, 1979). These methods, especially capillary-column gas chromatography, provide specific information about the patterns of fatty acids, although sample preparation time is considerable and chromatographic analysis is slow, requiring about 2 hours per sample by capillary-column gas chromatography.

Considerable interest exists with respect to the content of *trans* fatty acid isomers and the omega-3 family of fatty acids in foods. The formation of the *trans* fatty acid isomer occurs spontaneously in the hydrogenation of fats and oils, and naturally occurring *trans* fatty acids are present in small quantities in animal tissues and products. *Trans* fatty acid isomers can be determined in margarine and shortening samples by direct infrared spectrophotometry (AOAC, 1989, method 28.086) or in any other food product by capillary-column gas chromatography (Slover and Lanza, 1979). Similarly, in view of the uncertain nutritional benefit of omega-3 fatty acids versus those of other unsaturated fatty acids, the additional expense of providing omega-3 fatty acid data on nutrition labels does not appear to be warranted at this time.

Several methods are available for the measurement of cholesterol in foods, with selection based on the type of sample and the equipment that are available. A gas chromatographic method, if properly calibrated, provides the most specific measurement of cholesterol in the presence of other sterols (AOAC, 1989, method 43.283). Less specific enzymatic methods require careful validation if accurate results are to be obtained (Newman, 1989).

Protein   Methods for the measurement of protein in foods are highly reliable. In addition, most foods exhibit relatively little variation with respect to their protein content. Thus, nutrition labeling of the protein component of foods can be accomplished with less difficulty than is encountered for other food components.

Vitamins and Minerals   Suitable methods appear to exist for the individual or simultaneous measurement of most minerals of interest (Beecher and Vanderslice, 1984). However, further efforts in the standardization and validation of methods, along with the further implementation of analytical quality control procedures (e.g., the use of standard reference materials), are needed. As summarized by Beecher and Vanderslice (1984), considerable development of reliable analytical methods for many of the vitamins is required, including the need for improved methods both for the actual measurement of various nutrients and for the extraction of vitamins from the food prior to analysis.

Of the methods applied to vitamins designated as having current or potential public health significance, including folate and vitamins A, B_6, and C (LSRO, FASEB, 1989), only the method used to analyze vitamin C has been judged to be reliable. Considerable improvement has been made recently in the measurement of vitamin A in foods, although substantial uncertainty exists in the selection of appropriate methods (Parrish et al., 1985). Several suitable liquid chromatographic methods have been developed for the measurement of vitamin B_6, but how well those methods compare with traditional microbiological assay procedures (e.g., AOAC) is uncertain (Gregory, 1988). Certainly, the AOAC methods for analyzing vitamins A and B_6 do not reflect recent advances in analytical methodologies.

Of all of the methods for analyzing vitamins of current interest in nutrition labeling and public health, the poorest are those available for folate analysis.

Recent improvements in methods for folate analysis have been made, although questions regarding the factors that affect the responses of the various types of assays (i.e., chromatographic, microbiological, or ligand binding) have not been fully resolved (Gregory, 1989). The Surgeon General's report (DHHS, 1988) indicated that research should be directed toward the development of improved methods for the measurement of folate in foods. The AOAC methods for analyzing folate (AOAC, 1989, methods 43.183–43.190) are designed such that they cannot be applied to the measurement of total folate in foods. The organism used in AOAC assays for folate analysis, *Streptococcus faecalis,* does not respond to methyl folates, the major form of the vitamin found in foods. The method also does not provide for the deconjugation of food folates, and thus would grossly underestimate the amount of the vitamin in foods.

In *Nutrition Monitoring in the United States* (LSRO, FASEB, 1989), carotenes were proposed as a class of nutrients having potential public health significance. Currently, there appears to be little justification for the inclusion of data regarding total carotenes in nutrition labeling on analytical grounds. The AOAC method for carotene analysis is based on cumbersome open-column chromatography, and its validity is questionable for samples containing complex mixtures of carotenes, as present in most foods (Simpson et al., 1985). Recent advances have been made in high-performance liquid chromatographic methodology, but individual quantitation of the many naturally occurring carotenes requires considerable effort to adapt the procedures to each different type of food sample analyzed (Khachik et al., 1989). The existence of *cis* and *trans* isomers of carotenes further complicates the analysis.

Ability of Analytical Laboratories To Accommodate Expanded Nutrition Labeling

There is some question among industry representatives concerning the ability of analytical laboratories to manage the increased analytical demand imposed by expanded nutrition labeling requirements. This burden may be as serious for small companies with limited laboratory capabilities as it is for larger manufacturers with diverse product lines. The services of private analytical laboratories are commonly used by all segments of the food industry, particularly with respect to analyses involving nutrition labeling which are frequently not performed in-house on a routine basis, as is the case for quality control analyses used to monitor the formulation and processing of food products. Private analytical laboratories appear to be able to expand to the analytical demands of the marketplace (as influenced, in this case, by nutrition labeling requirements). For laboratories that already provide the analyses required for nutrition labeling, accommodating a greater volume of samples would be feasible but would require the addition of equipment and technical personnel. Regulatory agencies would also require additional resources (personnel, equipment, and laboratory space) to monitor compliance.

Nutrition Labeling of Nonpackaged Foods: Application of Food Composition Data Bases

The application of current labeling procedures based principally on direct analytical data appears to be impractical for fresh foods, including meat, poultry, seafood, and produce and foods sold in restaurants. In view of the need for expansion of public access to food composition information; however, the use of information from appropriate data bases may be a useful alternative. However, the validity, analytical basis, and completeness of existing data must be examined.

The most complete food composition data base for unprocessed foods is the National Nutrient Data Bank, which is maintained by the Human Nutrition Information Service, USDA. This system contains reasonably complete data concerning the proximate composition of foods, although the data are less complete and potentially less reliable for nutrients for which sound analytical methods are lacking, especially dietary fiber and folate (Hepburn, 1987). This data base needs to be completed and updated; some values are woefully out of date. Table 4-1 illustrates the comparatively incomplete state of the USDA data base as of 1987. Since then, progress has been made with respect to the inclusion of additional foods and modest increases in the percentage of foods for which actual analytical data are available for each nutrient (Ruth Matthews, Human Nutrition Information Service, USDA, personal communication, 1990).

The accuracy of information in the USDA data base has not been examined systematically. This is very important, especially for the micronutrients that are subject to considerable natural variation, inadequate sampling, analytical uncertainty, or to which obsolete methods are applied (e.g., cholesterol and iron). With respect to the USDA data base concerning folates in foods, Subar et al. (1989) recently reported on a preliminary comparative study of the content of folate in foods. It was concluded that, despite potential underestimation and overestimation of the actual folate content in foods, overall assessments of dietary folate may be reasonably accurate when the USDA data base is used.

As discussed previously, the composition of food is subject to a high degree of variability. This is particularly true of vitamins and minerals. In addition, the amounts of certain major constituents, including dietary fiber, total fat, and the pattern of individual fatty acids, vary across different samples of the same food. To generate information for use in data bases, appropriate sampling protocols would involve selection of samples from various sources to compensate for geographic and seasonal variation. Data bases currently in use may be biased if values are based on inappropriate sampling procedures or have been imputed without consideration of these variables.

TABLE 4-1 Percentage of Analytical Data for a Given
Nutrient in USDA Primary Data Set

Nutrient	Percentage All Foods	Best Sources
Calcium	97	
Protein	97	
Fat	96	
Thiamin	91	
Riboflavin	91	
Niacin	91	
Sodium	90	
Potassium	90	
Phosphorus	90	
Iron	90	
Vitamin C	83	92
Vitamin A (IU)	80	89
Cholesterol	80	
Magnesium	75	72
Zinc	73	79
Copper	67	71
Vitamin B_6	64	72
Vitamin B_{12}	64	79
Vitamin A (RE)	61	73
Folate	56	69
Carotene	54	88
Dietary fiber	29	40
α-Tocopherol	28	39

NOTE: The USDA Primary Data Set contains data on basic
foods, including ingredients of foods such as flour.
SOURCE: Adapted from Hepburn, F. 1987. Food con-
sumption/food composition interrelationships. Pp. 68–74 in Research on Survey Methodology, HNIS Report No. Adm–382. Human Nutrition Information Service, U.S. Department of Agriculture, Hyattsville, Md.

The information in a data base may indicate representative food composition, but there may be large differences between data base values and the actual
concentrations of certain nutrients in a single specimen of that food. It has been
suggested that information from appropriate data bases (e.g., USDA) could be
used as the basis for nutrition labeling of certain foods that cannot be readily analyzed during distribution (e.g., fresh meat, poultry, seafood, fruits, and
vegetables). If this data base is to be used to provide nutrient composition data

for nonpackaged foods, this potential for substantial variability with respect to micronutrient content must be recognized.

In addition to the USDA data base, other sources of food composition data are available for use in nutrition labeling of foods. Although not actually formal data bases, analytical data provided by various trade associations clearly complement other sources of information for nutrition labeling. Some of these data bases are reviewed by FDA, although no formal certification procedure currently exists.

Data bases may serve as a mechanism for providing reasonably representative nutrient content data for foods sold in restaurants, particularly those providing packaged products in a highly standardized format (i.e., for foods sold in limited-menu restaurants). At present, there appears to be no means of analytical verification of the nutrient content of foods sold in other restaurants and noncommercial food service settings, although the nutrient composition of recipe menus could be calculated by using food composition data from nutrient data bases.

Committee Recommendations

All nutrition labeling is predicated on acceptable accuracy and precision of the information provided, whether obtained by direct analysis or indirectly from a food composition data base. Thus, the validity of nutrition labeling ultimately depends on the adequacy of analytical methods used in food analysis and their appropriate application. Because of the key role of food analysis in nutrition labeling and in view of the analytical limitations described in this section, the Committee recommends that:

- Label verification by analysis of composite samples should be made at least twice each year to ensure reasonable accuracy of nutrition labels without imposing the burden of a complete quarterly analysis. Although there are clear merits of the USDA system of label verification in terms of ensuring accuracy, management of the FDA system seems much less costly.
- FDA and USDA should certify data from the National Nutrient Data Bank or other appropriate sources regarding the nutrient content of fresh foods and foods sold in restaurants.
- FDA and USDA should allow considerable flexibility in the selection of analytical methods for label verification. The limitations of certain official methods hinder the analytical process, given the volume of analyses performed.
- In proposing an alternative (nonofficial) analytical method, suitable verification must be required (e.g., recovery of samples and analysis of reference materials), and appropriate quality control procedures should be used in each analysis. A mechanism should be developed to verify the quality

control measures that are used whenever analytical data are submitted to a regulatory agency.

- Development of additional standard reference materials for use in food analysis should be encouraged.
- Funding should be provided for the development of improved analytical methods, establishment of programs for the testing of methods through interlaboratory studies, and development of additional standard reference materials.
- Completion and expansion of the USDA National Nutrient Data Bank should be continued. It is recommended that the relative merits of the various alternative food composition data bases be examined and that efforts toward the consolidation of data bases be supported.

REFERENCES

Achterberg, C. 1990. Information presented at the Workshop on Consumer Understanding and Use of Food Labels, Committee on the Nutrition Components of Food Labeling, Food and Nutrition Board, Institute of Medicine, Washington D.C. March 13.

Achterberg, C., G. Auld, V. Getty, and J. Durrwachter. 1990. Misconceptions about fat and cholesterol in a sample of Pennsylvania men and women. Unpublished draft paper. Pennsylvania State University, University Park.

ADA (American Dietetic Association). 1990. Position of the American Dietetic Association: Nutrition education for the public. J. Am. Diet. Assoc. 90:107–110.

Alvarez, R. 1984. NBS standard reference materials for food analysis. Pp. 81–99 in Modern Methods of Food Analysis, K.K. Stewart and J.R. Whitaker, eds. AVI Publishing Co., Westport, Conn.

AOAC (Association of Official Analytical Chemists). 1989. Official Methods of Analysis, 15th ed. AOAC, Washington, D.C. 1298 pp.

Asam, E.H., and L.P. Bucklin. 1973. Nutrition labeling for canned goods: A study of consumer response. J. Marketing 37:32–37.

Babcock, M.J., and M.M. Murphy. 1973. Two nutrition labeling systems. J. Am. Diet. Assoc. 62:155–161.

Beecher, G.R., and J.T. Vanderslice. 1984. Determination of nutrients in foods: Factors that must be considered. Pp. 29–56 in Modern Methods of Food Analysis, K.K. Stewart and J.R. Whitaker, eds. AVI Publishing Co., Westport, Conn.

Bettman, J.R. 1979. An Information Processing Theory of Consumer Choice. Addison-Wesley, Reading, Mass. 402 pp.

CNI (Community Nutrition Institute). 1988. FDA, private surveys disagree on diet trends. Nutr. Week. June 23. 18(23):1

Daly, P. 1976. The response of consumers to nutrition labeling. J. Consumer Affairs 10:170–178.

DHEW/USDA/FTC (U.S. Department of Health, Education, and Welfare; U.S. Department of Agriculture; and Federal Trade Commission). 1979. Food Labeling Background Papers. Government Printing Office, Washington, D.C. 124 pp.

DHHS (U.S. Department of Health and Human Services). 1988. The Surgeon General's

Report on Nutrition and Health. Government Printing Office, Washington, D.C. 727 pp.

DHHS/USDA (U.S. Department of Health and Human Services and U.S. Department of Agriculture). 1986. Nutrition Monitoring in the United States: A Report from the Joint Nutrition Monitoring Evaluation Committee. Government Printing Office, Washington, D.C. 356 pp.

DOC (U.S. Department of Commerce). 1990. 1990 U.S. Industrial Outlook (January). Government Printing Office, Washington D.C. 534 pp.

Fanelli, M., and M. Abernathy. 1986. A nutritional questionnaire for older adults. Gerontologist 26:192–197.

FMI (Food Marketing Institute). 1989. Trends. Consumer Attitudes and the Supermarket. FMI, Washington D.C. 65 pp.

FMI (Food Marketing Institute). 1990. Trends. Consumer Attitudes and the Supermarket. FMI, Washington D.C. 70 pp.

Frattali, V.P., J.E. Vanderveen, and A.L. Forbes. 1988. The role of the United States government in regulating the nutritional value of the food supply. Pp. 687–705 in Nutritional Evaluation of Food Processing, 3rd ed., E. Karmas and R.S. Harris, eds. Van Nostrand Reinhold Co., New York.

Friedman, M., ed. 1990. Gorman's New Product News. Gorman Publishing Co., Chicago. January 5, vol. 25, no. 12. 46 pp.

Froning, G.W. 1988. Effects of agricultural practices on poultry and eggs. Pp. 225–244 in Nutritional Evaluation of Food Processing, 3rd ed., E. Karmas and R.S. Harris, eds. Van Nostrand Reinhold Co., New York.

Geiger, C.J., B.W. Wyse, C.R.M. Parent, and R.G. Hansen. 1990. The use of adaptive conjoint analysis (ACA) to determine the most useful nutrition label for purchase decisions. Abstract 4587. Annual Meeting of the Federation of American Societies for Experimental Biology, Washington, D.C.

Glanz, K., and R. Mullis. 1988. Environmental interventions to promote healthy eating: A review of models, programs, and evidence. Health Ed. Q. 15(4):395–415.

Glanz, K., J. Rudd, R.M. Mullis, and P. Snyder. 1989. Point of choice nutrition information, federal regulations and consumer health education: A critical view. J. Nutr. Ed. 21(2):95–100.

Glascoff, M.A., S. Taylor, and D.W. Glascoff. 1986. A social marketing approach to reducing salt intake. Health Ed. 17(2):11–14.

Gregory, J.F. 1988. Methods for determination of vitamin B_6 in foods and other biological materials: A critical review. J. Food Comp. Anal. 1:105–123.

Gregory, J.F. 1989. Chemical and nutritional aspects of folate research: Analytical procedures, methods of folate synthesis, stability, and bioavailability of dietary folates. Pp. 1–101 in Advances in Food and Nutrition Research, vol. 33. J. Kinsella, ed. Academic Press, Orlando, Fla.

Hall, R.L. 1977. Food additives: An industry view. FDA Consumer 11(10):6–11.

Hammonds, T. 1978. Testimony before the Subcommittee on Nutrition and Investigations, Committee on Agriculture, Nutrition, and Forestry, U.S. Senate, Washington D.C. August 9–10.

Hansen, R.G., C.T. Windham, and B.W. Wyse. 1985. Nutrient density and food labeling. Clin. Nutr. 4:164–170.

Harris, S., and S. Welsh. 1989. How well are our food choices meeting our nutrition needs? Nutr. Today 24:20–28.

Heimbach, J.T. 1982. Public Understanding of Food Label Information. Food and Drug Administration, Washington, D.C. 24 pp.

Heimbach, J.T. 1985. Cardiovascular disease and diet: The public view. Public Health Rep. 100:5.

Heimbach, J.T. 1986. The growing impact of sodium labeling of foods. Food Technol. 40(12):102.

Heimbach, J.T. 1987. Risk avoidance in consumer approaches to diet and health. Clin. Nutr. 6:159.

Heimbach, J.T., and R.C. Stokes. 1979. Food and Drug Administration, 1978 Consumer Food Labeling Survey. Food and Drug Administration, U.S. Department of Health and Human Services, Washington, D.C. 133 pp.

Hepburn, F. 1987. Food consumption/food composition interrelationships. Pp. 68–74 in Research on Survey Methodology, HNIS Report No. Adm-382. Human Nutrition Information Service, U.S. Department of Agriculture, Hyattsville, Md.

Hixson, M.L., R.C. Lefebre, and S. Banspach. 1988. Evaluation of a grocery store point of purchase nutrition intervention program. Paper presented at the 1988 Annual Meeting of the Society for Behavioral Medicine, Boston.

Hochbaum, G. 1981. Strategies and their rationale for changing people's eating habits. J. Nutr. Ed. 13(Suppl):59–65.

Houston, D.L. 1985. USDA's regulation of food claims. Food, Drug, Cosmetic Law J. 40:238–243.

Hutt, P.B. 1985. The importance of analytical chemistry to food and drug regulation. Vanderbilt Law Rev. 38:479–493.

IFIC/ADA (International Food Information Council and The American Dietetic Association). 1990. How Are Americans Making Food Choices? Results of a Gallup Survey. IFIC, Washington D.C. 27 pp.

Jacoby, J., R.W. Chestnut, and W. Silberman. 1977. Consumer use and comprehension of nutrition information. J. Consumer Res. 4:119–128.

Jacoby, J., J.C. Olson, G.J. Szybillo, and E.W. Hart. 1979. Behavioral science perspectives on conveying nutrition information to consumers. P. 2a in Criteria of Food Acceptance: How Man Chooses What He Eats, J. Solms and R.L. Hall, eds. Forster, Zurich. 461 pp.

Kessler, D.A. 1989. The federal regulation of food labeling. Promoting foods to prevent disease. N. Engl. J. Med. 321:717–725.

Khachik, F., G.R. Beecher, and W.R. Lusby. 1989. Separation, identification, and quantification of the major carotenoids in extracts of apricots, peaches, cantaloupe, and pink grapefruit by liquid chromatography. J. Agric. Food Chem. 37:1465–1473.

Klein, B.P., and A.K. Perry. 1982. Ascorbic acid and vitamin A activity in selected vegetables from different geographical areas of the United States. J. Food Sci. 47:941–945.

Krzynowek, J. 1988. Effects of handling, processing, and storage on fish and shellfish. Pp. 245–265 in Nutritional Evaluation of Food Processing, 3rd ed., E. Karmas and R.S. Harris, eds. Van Nostrand Reinhold Co., New York.

Kushner, G.J., R.S. Silverman, S.B. Steinborn, and R.A. Johnson. 1990. A Guide to Federal Food Labeling Requirements. Prepared for the U.S. Department of Agriculture and the U.S. Department of Health and Human Services, Washington, D.C. 42 pp.

Lanza, E., and R.R. Butrum. 1986. A critical review of food fiber analysis and data. J. Am. Diet. Assoc. 86:732–743.

Lecos, C. 1988. Food labels—test your food label knowledge. FDA Consumer 22(2):16–21.

Lenahan, R.J., J.A. Thomas, D.A. Taylor, D.L. Call, and P.I. Padberg. 1972. Consumer reaction to nutrition information on food product labels. Search Agric. 2(15):1–26.

Leung-Chung, E., L.S. Sims, and J. Olson. 1985. Assessing consumers' comprehension of nutrition information on food labels. Unpublished working paper. Pennsylvania State University, University Park.

Levy, A.S., and M. Stephenson. 1990. Nutrition knowledge levels about dietary fats and cholesterol: 1983–1988. Unpublished paper. Food and Drug Administration, Washington, D.C. 20 pp.

Levy, A.S., and R.C. Stokes. 1987. Effects of a health promotion advertising campaign on sales of ready-to-eat cereals. Public Health Rep. 102:398–403.

Levy, A.S., O. Mathews, M. Stephenson, J.E. Tenney, and R.E. Schucker. 1985. The impact of a nutrition information program on food purchases. J. Marketing Public Policy 4:1–3.

Li, B.W., M.W. Marshall, K.W. Andrews, and T.T. Adams. 1988. Analysis of individual foods for the validation of sugars and starch contents of composited diets. J. Food Comp. Anal. 1:152–158.

Light, L., B. Portnoy, J.E. Blair, J.M. Smith, A.B. Rodgers, E. Tuckermanty, J. Tenney, and O. Mathews. 1989. Nutrition education in supermarkets. Family and Community Health: J. Health Promotion Maintenance 12(1):43–52.

LSRO, FASEB (Life Sciences Research Office, Federation of American Societies for Experimental Biology). 1984. Assessment of the Folate Nutritional Status of the U.S. Population Based on Data Collected in the Second National Health and Nutrition Examination Survey, 1976–1980, F.R. Senti and S.M. Pilch, eds. FASEB, Bethesda, Md. 96 pp.

LSRO, FASEB (Life Sciences Research Office, Federation of American Societies for Experimental Biology). 1989. Nutrition Monitoring in the United States: An Update Report on Nutrition Monitoring. Prepared for the U.S. Department of Agriculture and the U.S. Department of Health and Human Services. Government Printing Office, Washington, D.C. 408 pp.

Marlett, J.A., and D. Navis. 1988. Comparison of gravimetric and chemical analyses of total dietary fiber in foods. J. Agric. Food Chem. 36:311–315.

Marlett, J.A., J.G. Chesters, M.J. Longacre, and J.J. Bogdanske. 1989. Recovery of soluble dietary fiber is dependent on the method of analysis. Am. J. Clin. Nutr. 50:479–485.

Mazis, M.B., and R. Staelin. 1982. Using information-processing principles in public policymaking. J. Marketing Public Policy 1:314.

McCullough, J., and R. Best. 1980. Consumer preference for food label information: A basis for segmentation. J. Consumer Affairs 14(1):180–192.

McGuire, W.J. 1969. The nature of attitudes and attitude change. Pp. 136–314 in

Handbook of Social Psychology, vol. 3, 2nd ed., G. Lindzey and E. Aronson, eds. Addison-Wesley, Reading, Mass.

McGuire, W.J. 1976. Some internal psychological factors influencing consumer choices. J. Consumer Res. 2:302.

Mohr, K.G., B.W. Wyse, and R.G. Hansen. 1980. Aiding consumer nutrition decisions: Comparison of a graphical nutrient density labeling format with the current food label system. Home Econ. Res. J. 8(3):162–172.

Muller, T.E. 1985. Structural information factors which stimulate the use of nutrition information: A field experiment. J. Marketing Res. 22(2):143–157.

Mullin, W.J., D.F. Wood, and S.G. Howsam. 1982. Some factors affecting folacin content of spinach, Swiss chard, broccoli and Brussels sprouts. Nutr. Rep. Int. 26:7–16.

Mullis, R.M., M.K. Hunt, M. Foster, L. Hachfeld, D. Lansing, P. Snyder, and P. Pirie. 1987. The Shop Smart for Your Heart grocery program. J. Nutr. Ed. 19(5):225–228.

Nagy, S., and W.F. Wardowski. 1988. Effect of agricultural practices, handling, processing, and storage on fruits. Pp. 73–100 in Nutritional Evaluation of Food Processing, 3rd ed., E. Karmas and R.S. Harris, eds. Van Nostrand Reinhold Co., New York.

Newman, A.R. 1989. Measuring the fat of the land. Anal. Chem. 61:663A–664A.

NRC (National Research Council). 1989. Diet and Health: Implications for Reducing Chronic Disease Risk. Report of the Committee on Diet and Health, Food and Nutrition Board, Commission on Life Sciences. National Academy Press, Washington, D.C. 749 pp.

Ockerman, H.W. 1988. Effects of agricultural practices, handling, processing, and storage on meat. Pp. 153–202 in Nutritional Evaluation of Food Processing, 3rd ed., E. Karmas and R.S. Harris, eds. Van Nostrand Reinhold Co., New York.

Olson, J., and L.S. Sims. 1980. Assessing nutrition knowledge from an information processing perspective. J. Nutr. Ed. 12(3):157–161.

ORC (Opinion Research Corporation). 1990. Food Labeling and Nutrition: What Americans Want. Survey conducted for the National Food Processors Association. ORC, Washington D.C. 178 pp.

Parrish, D.B., R.A. Moffitt, R.J. Noel, and J.N. Thompson. 1985. Vitamin A. Pp. 153–184 in Methods of Vitamin Assay, 4th ed., J. Augustin, B.P. Klein, D. Becker, and P.B. Venugopal, eds. John Wiley & Sons, New York. 590 pp.

Prosky, L., N.-G. Asp, I. Furda, J.W. DeVries, T.F. Schweizer, and B.F. Harland. 1985. Determination of total dietary fiber in foods and food products: Collaborative study. J. Assoc. Off. Anal. Chem. 68:677–679.

Prosky, L., N.-G. Asp, T.F. Schweizer, J.W. DeVries, and I. Furda. 1988. Determination of insoluble, soluble, and total dietary fiber in foods and food products: Interlaboratory study. J. Assoc. Off. Anal. Chem. 71:1017–1023.

Putnam, J.J., and J. Weimer. 1981. Household diet changes linked to nutrition concerns. Staff paper of Economic and Statistics Service, U.S. Department of Agriculture, Washington, D.C. 11 pp.

Quelch, J.A. 1977. The role of nutrition information in national nutrition policy. Nutr. Rev. 35(11):289–293.

Rahn, M.J. 1980. Nutrition knowledge of a sample of urban women. Unpublished M.S. thesis. Faculty of Graduate Studies, University of Guelph, Guelph, Ontario, Canada.

Renner, E. 1988. Effects of agricultural practices on milk and dairy products. Pp. 203–

224 in Nutritional Evaluation of Food Processing, 3rd ed., E. Karmas and R.S. Harris, eds. Van Nostrand Reinhold Co., New York.

Robinson, J.P. 1990. Thanks for reading this. Am. Demogr. 12(2):6–7.

Rudd, J. 1986. Aiding consumer nutrition decisions with the simple graphic label format. Home Econ. Res. J. 14(3):342–346.

Rudd, J. 1989. Consumer response to calorie base variations on the graphical nutrient density food label. J. Nutr. Ed. 21:259–264.

Rudd, J., and K. Glanz. 1990. How individuals use information for health action: Consumer information processing. In Health Behavior and Health Education, K. Glanz, F.M. Lewis, and B.K. Rimer, eds. Jossey-Bass, San Francisco.

Russo, J.E., R. Staelin, C.A. Nolan, G.J. Russell, and B.L. Metcalf. 1986. Nutrition information in the supermarket. J. Consumer Res. 13:48–70.

Salunkhe, D.K., and B.B. Desai. 1988. Effects of agricultural practices, handling, processing, and storage on vegetables. Pp. 21–71 in Nutritional Evaluation of Food Processing, 3rd ed., E. Karmas and R.S. Harris, eds. Van Nostrand Reinhold Co., New York.

Sansolo, M., ed. 1990. Progressive Grocer. April. MacLean Hunter Media, Stamford, Conn. 66 pp.

Scammon, D. 1978. Information load and consumers. J. Consumer Res. 4(3):148–155.

Sempos, C., R. Fulwood, C. Haines, M. Carroll, R. Anda, D.F. Williamson, P. Remington, and J. Cleeman. 1989. The prevalence of high blood cholesterol levels among adults in the United States. J. Am. Med. Assoc. 262(1):45–52.

Shepherd, S.K. 1990. Nutrition and the consumer: Meeting the challenge of nutrition education in the 1990s. Food Nutr. News 62(1):1–3.

Shepherd, S.K., L.S. Sims, F.J. Cronin, A. Shaw, and C.A. Davis. 1989. Use of focus groups to explore consumers' preferences for content and graphic design of nutrition publications. J. Am. Diet. Assoc. 89(11):1612–1614.

Simpson, K.L., S.C.S. Tsou, and C.O. Chichester. 1985. Carotenes. Pp. 185–220 in Methods of Vitamin Assay, 4th ed. J. Augustin, B.P. Klein, D. Becker, and P.B. Venugopal, eds. John Wiley & Sons, New York.

Sims, L.S. 1981. Further thoughts on research perspectives in nutrition education. J. Nutr. Ed. 13(1):S70–S75.

Sims, L.S., and Sheperd, S.K. 1985. Further Exploration of Formatting, Structuring, and Sequencing of Nutrition Information for Household Food Managers. Final report submitted in partial fulfillment of FNS contact no. 53–3198–4–66. U.S. Department of Agriculture, Washington, D.C. 97 pp.

Sloan, A.E. 1987. Educating a nutrition-wise public. J. Nutr. Ed. 19:303–305.

Slover, H.T., and E. Lanza. 1979. Quantitative analysis of food fatty acids by capillary gas chromatography. J. Am. Oil Chem. Soc. 56:933–943.

Snider, S., P. Kendal, W. Hurst, C. Bueso, and E. Burns. 1990. Regional Communicators' Focus Group Summary. Institute of Food Technologists, Chicago. 24 pp.

Stewart, K.K. 1981. Nutrient analyses of food: A review and a strategy for the future. In Beltsville Symposia in Agricultural Research [4] Human Nutrition Research, G.R. Beecher, ed. Allanheld, Osmun Publishers, Totowa, N.J.

Stewart, K.K. 1985. Method choice and development. Pp. 1–15 in Methods of Vitamin

Assay, 4th ed., J. Augustin, B.P. Klein, D. Becker, and P.B. Venugopal, eds. John Wiley & Sons, New York.

Stewart, K.K. 1988. Improvement of food composition data. Needs for analytical training. Editorial. J. Food Comp. Anal. 1:291–292.

Stewart, K.K. 1989. Data validation. Editorial. J. Food Comp. Anal. 2:91–92.

Subar, A.F., G. Block, and L.D. James. 1989. Folate intake and food sources in the US population. Am. J. Clin. Nutr. 50:508–516.

Timmer, C.P., and M.C. Nesheim. 1979. Nutrition, product quality, and safety. Pp. 155–203 in Consensus and Conflict in U.S. Agriculture: Perspectives from the National Farm Summit, B.L. Gardner and J.W. Richardson, eds. Texas A&M University Press, College Station. 280 pp.

USDA (U.S. Department of Agriculture). 1979. Chemistry Laboratory Guidebook. Food Safety and Quality Service, Science. Government Printing Office, Washington, D.C.

USDA (U.S. Department of Agriculture). 1988. FSIS Policy Memorandum 085B. Food Safety and Inspection Service, Washington, D.C.

USDA (U.S. Department of Agriculture). 1989a. Food Cost Review. Agricultural Economic Report No. 615 (July). Economic Research Service, Washington, D.C. 54 pp.

USDA (U.S. Department of Agriculture). 1989b. National Food Review 1989 Yearbook: Food Beyond the Farm Gate (April-June). Economic Research Service, Washington, D.C. 52 pp.

Venkatesan, M. 1977. Providing nutritional information to consumers. Paper presented at Special National Science Foundation/Massachusetts Institute of Technology Conference on Consumer Research for Consumer Policy, Cambridge, Mass., July.

Venkatesan, M., W. Lancaster, and K.W. Kendall. 1986. An empirical study of alternate formats for nutritional information disclosure in advertising. J. Public Policy Marketing 5:29–43.

Woolcott, D.M. 1983. Nutrition concerns and information seeking behavior of rural and urban women. Paper presented at the Society for Nutrition Education, Denver.

Yankelovich, Inc. 1971. Nutrition labeling: A consumer experiment to determine the effects of nutrition labeling on food purchases. Chain Store Age (January):57–77.

PART II
REFORMING FOOD LABELS

5

Labeling Coverage

Health professionals have achieved a consensus on the characteristics of foods Americans should choose to have both a healthier diet and reduce the risk factors for chronic diseases and conditions. *The Surgeon General's Report on Nutrition and Health* (DHHS, 1988) and the National Research Council (NRC) report, *Diet and Health: Implications for Reducing Chronic Disease Risk* (NRC, 1989), set forth the scientific findings and recommended changes that should be made in dietary intake patterns and the need for expanded nutrition labeling described in this report. In addition, the *Year 2000 Objectives for the Nation* propose that there be an increase in nutrition labeling that provides information to facilitate choosing foods consistent with the Dietary Guidelines for Americans to at least 80 percent of processed foods and 40 percent of fresh meat, poultry, fruits, vegetables, baked goods, and ready-to-eat carry-away foods (DHHS, 1989).

MANDATORY NUTRITION LABELING

If consumers are to make the dietary adjustments recommended by the health care community, they must be able to make informed judgments across the full spectrum of their daily shopping, cooking, and eating decisions. It is extremely unlikely that significant advances in consumer application of current dietary guidelines to everyday purchase and consumption decisions can be made if each label poses a new challenge to consumers. The lack of relevant information and the inconsistency of label formats among products are significant deterrents to making informed choices. Other issues include the quantity and complexity of information and comprehension issues (see Chapter 4). Mandatory nutrition labeling requirements for most packaged foods and foods sold at various eating locations would present consumers with a consistent set of information in a uniform format.

Committee Recommendations

The Committee recommends that:

- The Food and Drug Administration (FDA) and the U.S. Department of Agriculture (USDA) should promptly adopt regulations to institute mandatory and uniform nutrition labeling requirements for all packaged foods under their respective jurisdictions, with some exemptions as outlined in the next section. The agencies' legal authority to implement this recommendation is discussed in Chapter 8.

Exemptions

Exemptions could be provided for products that make no significant nutritional contribution per serving or that are physically unsuited to carry the nutrition panel. No exemption should be allowed for any food for which a nutrition claim is made. Additionally, no exemption should be made unless all alternatives to nutrition labeling have been considered and found unreasonable, impractical, and/or costly.

No Nutritional Significance If a food does not make, and is not generally expected to make, a significant nutritional contribution, nutrition labeling should be optional, not required. Examples include tea bags, flavors, spices, and bottled water. However, the Committee recommends that:

- The agencies should establish criteria for determining nutritional significance, such as a threshold for the number of calories (and/or other nutrients) per serving below which nutrition labeling would be optional.

Package Size Foods sold in small packages also warrant consideration of exemption. If a package is too small to accommodate nutrition labeling and the package cannot reasonably accommodate a larger label, it would not be cost-effective, even if theoretically possible, to require mandatory labeling. However, the Committee recommends that:

- Alternatives such as nutrition labeling on larger packages containing multiple individually wrapped servings or other point-of-purchase alternatives be required for foods sold in small packages.

Baby Food

The recommendations of recent reports linking nutrition and long-term health have been proposed for adults and children over age 2. The dietary needs of infants and toddlers up to age 2 differ from those of adults and older children. Although the labeling and minimum nutrient content of infant formulas are defined by specific FDA regulations (21 CFR Part 107), the labeling of commercial baby foods and products intended for children under age 2 can be considered a special case in the revision of nutrition labeling policy.

Because of the high rate of growth and organ development of infants up to age 2, their requirements for essential nutrients and energy differ markedly from those of adults, especially with respect to calories, protein, fat, cholesterol, and dietary fiber (AAP, 1985). Consumption of foods that provide adequate caloric intake is essential for maintaining appropriate rates of growth and development. In particular, fat is an important food component for infants and toddlers because of its high caloric density. However, fat does not need to be saturated or come from sources rich in cholesterol. Sugars and other carbohydrates represent additional sources of energy, although the relationship between sugar intake and dental caries is well recognized. Consumption of high-fiber diets is not beneficial for infants and young children; the immature intestinal tract may not tolerate excessive amounts of dietary fiber. Although not well documented in young children, impaired absorption of trace minerals may also occur when they consume diets high in fiber.

It should be emphasized that these considerations apply only to foods intended for infants and children under age 2. The present scientific evidence indicates that the same dietary recommendations developed for adults generally apply to children over age 2 (NRC, 1989). Despite earlier concern about the possible special needs of older children and adolescents for fat, cholesterol, and sodium, the best evidence now indicates that diets lower in saturated fatty acids, cholesterol, and sodium, as recommended for adults, are safe and also likely to be beneficial for children in those age groups.

Current regulations require nutrition labeling to be provided on foods for children under age 4 (21 CFR § 101.9(h)(1)) using the U.S. Recommended Daily Allowances (U.S. RDA) for that group and in compliance with the other rules for nutrition labeling.

Committee Recommendations

Nutrition labeling of foods intended for children under age 2 should reflect the dietary principles discussed above. Nutrition labeling based on recommendations for adults (e.g., U.S. RDA) with respect to fat, cholesterol, and dietary fiber could be misleading to consumers (e.g., parents) who are not familiar with the special nutritional needs of infants and young children, promoting the selection of nutritionally inappropriate diets for their children.

The Committee recommends that:

- Labeling of calories, fat, cholesterol, protein, carbohydrate, dietary fiber, and sodium content should be required, by weight in grams or milligrams per serving, on foods designed for children under age 2.
- Declaration of calcium and iron content should be mandatory for baby food. In the absence of compelling nutritional justification with respect to other vitamins and minerals, label information on these nutrients should be provided on an optional basis as a percentage of the U.S. RDA for children under age 2 for which the food is intended.

Institutional Packages and Commodity Foods

Food packages used by commercial food service and the larger food packages used by institutions are currently exempted from nutrition labeling regulations (21 CFR § 101.9(h)(8)). Nutrition labeling of large containers or provision of nutrition information through product specification sheets used by institutions makes nutrition information more accessible, and since containers are generally larger than those for foods purchased in grocery stores, nutrition labeling can easily be provided and can even be expanded. Specification sheets that include nutrition information are usually provided by suppliers; thus, food costs are not expected to rise if nutrition labeling is also required.

The Commodity Distribution Reform Act of 1987 (P.L. 100-237) commissioned the National Advisory Council on Commodity Distribution to be formed to recommend changes through an annual report to the Secretary of USDA and the U.S. Congress. The purpose of the Council is to advise the Secretary on regulations and policy development with respect to specifications for commodities and other issues. In its first annual report, the Council recommended that:

> Nutrition analysis or nutritional labeling should be investigated for all USDA commodities, especially items used in the Commodity Supplemental Food Program and the Food Distribution Program on Indian Reservations (USDA, 1989b, p. 4).

Committee Recommendations

The Committee recommends that:

- FDA and USDA should require nutrition labeling on packages or specification sheets for products used by institutional food services.
- USDA should require nutrition labeling on commodities distributed through the agency's food programs.

PRODUCE, SEAFOOD, AND MEAT AND POULTRY

Overview of the Issues in Labeling of Fresh Foods

A strong argument for point-of-purchase nutrition information for fresh food products is to provide consumers with sufficient information to promote the consumption of more fruits and vegetables and to be able to choose leaner meats. In general, fruits and vegetables (referred to here as produce) are major sources of vitamins, minerals, and dietary fiber. They do not contain cholesterol and are typically low in fat. Meat, poultry, and seafood (referred to here as muscle-based foods) are important dietary sources of high-quality protein and B vitamins. Both meat and seafood are sources of minerals (e.g., iron and zinc in beef and copper in seafood). Seafood is typically low in fat. Current dietary recommendations suggest that Americans should cut back their intakes of total fat, saturated fatty acids, and cholesterol; eat more fruits and vegetables; eat smaller portions of meat; choose leaner cuts of meat; and remove skin from poultry (DHHS, 1988; NRC, 1989).

Nutrition labeling of fresh foods should be an effective aid for health-conscious consumers, but the most appropriate method of labeling remains to be determined. Producers and retailers face special challenges in providing nutrition information on fresh produce. Before recommending a program for nutrition labeling of all produce, meat, poultry, and seafood, policymakers must consider the heterogeneity of foods, whether to list nutrient content data for the food in the manner in which it is purchased or prepared, the adequacy of the nutrient data bases, and potential technical problems.

Heterogeneity of Foods

As discussed in the section on analytical issues (see Chapter 4), foods are inherently heterogeneous, which is particularly true in the case of produce and muscle-based foods. This is in contrast to "pooled foods," such as flour or frozen orange juice, or formulated foods, which are more uniform in their composition and are batch tested.

Variabilities in the nutrient content of plant-derived foods are due to factors such as biological variability, including genetic characteristics; climatic and seasonal effects, such as precipitation and photoperiod; type of soil; and agricultural practices, such as the fertilization regimen, stage of maturity at the time of harvest, and postharvest handling. The nutrient composition of animal-derived foods varies as a function of genetic and nutritional factors, stage of maturity at the time of slaughter, and animal husbandry methods. Seafood is subject to an even higher degree of nutrient variability both within and between species.

Effects of Storage, Preparation, and Cooking

Fruits and vegetables are eaten both raw and cooked; muscle-based foods are primarily eaten cooked. In addition, many of these foods may be frozen or stored in the home for extended periods of time prior to consumption. All forms of food storage and preparation, whether commercial or in the home, cause some loss of nutrients (Adams and Erdman, 1988). Changes in food composition occur during cooking; for example, fat, water, and soluble nutrients are lost in drippings when meats are cooked, and leaching and various other modes of degradation of vitamins and minerals occur when fruits and vegetables are cooked. Changes in the bioavailabilities of certain vitamins, minerals, and amino acids may also occur during commercial or home preparation.

The magnitude of differences between the effects of commercial processing and home preparation of foods is not clear given the wide range of cooking conditions used. However, commercial processing is generally conducted under controlled conditions to minimize the loss of labile nutrients (Lund, 1988). In fact, greater losses of nutrients may occur during cooking in the home (Adams and Erdman, 1988). Variability in the effects of home preparation of foods, along with natural variations in food composition, pose obstacles to the provision of reasonably accurate data for a mandatory nutrition labeling program for all foods.

Fruits and Vegetables   Produce is eaten either raw or cooked. Storage, preparation, and cooking methods affect the nutrient composition of fruits and vegetables. These effects are not reflected in the nutrient composition data on raw produce.

The level of maturity at the time of harvest and storage methods affect nutrient changes over time. For example, the vitamin A content of carrots and sweet potatoes increases with maturity (USDA, 1984a). Thus, because canned and frozen carrots are usually more mature than fresh carrots, they may have higher levels of vitamin A. The caloric value of Jerusalem artichokes actually increases with storage. A significant portion of their carbohydrates is in the form of inulin which has limited bioavailability. Over time, the inulin is converted to sugar (USDA, 1984a). Avocados harvested at different times display fat contents that range from 8 to over 20 percent. This change strongly affects the caloric content. Half of an avocado (Fuerte variety) has 80 kcal if harvested when it has 8.3 percent fat and 237 kcal if harvested when it has 22.8 percent fat (Slater et al., 1975).

Losses of certain vitamins begin with harvesting and can be accelerated by the method and/or length of storage and processing. Freshly harvested potatoes contain about 26 mg of vitamin C per 100 g. After 3 months of storage, the vitamin C content decreases to about 13 mg, and after 6 months it decreases to about 8 mg/100 g. During cooking or processing, nutrient composition values are altered by the addition of fat, sodium (as salt), and carbohydrates (as sugar) and by the leaching of vitamins and minerals when foods are boiled. Most fruits and vegetables are naturally low in sodium. Thus, the amount of sodium in cooked vegetables reflects the amount of sodium or salt used in the cooking water, which is usually tap water (USDA, 1984a). This is true for all foods prepared in or with tap water. Food composition values for fruits and vegetables given in data bases may also overestimate the actual amounts of vitamins because of losses during food preparation. For example, chopping, shredding, and cutting of vegetables such as cabbage, lettuce, and squash result in the loss of vitamin C activity because of oxidation.

Meat, Poultry, and Seafood   Methods of home cooking have different effects on the nutrient composition of muscle-based foods. The different levels of fat in various grades of muscle-based foods, the trimming of fat or removal of skin during preparation, and the method of preparation affect the final fat content of those foods after they are cooked. The contents of those other nutrients also change during preparation and cooking, most notably through the addition of salt.

For meat, the percent change in fat content during cooking differs between grades. The total amount of fat in the cooked product, if prepared by similar methods, would be greater in those that exhibit the highest initial fat content. Large differences in the fat content of fried and other broiled or steamed seafood have been reported (NRC, 1989). In addition, breading may result in up to a fourfold increase in sodium content. The fat, carbohydrate, and sodium content of poultry products are affected by the method of cooking, removal of skin, breading, and seasoning. These factors clearly would not be reflected by nutrition labeling of raw muscle-based foods.

Adequacy of Food Composition Data Bases

The use of data bases would be a more practical alternative to routine laboratory analysis of fresh foods. Issues related to the use of data bases include whether the existing ones contain valid composition data and whether sampling has been adequate to ensure representative data. Variability among samples is a factor in determining the final data that should be included in data bases. An additional issue concerns the accuracy of data bases that could serve as the basis for nutrition information in food labeling.

USDA Primary Data Set   The USDA National Nutrition Data Bank is the authoritative source of data on the nutrient composition of foods in the United States. This data base provides representative data for many raw, processed, and prepared foods. It is not complete, however, in the case of many species of seafood and certain varieties of fruits and vegetables. Additionally, data for many foods that have undergone some form of preparation are not included. The data base is continually being expanded and periodically reevaluated and this improvement must continue. The current update began in 1976, and to date, 19 of the 22 volumes of data have been completed (Ruth Matthews, Human Nutrition Information Service, USDA, personal communication, 1990).

Other food composition data bases exist in the United States and throughout the world. Many non-USDA data bases are based on specialized analytical data, cover selected foods that are not covered in the USDA data base, or offer commercial calculations of nutrient intakes. Bergstrom (1988) reviewed the use of data bases and conducted limited comparisons of the USDA data base with those of four European countries. Although the values for water, protein, and energy were similar, wide variations were reported for total fat, fatty acids, vitamins, and minerals. These discrepancies are presumably due to both the limitations of analytical methods and the heterogeneities of the foods that were evaluated. Information from data bases cannot be as precise as that from direct laboratory analysis of a specific lot, but such laboratory analytical data also can be misleading because of wide lot-to-lot variation. Certainly the use of the USDA and other data bases can provide representative data for nutrition labeling.

Data Bases for Meat and Poultry   USDA composition data are relatively complete for a variety of cuts and grades of beef subjected to representative cooking methods (USDA, 1990). The data are presented for separate lean, edible portions and assume that there is some trimming prior to consumption. In addition, USDA composition data are fairly complete for poultry products (USDA, 1979); pork products (USDA, 1983); and lamb, veal, and game (USDA, 1989a).

Data Bases for Seafood   The creation of food composition data bases for seafood required considerable effort with respect to the diversity of domestically harvested species, the natural variabilities in their composition, and the further influence of cooking methods on nutrient content. An additional complication is the fact that approximately 70 percent of seafood eaten in the United States is imported (IOM, 1990). Currently, there are composition data for 92 raw and 82 prepared seafood products (USDA, 1987). Few other systematic sources of seafood composition data are available. However, a compilation of data on seafood harvested and consumed in the southeastern United States has been assembled by Sullivan and Otwell (1990).

As indicated previously, the validity of much of the published nutrient composition data for seafood is frequently uncertain due to the high degree of natural variability of these products. Within most species, composition is influenced by various factors, including geographic location, season, stage of the reproductive cycle, age, and diet. One of the most variable aspects of seafood composition is the quantity of total fat and the distribution of fatty acids. Studies of the seasonal and geographic variabilities of the fatty acid distribution of finfish have indicated wide variations even when samples involved thousands of finfish to minimize effects of within-group differences (Stansby, 1981). For example, the percentage of eicosapentanoic acid, a major omega-3 fatty acid, ranged from 11.4 to 15.2 percent in herring oil from finfish caught off Alaska and from 3.9 to 8.8 percent in herring oil from finfish caught off Nova Scotia. Substantial variation in the total content of lipid (fat or oil) also occurs. These findings illustrate the difficulty in determining "representative" data for seafood lipids.

Stansby (1982) further examined the problems of within-species variability and proposed a classification system for seafood that was based on only five categories, by total fat and protein content. With approximately 85 percent of the seafood eaten in the United States being in the low-oil and high-protein category, such data could provide the starting point for developing a system of presentation of seafood composition data.

Data Bases for Fresh Produce   The average supermarket has approximately 240 items in its produce department (PMA, 1988). The primary issue is whether current data bases are sufficient and appropriate for nutrition labeling of fruits and vegetables.

Although available for most produce, data are incomplete for many varieties for the assessment of differences in nutrient content due to maturity, growing location, season, and environmental factors (USDA, 1982, 1984a,b). Where data are available for different varieties of fruits, weighted values for a given nutrient may be available based on production and marketing statistics. For example, California Valencia oranges are reported to have more vitamin A (23 retinol equivalents, RE) than Florida oranges (20 RE). Both have relatively less than the average orange (25 RE), a value derived from composite sampling based on marketing statistics for fresh oranges (i.e., California navel and Valencia oranges and Florida oranges). The nutritional and statistical significance of using average values is unclear.

The differences in nutrient composition of different varieties of the same vegetable are generally too small to justify separate entries (USDA, 1984a). For example, the nutrient values given for raw potatoes represent a composite of Russet Burbank (35.8 percent), Kennebec (4.2 percent), Katahdin (30.3 percent), Superior (5.8 percent), Norgold (12.8 percent), Pontiac (5.6 percent), and White Rose (5.4 percent) (USDA, 1984a).

The nutrient content of fruits and vegetables can vary depending on the soil in which the plants are grown (Leveille, 1983). This variation can be a special problem when reporting values for trace mineral content, because there can be huge differences in the same type of food. For example, the selenium content of New England–grown wheat may be quite different than that of Iowa-grown wheat.

There are concerns about the adequacy of much of the published data on the fiber content of foods. Insoluble dietary fiber was frequently determined by the neutral detergent fiber method in the development of data between 1977 and 1988. Various applications of this method have been reviewed by Lanza and Butrum (1986). Originally developed for animal forages, the neutral detergent fiber method underestimates the total fiber in the human food supply. The soluble fiber in most fruits and vegetables in the USDA data base is measured as pectin, which underestimates the amount of soluble fiber, and data are not complete for all fruits and vegetables. The Prosky method, which was approved by the Association of Official Analytical Chemists (AOAC) in 1988, is currently the preferred method for determining total dietary fiber (see Chapter 4). However, the USDA-provided fiber contents of fruits and vegetables that were published prior to 1988 (USDA, 1982, 1984a,b) were not derived by the Prosky method.

The Produce Marketing Association (PMA) is another source of data. It has established a national nutrient data base for a number of different produce commodity groups in the United States. Data are collected so that information may be given for individual fruits and vegetables at the point of purchase in compliance with FDA guidelines. FDA has argued that the data base information may not be representative of the items sold. PMA has argued that the numbers that it has generated represent up-to-date information for specific items.

The PMA Nutrition Labeling Program has been extended to include artichokes, asparagus, bell peppers, broccoli, cabbage, California dates, cantaloupes, carrots, cauliflower, celery, cucumbers, honeydew melons, iceberg lettuce, kiwi fruit, Le Rouge Royale (red) peppers, mushrooms, onions, papayas, pineapples, potatoes, radishes, spinach, strawberries, tomatoes, and watermelon. In contrast, the USDA data base responds more slowly to changes in the composition of foods sold in the marketplace because of technological and funding constraints. USDA updates its data on a moving average, and it may be a number of years for the data base to reflect new information. These apparently troublesome sources of variability recede somewhat in importance when considered in the context of a total diet eaten over many years. The nutrient content of a specific lot is thus of less critical importance.

Point-of-Purchase Nutrition Information
Programs for Produce and Meat

Within the past 10 years, several point-of-purchase nutrition information programs have been conducted in supermarkets. When signs containing nutrition information were provided in the produce departments of 300 stores of a major national supermarket chain, the signs seemingly had no effect on the in-store purchasing behavior of customers during the 1-month study period (Achabal et al., 1987). The limited number of produce items carrying information, the small size and physical placement of the signs, and the short time frame for the study were suggested as reasons why the signs had no effect on sales.

In 1984, the Minnesota Heart Health Program, in collaboration with the Minnesota Beef Council and the Minnesota Pork Producers Council, began a program to teach consumers how to select and prepare lean cuts of meat and choose appropriate portion sizes (Mullis and Pirie, 1988). Labels on individual meat packages and rail strips identified and promoted various lean cuts at the meat case. On the basis of sales data, the program appeared to have an effect on purchases of specific lean cuts of meat; for example, 80 percent lean ground beef outsold 70 percent lean ground beef in participating stores, whereas the opposite was true in control stores (presumably due to cost differences).

The Meat Nutri-Facts program, sponsored jointly by the American Meat Institute, the Food Marketing Institute, and the National Live Stock and Meat Board, was designed to provide consumers with accurate, up-to-date nutrition information on 3-ounce portions of trimmed and cooked red meat (NLMB, 1990). The Nutri-Facts program used cards with detailed nutrient data on over 30 cuts of beef, pork, and lamb; rail strips with calories; stickers for individual meat packages; and take-home brochures with nutrition and recipe information. The program was evaluated through consumer, meat manager, consumer affairs, and supermarket business surveys. About two-thirds of consumers surveyed reported using Nutri-Facts materials in making meat selections, and approximately 80 percent of respondents found the graphs and brochures to be "just about right" in terms of complexity and the content of information displayed. Meat managers and consumer affairs officials judged the information to be very or somewhat helpful for consumers; however, they both cited the amount of time needed to maintain the program as the main deterrent for continuation of the program beyond the study period. In a 1-year followup survey, responses from retailers revealed that over 60 percent had continued the Nutri-Facts program. Poultry and Seafood Nutri-Facts programs were subsequently initiated, but have not yet been formally evaluated. Additional consumer education and a longer evaluation period in studies such as these may reveal greater effectiveness.

Current FDA Guidelines for Labeling of Fresh Fruits and Vegetables

Although nutrition information for fresh produce is not currently required at the point of purchase, FDA requires that, when it is provided, it be based on up-to-date information about the item that the consumer purchases at the store. This requirement precludes the use of information from the USDA nutrient data bank if current laboratory methods and sampling procedures are not used.

FDA's regulatory compliance assurance standards for nutrition labeling do not currently allow average values, such as those given in the USDA data base.

For example, if a producer wants to give nutrition information for an apple, FDA requires that the values for vitamins, minerals, and dietary fiber on the label reflect the apple that a consumer selects 95 percent of the time, representing the lower end of the sampling distribution. For calories, fat, and sodium, the upper end of the sampling distribution is reported. In order to construct a randomized composite sample that is in compliance with FDA requirements and, therefore, that is representative of the large variations in nutrition content of individual items, a market-basket sampling approach is typically used.

Enforcement Issues in Labeling of Fresh Foods

For FDA-regulated foods, strict enforcement of nutrition labeling requirements is difficult. This problem does not exist for USDA with its prior approval program for labels. However, mandatory labeling of fresh foods would involve FDA and USDA verification of compliance. The additional analytical burden and staffing requirements would be greater than current programs require. Current regulations regarding packaged foods indicate that the actual contents of the components must be no more than 20 percent greater than the label claim for fat, calories, sodium, and cholesterol and no more than 20 percent less than the label claim for vitamins and minerals. Given the variations in composition of fresh food products, adherence to this 20 percent tolerance would, in effect, require that labeling grossly distort the actual average composition of the product in order to be in regulatory compliance. Regulatory compliance could be accomplished through less stringent regulations that permit the use of representative data (e.g., the mean or the mean ± one standard deviation) instead of the tolerances currently applied to nutrition labeling of packaged foods.

Committee Recommendations

Fresh foods make up an important part of the average American's diet. Although the Committee in principle favors nutrition labeling of all foods, in consideration of the issues related to nutrition labeling of fresh foods, a structured, yet flexible, approach is necessary.

The Committee recommends that:

- Retailers should be required to provide point-of-purchase nutrition labeling information for produce and for fresh and frozen meat, poultry, and seafood (e.g., 20 to 30 top items in each category using data base information, rather than lot-by-lot analysis). After the first 3 years, the program should be evaluated for consumer reaction, use, and understanding, and modified accordingly.
- FDA and USDA should allow flexibility in the format and nutrition information required for labeling of fresh foods.

- FDA and USDA should establish a joint committee to certify the data bases and acceptable methodologies for providing nutrient composition data on fresh foods.
- FDA and USDA should continue to improve the USDA's National Nutrient Data Bank, particularly in the area of fresh foods, in harmony with the above recommendations.

FOODS SOLD BY RESTAURANTS

As the 1990s commence, Americans continue to eat an increasing number of their meals away from home, albeit at a somewhat slower growth rate than in the 1980s (Claire Regan, National Restaurant Association, personal communication, 1990). In 1955, about 25 percent of the food dollar was spent on meals that were eaten away from home. By 1988, the share of the food dollar spent away from home had grown to 42.7 percent (NRA, 1990a). With one of every five meals being eaten away from home (Sweet, 1989), Americans were expected to spend about $156.4 billion on food eaten away from home in 1990 (NRA, 1990b). It is anticipated that as much as 50 percent of the food dollar may be spent on food eaten away from home by the year 2000.

Restaurant Segment of the Industry

The commercial food service industry is multifaceted. In 1989, commercial food service sales totaled $227.2 billion. Eating place sales totaled $147 billion in 1989 and accounted for 65 percent of total food service sales. Eating places include restaurants, lunchrooms, refreshment places, commercial cafeterias, social caterers, and ice cream and frozen custard stands. Federal definitions of eating and drinking places describe *restaurants* and *lunchrooms* as establishments engaged in serving food and beverages where patrons are served at tables and the operations have seating capacities for at least 15 people (DOC, 1987). *Refreshment places* consist of establishments that primarily sell limited lines of refreshments and prepared foods, including single-item establishments such as chicken, hamburger, and pizza places where food is either eaten on the premises or taken out. This latter definition is the closest to the type of restaurants considered to be limited-menu or fast food restaurants. In 1989, these two segments of the industry (restaurants, lunchrooms, and refreshment places) were estimated to represent about $73 billion in sales, and limited-menu restaurants had about $57 billion in sales (NRA, 1990b).

In 1986, the National Restaurant Association (NRA) estimated that as many as 45.8 million Americans (20 percent) are served at limited-menu restaurants each day (Massachusetts Medical Society, 1989). This segment of the industry has experienced phenomenal growth. From 1970 to 1980, sales at limited-menu restaurants increased 300 percent. Part of that growth has included expansion to public schools, colleges, military bases, and foreign countries. Menus have become more varied, and the hours of operation have expanded to include breakfast. Sales at limited-menu restaurants rose 8.8 percent in 1987, reaching $61.3 billion and grew from 14.7 percent of total industry food and drink sales in 1970 to 28.2 percent in 1988 (NRA, 1990a). This segment of the industry accounts for 44.2 percent (1,311,446 units) of total eating place sales.

Restaurant Eating Trends and Attitudes

The growing consumption of food outside the home can be attributed to several factors, including the increasing number of people who live alone, smaller families, the growing number of women employed outside the home, the prevalence of less formal life-styles, increases in disposable income, and consumers' desire for convenience. The fast pace of today's society means that the trend in away-from-home food consumption will continue to be a permanent part of the American life-style. This situation, in turn, leads to concerns about the impact of such eating patterns on long-term health.

In 1989, NRA conducted a nationwide survey to assess consumer awareness of and attitudes toward health and nutrition issues and their influence on the choice of foods and restaurants (Riehle, 1990). Consumers were asked questions about describe their eating habits, including their interest in low-fat foods when eating out, whether more restaurants should offer menu items cooked without salt, and whether they are less concerned about nutrition when dining out for a special occasion. The survey population fell into three distinct groups. *Unconcerned patrons* tended to describe themselves as meat and potato eaters, choosing whatever foods they want. *Committed patrons* believed that a good diet plays a role in the prevention of illness and said that when they eat out their dining behavior is generally consistent with their commitment to good nutrition. The *vacillating group* described themselves as concerned about nutrition and health, but said that their food choices were driven by taste and occasion when they eat out. Compared with the results of a similar 1986 survey, committed patrons grew from 35 percent in 1986 to 39 percent in 1989, whereas unconcerned patrons shrank from 38 to 32 percent. Table 5-1 gives the behavioral characteristics of the various groups and the foods they are most likely to order in restaurants.

Restaurant Attention to Dietary Recommendations

A 1986 Gallup survey conducted for NRA found that about 40 percent of the consumers polled claimed to be changing their away-from-home eating habits by consuming more vegetables and fewer fats, meat, and fried foods.

TABLE 5-1 Characteristics of Consumer Groups Regarding Attitudes Toward Health and Nutrition, 1989

Characteristics	Unconcerned Patrons	Committed Patrons	Vacillating Patrons
Percent of U.S. adult population	32	39	29
Percent of total eating-out occasions	39	32	29
Demographic characteristics[a]	Men; ages 18 to 24; average income; single/never married; work full time; high school education; live in urban areas; East North Central, West North Central, and Mountain states	Women; ages 35 to 54; higher than average income; married; work part time; college graduate; live in suburban areas; New England and Pacific states	Women; ages 65 years and older; below average income; widowed or separated/ divorced; do not work; high school education; live in rural areas; West South Central, East South Central, and South Atlantic states
Behaviorial characteristics[a]	Patronize limited-menu restaurants; do not diet or exercise; do not restrict use of salt, additives, sugar, fat, or cholesterol; drink alcoholic beverages; do not consume foods high in fiber, calcium, or starch	Patronize moderately priced and fine-dining restaurants; diet and exercise; restrict use of salt, additives, sugar, fat, and cholesterol; consume foods high in fiber, calcium, and starch	Patronize limited-menu and fine-dining establishments; diet to control blood cholesterol and pressure; are average in their attempts to restrict use of salt, additives, sugar, fat, and cholesterol; do not drink alcoholic beverages; consume foods high in calcium and starch
Foods likely to be ordered in restaurants[b]	Steak or roast beef; fried chicken or fish; regular soft drink; premium ice cream; rich, gooey, or chocolate desserts	Broiled or baked seafood; poultry without skin; raw vegetable appetizers; fresh fruit; vegetables seasoned with only herbs or lemon juice; whole-grain muffins; low-fat frozen yogurt	Lean meats; steak or roast beef; broiled or baked seafood; fried chicken or fish; food cooked without salt; regular soft drink; caffeine-free coffee; premium ice cream; rich, gooey, or chocolate desserts

[a] Members of all three groups come from all demographic and behavior segments. The characteristics presented here represent those in which a greater proportion than average occurs.

[b] Members of all groups are likely to order any of the foods covered by the survey. The ones presented here represent those foods that an above-average proportion of group members was likely to order.

SOURCE: Adapted from Riehle, H. 1990. Consumer commitment to nutrition increases. Restaurants USA March:36–38.

The survey also found that 23 percent of restaurant operators featured health and nutrition promotions, and nearly 75 percent said they would alter food preparation methods upon request (NRA, 1986). By 1989, approximately 40 percent of the food chain operators surveyed reported that they offered special nutritional menu items that were lower in calories, fat, salt, and cholesterol (Table 5-2). In the same survey, 75 percent of limited-menu and family restaurant chains reported that they provide nutrition information for patrons who request it, and 62 percent provide ingredient information available by the use of symbols (e.g., apples, doves, or hearts) for foods that meet some criteria for being low in fat, cholesterol, salt, and/or calories (NRA, 1989).

Restaurants can subscribe to programs that provide an evaluation of all or part of their recipes. Examples of this type of service are the American Heart Association's Healthy Heart program, Denver's Health Mark program, and the American Heart Association's Restaurant Guide prepared for consumers in Washington, D.C.

The proliferation of computer software to provide nutrient information at relatively low cost means that most establishments could afford evaluation of menus if they used these software programs rather than more expensive direct laboratory analyses. NRA has started a recipe evaluation service that members as well as other operators can use to determine the nutrient content of their recipes. The NRA recipe evaluation service provides nutrient information on calories, protein, carbohydrate, sugar, dietary fiber, sodium, fat (by level of saturation), and cholesterol. In addition, caloric distribution, diabetic exchanges, graphic analysis compared with dietary recommendations, and ingredients sorted by nutrients are provided. Other recipe and menu components can be evaluated

TABLE 5-2 Nutrition or Dietary Modifications to Foods Served by Food Chain Operators

Food Served	Number	Percent
Decaffeinated coffee	16	76
Low-fat milk	16	76
Entree salads and/or salad bars	15	71
Fruit juice	15	71
Reduced- or low-calorie salad dressing	15	71
Grilled chicken sandwich	11	52
Fresh fruit (including that on salad bar)	6	29
Low-fat frozen yogurt	6	29
Skim milk	5	24
Grilled fish sandwich	1	5

SOURCE: Adapted from National Restaurant Association. 1990. Current Issues Report: Nutrtion Awareness and the Foodservice Industry. NRC, Washington, D.C. 20 pp.

upon request. NRA's recipe evaluation service costs $10 per recipe ($20 for nonmembers), with the per recipe cost decreasing as the quantity of recipes increases. To date, use of the NRA service has exceeded original expectations (Claire Regan, NRA, personal communication, 1990).

Many restaurants include a statement on their menus that encourages special requests, such as to cook foods without the use of added salt or to provide sauces on the side. In addition, many menus describe the manner of food preparation, such as broiled, grilled, or poached, which can aid consumers in selecting foods that better meet their nutritional desires.

Table 5-3 shows the various methods used by NRA members to disseminate nutrient and ingredient information.

Current Regulatory Requirements

No specific federal laws or regulations require that the commercial food service industry provide nutrition information to consumers. However, FDA has taken the position that if nutrition labeling is provided, it must follow current agency regulations.

A nutrition claim or nutrition information concerning a combination of restaurant foods, e.g., the total nutritional value of a meal consisting of a hamburger, french fries, and milk shake, may be included in advertising and/or in labeling (other than labels) without causing nutrition information to be required on the label(s) of each article of food: *Provided,* That complete nutrition information for the combination of foods (the combination as an entity without the nutritional value of each article being specified) in the format established by 21 CFR § 101.9(c) is

TABLE 5-3 Method of Dissemination of Nutrition and Ingredient Information by Food Chain Operators

Method of Dissemination	Nutrition Information		Ingredient Information	
	Percent	Number	Percent	Number
Operators with information	76	16	62	13
Through corporate headquarters	67	14	52	11
In printed material (booklets, pamphlets, etc.)	57	12	33	7
In units	29	6	10	2
Toll-free telephone request	14	3	10	2
Wall posters	10	2	0	
On package	0		14	3
Interactive computer program	5	1	0	

SOURCE: Adapted from National Restaurant Association. 1990. Current Issues Report: Nutrtion Awareness and the Foodservice Industry. NRC, Washington, D.C. 20 pp.

effectively displayed to the customer both when he orders the food and when he consumes the food. This statement of policy does not apply to food dispensed in automatic vending machines (21 CFR § 101.10).

There is little evidence that this policy has been used or enforced.

In 1979, the U.S. Department of Health, Education, and Welfare (DHEW), USDA, and the Federal Trade Commission (FTC) considered the possibility of requiring ingredient labeling for restaurant foods (DHEW/USDA/FTC, 1979). The agencies asserted that they had the legal authority to require ingredient listings on foods sold in limited-menu establishments, where food is generally served in individually wrapped portions, but they were concerned about enforcement of such a requirement. FDA and USDA (FTC was not involved in this issue) expressed serious doubt about their authority to require ingredient information for foods sold unpackaged on plates. Neither agency took steps to implement labeling of any type for foods sold in restaurants.

In 1985, USDA and FDA were petitioned to require ingredient labeling on food packages in limited-menu restaurants. The petitioners claimed that the lack of ingredient labeling of these foods was a violation of existing laws and regulations. They viewed the highly standardized nature of the food products, the limited number of items offered on the menu, and the use of serving wrappers as easily accommodating the ingredient information being requested. Both agencies subsequently denied the petition. In general, they concluded that the petition failed to demonstrate that a change from the current policy was necessary, and expressed doubt that a definition of fast food was practicable, that enforcement against a single segment of the food service industry was equitable, or that the costs incurred would yield a real benefit to consumers. Both agencies also said that they regarded the regulation of the food service industry to be the responsibility of state and local regulatory authorities.

When the petition was denied, the attorneys general of several states threatened suit against five limited-menu restaurant chains to persuade them to provide ingredient and nutrition information about their products. In a negotiated settlement, McDonald's, Burger King, Jack in the Box, Kentucky Fried Chicken, and Wendy's agreed to distribute printed materials containing this information to consumers. The printed material was to be provided free at the point of purchase upon request; however, subsequent practice has shown that materials were not always available (Chicago Tribune, March 6, 1990). Recently, McDonald's has begun distributing posters and placemats containing nutrition information on foods sold at the point of selection in their restaurants (Michael Goldblatt, Nutrition Division, McDonald's Corporation, personal communication, 1990). Legislation to require nutrition and ingredient labeling in such restaurants has been introduced in several states but has not yet been enacted in any jurisdiction. Federal legislation to require nutrition information on the packaging of foods sold in limited-menu restaurants has been introduced in the past three sessions of Congress, but it has yet to be passed.

Current Status of Nutrition Labeling of Restaurant Foods

Some health and consumer groups have urged that information be provided on the ingredients and nutrient composition of foods sold in restaurants. Concerns about the consumption of salt, fat, sugar, and substances that cause allergic reactions in some people have led to increased attention to the nutritional profiles of foods sold in restaurants. Although current attention has focused chiefly on the limited-menu segment of the industry, there is no evidence that meals served by the restaurant and lunchroom segment of the industry are more (or less) nutritious or likely to meet the guidelines provided in dietary recommendations.

Although the Committee believes that improvements in nutrition labeling of foods purchased in grocery stores is the primary goal, it recognizes that Americans now spend almost half of their food dollar on meals consumed away from home. The Committee applauds the efforts of restaurants that are providing more nutrition information for the foods on their menus.

The Committee does not consider direct laboratory analysis–based labeling to be feasible for foods sold in most restaurants, but foods sold in limited-menu restaurants represent a special case. Reports on the fat, salt, sugar, and caloric composition of meals served in these establishments have led to numerous proposals to require nutrition labeling in limited-menu restaurants (Massachusetts Medical Society, 1989; Shields and Young, 1990). Several of these proposals would require the provision of nutrition information on preprinted food packages. Representatives of the industry oppose the requirement of nutrition information on food wrappers and cups, primarily for economic reasons. The Committee believes that there is a convincing case for providing consumers of meals at limited-menu restaurants with information about the nutrient composition of those meals. Their consumers consist largely of people on the go, as well as many children and young adults who are experiencing rapid growth and who are beginning to learn about long-term health. Furthermore, many of the foods served in vast quantities are high in fat, cholesterol, and sodium, and low in fiber.

The entire restaurant industry deserves credit for improving the nutritional quality of its product lines, but such innovations will be hastened if nutrition labeling is required. Consumers should come to expect and ask for this nutrition information in all restaurants. Many menu items become standard fare for the restaurants that serve them. Problems that make general labeling impractical for all restaurants at this time are less formidable in the context of limited-menu restaurants. Menu items are standardized, and their nutrient compositions are well characterized and carefully controlled across the country. In addition, many of the foods are already served in packages or wrappers designed for a particular food item on which the nutrition information could be placed. Furthermore, there are numerous other options for the presentation of nutrition information at the point of selection. The serving size for foods in these restaurants would be standardized, and therefore, nutrient content information would be based on these portion sizes. For other restaurants, where food is not preportioned, nutrient content information will need to be based on a normative-sized portion determined by the agencies.

The Committee believes that FDA and USDA should determine precisely how nutrition labeling should be provided in limited-menu restaurants. The Committee suggests that these agencies explore the most appropriate options with the affected industry, recognizing that nutrition labeling for some foods can be provided on the outside of the container or wrapper, whereas for others, placards at the point of selection may be appropriate.

Committee Recommendations

Considering the extent to which U.S. consumers are eating meals away from home, with nearly 50 percent of the food dollar being spent in these settings, the Committee believes that more complete nutrition information needs to be available to consumers at the point of selection. The Committee recommends that:

- All restaurants should be required to have standard menu items evaluated for their nutritional profiles and provide this information to patrons upon request. This evaluation can be performed by using the service provided by NRA, a comparable service, or computer software that is readily available and inexpensive. Laboratory analysis should not be required.
- Restaurant menus should be required to state that "nutrient evaluation is available upon request," so that consumers can, if they desire, obtain such information.
- FDA and USDA should, through regulations, allow the use of nutrient data bases to provide nutrient evaluation of menu items.
- Food service establishments above a specified size and/or volume (limited-menu and regional/national restaurant chains) should be required to provide nutrition analysis of food items at the point of purchase. This requirement can be met by placing the information either on package wrappers and containers or at some other point-of-purchase location that allows consumers easy access and use.
- Restaurants should be encouraged to participate in programs and/or otherwise provide for appropriate symbols or descriptors on menu items that identify foods that meet criteria for low-calorie, low-fat, low-cholesterol, and/or

low-sodium. Comparable definitions for symbols and descriptors should be established by FDA and USDA.

- FDA and USDA should define the categories and size of restaurant operations for which regulations based on the above recommendations are applicable.

FOODS SOLD BY NONCOMMERCIAL FOOD SERVICES

The Committee divided food service operations into two categories: commercial and noncommercial. Noncommercial food services comprise operations in locations such as day-care programs, elementary and secondary schools, colleges and universities, prisons, military installations, and health care facilities such as hospitals and nursing homes. Food service operations in these various institutions are subject to multiple statutes, regulations, and guidelines under the jurisdiction of various agencies at the federal, state, and local levels. In many cases, individuals have no or very limited choices as to the meals and snacks provided at these institutions; however, programs generally must meet minimum guidelines for nutritional quality and variety.

Like restaurant operations, institutional food services have grown substantially in recent years (NRA, 1990b). People of all age groups are eating more meals prepared in institutional or congregate settings than in home kitchens. Children are eating more breakfasts as well as lunches at school. Long- and short-term-care facilities are feeding a larger percentage of elderly individuals. Military installations, correctional facilities, and colleges and universities are also feeding an increased number of people.

The DHHS *Year 2000 Objectives for the Nation* recommend an "increase to at least 75 percent the proportion of institutional food service operations with menus that are consistent with the Dietary Guidelines for Americans" (DHHS, 1989, p. 1-5).

Child Nutrition Programs

Child nutrition programs include the National School Lunch, Breakfast, and Milk programs and the Child Care and Summer Food programs. Lunches served as part of the National School Lunch Program (NSLP) must meet USDA minimum meal pattern requirements that are designed to provide one-third of the RDA for the age group (7 CFR § 210.10(b)). The NSLP operates in over 90 percent of the nation's schools, serving over 24 million children daily (ASFSA, 1989). Other child nutrition programs have minimum meal pattern guidelines for meals and snacks that are designed to provide a wide variety of nutritious foods (21 CFR Parts 220, 225, 226).

In 1990 the Special Supplemental Food Program for Women, Infants, and Children (WIC) is expected to serve over 4 million low-income, at-risk pregnant or lactating women, infants, and children through health services, food supplements, and nutrition education to improve nutritional status and pregnancy outcome (U.S. Congress, 1988). Foods offered through WIC include juices, milk, cheese, eggs, breakfast cereals, dry beans and peas, peanut butter, and infant formula and cereal. Many WIC foods are not labeled with nutrition information.

The Child Nutrition and WIC Reauthorization Act of 1989 (P.L. 101-147) requires the Secretaries of DHHS and USDA to develop nutrition guidance for child nutrition programs to help program managers construct menus and snacks consistent with current dietary recommendations. Legislation in several states has addressed additional requirements for nutrition content and education in child nutrition programs.

The DHHS *Year 2000 Objectives for the Nation* include an objective aimed at child nutrition programs: "Increase to at least 95 percent the proportion of school lunch and breakfast services with menus that are consistent with the Dietary Guidelines for Americans" (DHHS, 1989, p. 1-5).

Feeding Programs for Elderly Individuals

Congregate and home-delivered meal programs served over 337 million meals in 1988 (Mary Tonore, Louisiana Department of Aging, personal communication, 1990). These meal programs are regulated under provisions of Title III-C of the Older Americans Act (P.L. 100-175), which is administered by the Administration on Aging (AoA). The Act requires that all meals meet one-third of the RDA for people age 51 and older (OAA, Title III, Part C, § 331). Louisiana has additional restrictions that limit fat to 35 percent of total calories and sodium to 1,300 mg per meal. AoA does not have data on other states that may have adopted such similar requirements. Title III-C also requires a nutrition education component that provides information on nutrition and health. The quantity and quality of the nutrition education varies greatly, but at least the most basic information reaches some elderly participants.

Military Installations

All branches of the U.S. military have taken the initiative to provide healthy food alternatives for their personnel. NRA estimated that food and beverage sales and purchases for military food services were $2.4 billion in 1989. Garrison menus, which comprised 68.5 million meals in fiscal year 1989, are planned within standards set forth in the *Triservice Regulation on Nutrition* (DOD, 1989). Although there are no mandatory regulations for food service in the military, U.S. Department of Defense (DOD) Food Planning Board policies provide guidance on the purchase and selection of the special dietary products used in military menus.

The DOD Health Promotion Directive requires all branches of the military to implement a nutrition education program. Each branch's nutrition educator has the responsibility of educating the military community in its selection of healthful food products that are commonly available in military food service operations. The nutrition education materials used include posters, table tents, bulletin boards, and pamphlets displayed in dining halls. The army, for example, offers *Guide to Good Eating*, which provides personnel with information on calories, serving sizes, and levels of fat, sodium, and other nutrients in foods (Celia Adolphi, Office of the Deputy Chief of Staff for Logistics, U.S. Army, personal communication, 1990).

Correctional Institutions

In 1989, there were approximately 710,000 inmates in correctional institutions under state and federal jurisdiction and an additional 395,000 inmates at local and county detention facilities (U.S. Department of Justice, 1990a,b). Food service operations at correctional institutions provide over 3 million meals each day. Correctional facilities have generally been required, through internal policy and/or accreditation standards of the American Correctional Association, to provide a nutritionally balanced diet based on the RDAs, medically therapeutic diets, and diets to meet the requirements of religious preference.

College and University Food Services

There are no federal regulations governing college and university food services, but most adhere to policies set forth by the National Association of College and University Food Service (NACUFS, 1986). NACUFS guidelines require a nutrition education program that uses various forms of communication to reach students and staff.

Health Care Facilities

To participate in the Medicaid and Medicare programs, hospitals and acute care facilities must meet standards set by the Joint Commission on Accreditation of Healthcare Organizations (JCAHO), a private accreditation body comprising the American College of Physicians, American Medical Association, and American Hospital Association. There are currently 6,780 hospitals in the United States, of which 5,400 are accredited by JCAHO (1989). State licensing boards regulate hospitals that are not accredited by JCAHO.

The dietetic departments of accredited hospitals must be administered by an expert in food service management. JCAHO standards require that patients' nutrient intakes be assessed and recorded. Modified diets must be approved and monitored by a qualified dietitian, and menus must be planned to meet individual patients' nutritional requirements based on both the RDAs and medical factors. Patients on modified diets are required to receive written instructions and individualized counseling before they are discharged. Requirements for patients on regular diets are less stringent, but selection of menu items provides an opportunity for delivery of nutrition information.

Intermediate- and long-term-care facilities include skilled and intermediate nursing facilities and mental health, mental retardation, psychiatric, hospice, rehabilitation, and retirement centers. All must comply with federal (Medicare and Medicaid) and/or state requirements to receive reimbursement for care. The minimum federal standards require that meals be planned in accordance with each resident's individual nutritional needs, based on both the RDAs and medical factors (21 CFR §§ 483.10, 483.410).

Committee Recommendations

Institutions and other noncommercial food service operations present a distinctive set of characteristics when one considers proposals for food labeling. Almost all have program or menu requirements that provide some assurance that participants receive a proportion of a days' nutrition requirements. Several programs include nutrition education components, and food choices are restricted or nonexistent. However, nutrition information at point of purchase or point of selection for foods in such settings would be very valuable for nutrition education efforts.

On the basis of program requirements and the multijurisdictional nature of noncommercial food service operations, the Committee recommends that:

- The agencies at the federal, state, and local levels that oversee or support noncommercial food services encourage voluntary nutrition labeling of meals at the point of purchase or point of selection as part of overall nutrition education efforts.

REFERENCES

AAP (American Academy of Pediatrics). 1985. Pediatric Nutrition Handbook, 2nd ed. Committee on Nutrition. AAP, Elk Grove Village, Ill. 421 pp.

Achabal, D.D., S.H. McIntyre, C.H. Bell, and N. Tucker. 1987. The effect of nutrition P-O-P signs on consumer attitudes and behavior. J. Retailing 63:9–24.

Adams, C.E., and J.W. Erdman. 1988. Effects of home food preparation practices on nutrient content of foods. Pp. 557–605 in Nutritional Evaluation of Food Processing, 3rd ed., E. Karmas and R.S. Harris, eds. Van Nostrand Reinhold Co., Inc., New York.

ASFSA (American School Food Service Association). 1989. School Food Service Research Review, Fall 1989. ASFSA, Alexandria, Va. 191 pp.

Bergstrom, L. 1988. Nutrient data banks for nutrient evaluation in foods. Pp. 745–764 in Nutritional Evaluation of Food Processing, 3rd ed., E. Karmas and R.S. Harris, eds. Van Nostrand Reinhold Co., Inc., New York.

Chicago Tribune. March 6, 1990. Nutrition data on front burner; fast food chains broke pledge, consumer group says. Sec. 3, p. 5.

DHEW/USDA/FTC (U.S. Department of Health, Education, and Welfare, U.S. Department of Agriculture, and Federal Trade Commission). 1979. Food Labeling Background Papers. Government Printing Office, Washington, D.C. 124 pp.

DHHS (U.S. Department of Health and Human Services). 1988. The Surgeon General's Report on Nutrition and Health. Government Printing Office, Washington, D.C. 727 pp.

DHHS (U.S. Department of Health and Human Services). 1989. Promoting Health/Preventing Disease: Year 2000 Objectives for the Nation. Draft for Public Review and Comment. Public Health Service, Washington, D.C.

DOC (U.S. Department of Commerce). 1987. P. A-9 in 1987 Census of Retail Trade. Eating and Drinking Places (SIC Major Group 58). Government Printing Office, Washington, D.C.

DOD (U.S. Department of Defense). 1989. Triservice Regulation on Nutrition. DOD, Washington, D.C. 10 pp.

IOM (Institute of Medicine). 1990. Seafood Safety. Committee on Evaluation of the Safety of Fishery Products, Food and Nutrition Board. National Academy Press, Washington, D.C. In press.

JCAHO (Joint Commission on Accreditation of Healthcare Organizations). 1989. Joint Commission 1990 Accreditation Manual for Hospitals. JCAHO, Chicago.

Lanza, E., and R.K. Butrum. 1986. A review of food fiber analysis and data. J. Am. Diet. Assoc. 86:732–743.

Leveille, G.A. 1983. Nutrients in Foods. The Nutrition Guild, Cambridge, Mass. 291 pp.

Lund, D.B. 1988. Effects of heat processing on nutrients. Pp. 319–354 in Nutritional Evaluation of Food Processing, 3rd ed., E. Karmas and R.S. Harris, eds. Van Nostrand Reinhold Co., Inc., New York.

Massachusetts Medical Society Committee on Nutrition. 1989. Fast Food Fare: Consumer Guidelines. Prepared by Connie Roberts. N. Engl. J. Med. 321:752–756.

Mullis, R.M., and P. Pirie. 1988. Lean meats make the grade: A collaborative nutrition education program. J. Am. Diet. Assoc. 88(2):191–195.

NACUFS (National Association of College and University Food Service). 1986. Professional Standards Manual. NACUFS, E. Lansing, Mich.

NLMB (National Live Stock and Meat Board). 1990. In-Store Nutrition Information on Fresh Meat: Issues and Insights. Research Report No. 100-1. NLMB, Chicago. 18 pp.

NRA (National Restaurant Association). 1986. 1986 Gallup Poll results. NRA, Washington, D.C.

NRA (National Restaurant Association). 1989. Survey of Chain Operators. NRA, Washington, D.C. 16 pp.

NRA (National Restaurant Association). 1990a. Foodservice Industry: 1988 in Review. NRA, Washington, D.C. 12 pp.

NRA (National Restaurant Association). 1990b. Food Service Industry Forecast. NRA, Washington, D.C. 24 pp.

NRC (National Research Council). 1989. Diet and Health: Implications for Reducing Chronic Disease Risk. Report of the Committee on Diet and Health, Food and Nutrition Board, Commission on Life Sciences. National Academy Press, Washington, D.C. 749 pp.

PMA (Produce Marketing Association). 1988. Produce Retailing: Performance and Productivity. Food Marketing Institute and Produce Marketing Association, Wilmington, Del.

Riehle, H. 1990. Consumer commitment to nutrition increases. Restaurants USA March: 36–39.

Shields, J.E., and E. Young. 1990. Fat in fast foods—evolving changes. Nutr. Today 25(2):32–35.

Slater, G.G., S. Shankiman, J.S. Shepherd, and R.B. Alfin-Slater. 1975. Seasonal variation in the composition of California avocados. J. Agric. Food Chem. 23:468–474.

Stansby, M.E. 1981. Reliability of fatty acid values purporting to represent composition of oil from different species of fish. J. Am. Oil Chem. Soc. 58:13–16.

Stansby, M.E. 1982. Properties of fish oils and their applications to handling of fish and to nutritional and industrial use. Pp. 75–92 in Chemistry and Biochemistry of Marine Food Products, R.E. Martin, G.J. Flick, C.E. Hedbard, and D.R. Ward, eds. AVI Publishing Co., Westport, Conn.

Sullivan, A.L., and W.S. Otwell. 1990. A Nutrient Data Base for Southeastern Seafood: A Comprehensive Nutrient and Nomenclature Handbook for Selected Southeastern Species. Produced in cooperation between the Florida Department of Natural Resources and the University of Florida, Gainesville. In press.

Sweet, C.A. 1989. Rethinking eating out. FDA Consumer (November):8–13.

U.S. Congress. 1988. Subcommittee on Elementary, Secondary, and Vocational Education, Committee on Education and Labor. Child Nutrition Programs: Issues for the 101st Congress. 101st Cong., 2nd Sess., U.S. House of Representatives, Washington, D.C.

USDA (U.S. Department of Agriculture). 1979. Composition of Foods: Poultry Products. Agriculture Handbook No. 8-5. Government Printing Office, Washington, D.C. 330 pp.

USDA (U.S. Department of Agriculture). 1982. Composition of Foods: Fruit and Fruit Juices. Agriculture Handbook No. 8-9. Government Printing Office, Washington, D.C. 283 pp.

USDA (U.S. Department of Agriculture). 1983. Composition of Foods: Pork Products. Agriculture Handbook No. 8-10. Government Printing Office, Washington, D.C. 206 pp.

USDA (U.S. Department of Agriculture). 1984a. Composition of Foods: Vegetables and Vegetable Products. Agriculture Handbook No. 8-11. Government Printing Office, Washington, D.C. 502 pp.

USDA (U.S. Department of Agriculture). 1984b. Composition of Foods: Nut and Seed Products. Agriculture Handbook No. 8-12. Government Printing Office, Washington, D.C. 137 pp.

USDA (U.S. Department of Agriculture). 1987. Composition of Foods: Finfish and

Shellfish Products. Agriculture Handbook No. 8-15. Government Printing Office, Washington, D.C. 192 pp.

USDA (U.S. Department of Agriculture). 1989a. Composition of Foods: Lamb, Veal, and Game. Agriculture Handbook No. 8-17. Government Printing Office, Washington, D.C. 251 pp.

USDA (U.S. Department of Agriculture). 1989b. National Advisory Council on Commodity Distribution, 1989 Annual Report. First Report to the President and the Congress. Government Printing Office, Washington, D.C. 12 pp.

USDA (U.S. Department of Agriculture). 1990. Composition of Foods: Beef Products. Agriculture Handbook No. 8-13. Government Printing Office, Washington, D.C. 412 pp.

U.S. Department of Justice. 1990a. Prisoners in 1989. Office of Justice Programs, Bureau of Justice Statistics. U.S. Department of Justice, Washington, D.C. 11 pp.

U.S. Department of Justice. 1990b. Jail Inmates, 1989. Office of Justice Programs, Bureau of Justice Statistics. U.S. Department of Justice, Washington, D.C. 5 pp.

6

Nutrition Label Content

Beyond the issue of the specific foods to be covered by nutrition labeling requirements is the actual information that should be provided on food labels. The current nutrition information panel contains information on calories, protein, fat, carbohydrate, sodium, and percentage of the U.S. Recommended Daily Allowances (U.S. RDA) for protein and seven vitamins and minerals (21 CFR § 101.9; USDA, 1989). Other information about the nutrient content of foods frequently may be obtained from the ingredient listing and from nutrient descriptors found on the principal display panel of food labels (see Chapter 7). In light of the findings and recommendations in *The Surgeon General's Report on Nutrition and Health* (DHHS, 1988) and the National Research Council (NRC) report, *Diet and Health: Implications for Reducing Chronic Disease Risk* (NRC, 1989a), this information is at once incomplete and excessive. The Committee was directed to consider recommendations for food labeling reform based on the knowledge of nutrition in relation to long-term health contained in these reports. For nutrients and other food components currently included or proposed for inclusion on the nutrition information panel, this chapter describes their health relevance, dietary recommendations, current provision of labeling information, and the Committee's recommendations for nutrition labeling. Comprehensive information on dietary sources of nutrients and dietary intake patterns are provided in Chapter 4.

CALORIES

Health Relevance of Calories

Scientists, consumers, and food manufacturers all acknowledge that the information about calories per serving is one of the key elements of the nutrition information panel. Because of this consensus, only the highlights of current scientific evidence are provided in the discussion that follows.

There is consensus among health care professionals that obesity (defined as excess body fat) is associated with excess mortality. *Nutrition and Your Health: Dietary Guidelines for Americans* (USDA/DHHS, 1985), the Surgeon General's report (DHHS, 1988), the NRC *Diet and Health* report (1989a), and the *Report of the Dietary Guidelines Advisory Committee on the Dietary Guidelines for Americans* (USDA, 1990) emphasize the importance of maintaining a healthy or desirable weight to minimize the risk for chronic diseases such as diabetes, coronary heart disease (CHD), stroke, hypertension, and certain types of cancer. The causes of obesity include genetic factors, diet, and inactivity. In experimental animals, diets high in fat promote obesity (Schemmel et al., 1970). It is not clear how caloric density and diet composition influence obesity in humans.

An estimated 34 million American adults are obese (based on a standard of greater than 20 percent in excess of desirable body weight), and more than 80 million Americans are trying to control their weight (CCC, 1985). In order to maintain a stable body weight, caloric intake must be in balance with energy expenditure. Methods used to lose weight emphasize the need to decrease caloric intake and increase energy expenditure (Kayman et al., 1990). Provision of information on the caloric content of food products may be useful not only for obese individuals trying to lose weight but also for those who are trying not to gain excess weight. The number of calories in a food is the one component of the food label that consumers seem to understand.

Current Provision of Desired Information

Information about calories often is found in two places on the food label: the nutrition information panel and the principal display panel. On the nutrition information panel, the Food and Drug Administration (FDA) and the U.S. Department of Agriculture (USDA) require the disclosure of total calories per serving, expressed as kilocalories (21 CFR § 101.9(c)(3)).

The principal display panel may include nutrient descriptors that are regulated by FDA and/or USDA, such as *low calorie, reduced calorie, diet, sugar free,* and *no sugar,* with some minor differences (21 CFR § 105.66(c), (d), (f); USDA, 1982a). Some descriptors may be misinterpreted by the consumer to imply that a food is low in calories. There is a need for more uniform use of the terms *light* and *lite* with respect to the caloric content of foods to avoid consumer confusion (NRC, 1988), since four government agencies (FDA, USDA, the Federal Trade Commission [FTC], and the Bureau of Alcohol, Tobacco, and Firearms) have jurisdiction over products that carry these terms. The noncaloric use of these terms is discussed in Chapter 7.

For the purposes of marketing and nutrition education, some manufacturers are currently declaring calories in terms of the food's contribution to the total number of calories to be consumed in a day. One example is the increasing number of packaged foods designed to be eaten as a single meal and the use of various reference standards for total daily calories. The establishment of a single daily standard for calories for any purpose, including labeling, is difficult given the wide range of average caloric intakes for adults. However, if manufacturers are going to refer to the total number of calories to be consumed in a day, then a reference standard needs to be established.

Committee Recommendations

The Committee recommends that:

- FDA and USDA should continue to require the disclosure of calories expressed as kilocalories per serving on the nutrition information panel.
- If the manufacturer chooses to express nutrients as a percentage of total calories, 2,000 calories should be used and stated as the reference point for the average adult who engages in light physical activity. This amount will overestimate the needs for some individuals (e.g., many women) and underestimate the needs for others (e.g., many men). A daily reference standard based on a population average of 2,350 calories has been proposed by FDA (55 Fed. Reg. 29,476–29,533, July, 19, 1990), but a 2,000-calorie level would provide a standard that is both an amount closer to the average intakes of women and under the population average intake (which in general seems to consume more calories than are needed) as well as a round number for easier reference and use in calculations.
- Descriptors related to caloric content of foods that are currently defined by FDA and USDA should be continued.
- FDA and USDA should define and standardize the terms *light, lite,* and *diet* and other descriptors that can be interpreted as caloric claims.

FAT AND CHOLESTEROL

Health Relevance of Dietary Fat and Cholesterol

Current Dietary Recommendations for Fat and Cholesterol

Most health organizations in the United States that have examined the relationship between dietary fat and atherosclerotic disease have recommended that dietary saturated fatty acid intakes be reduced in order to reduce plasma cholesterol levels and thereby reduce the incidence of and mortality from CHD and related conditions. The specific recommendation has usually been to reduce total fat intake to 30 percent or less of total calories and saturated fatty acid intake to less than 10 percent of total calories (NRC, 1989a). Although it is widely believed that even lower total fat and saturated fatty acid intakes would be more beneficial, there has been concern about the palatability of foods with lower levels of fat content. Because no human populations that consume large proportions of polyunsaturated fatty acids (more than about 10 percent of total daily calories) have been adequately studied, and because some observations in experimental animals have suggested that polyunsaturated fatty acids might contribute to cancer, recommendations regarding fat intake usually include a limit on polyunsaturated fatty acid intake to about 10 percent of total calories.

The American Heart Association (AHA, 1986), the Surgeon General's report (DHHS, 1988), and the NRC *Diet and Health* report (NRC, 1989a) included recommendations to limit cholesterol intake to 300 mg daily as a means of lowering plasma cholesterol concentrations and thereby preventing atherosclerotic disease.

Roles of Fat and Cholesterol in the Body

Fats and Oils Fats and oils are complex organic molecules that are formed by combining three fatty acid molecules with one molecule of glycerol. Generally, fatty acids are straight chains of carbon atoms with two hydrogen atoms bound to most carbon atoms, but they vary in chain length and in the number of double bonds between carbon atoms. Generally, fatty acids in animal and plant tissues range from 4 to 24 carbon atoms. Those with no double bonds are called saturated fatty acids, those with one double bond are called monounsaturated fatty acids, and those with more than one double bond are called polyunsaturated fatty acids.

Fats containing predominantly saturated fatty acids are solid or viscous at room temperature; those containing predominantly monounsaturated or polyun-saturated fatty acids are liquid at room temperature. One polyunsaturated fatty acid, linoleic acid, which has 18 carbon atoms and two double bonds, is an es-sential nutrient because it is necessary for normal cellular function but the body cannot synthesize it; other fatty acids required by mammals can be synthesized by the body.

The principal function of fatty acids consumed in the mammalian diet is energy. Fats stored in adipose tissue provide a long-term reserve source of energy, because they produce about twice as much energy per unit of mass as protein or carbohydrate does. Fats and oils also greatly affect the taste, consistency, stability, and palatability of foods. Humans prefer foods containing more than 15 percent fat (by weight, about 30 percent of calories), even though 5 percent fat in the diet (by weight, 10 percent of calories) is nutritionally adequate. The U.S. population currently consumes about 36 percent of its calories from fat (LSRO, FASEB, 1989).

Fats and oils in Americans' diets are derived from plant and animal sources. Generally, saturated fatty acids are derived from meat and dairy products, whereas mono- and polyunsaturated fatty acids are derived from plant sources. Three exceptions are palm, palm kernel, and coconut oils, which are quite rich in saturated fatty acids.

Cholesterol   A quite different material than fats and oils, cholesterol is commonly classified among the lipids. It is a large molecule composed of several six-carbon rings joined together at their sides and with other structures joined to the outside rings. Cholesterol is an essential component of mammalian tissues, but it is synthesized in the body and is not an essential nutrient. Cholesterol is used to produce body hormones and cellular structures, but not for energy. It has no taste and its presence or absence does not affect the palatability of foods. Currently, U.S. intakes by men and women range between 304 and 435 mg/day (NCEP, 1990).

Health Effects of Dietary Fat and Cholesterol

Coronary Heart Disease   Evidence that dietary fat or cholesterol was involved in causing atherosclerosis and CHD first appeared early in the twentieth century, at about the same time that myocardial infarction was identified as a distinctive clinical syndrome and was found to be related to atherosclerosis and thrombosis of the coronary arteries. Almost no attention was directed toward diet as a possible cause of atherosclerosis or its major clinical sequela, CHD, until after World War II, when it became apparent that this disease had reached epidemic proportions in the industrialized countries.

In the Scandinavian countries, heart disease rates declined dramatically during World War II, a period when foods rich in fat were in short supply (Keys, 1975). Retrospective case-control studies also revealed that CHD was associated with serum cholesterol concentrations and that the serum cholesterol concentration was controlled, in part, by the amount and type of fat and cholesterol in the diet. International comparisons, studies of migrant populations, and observations of vegetarians showed that saturated fatty acid and cholesterol intakes were associated with CHD rates, but these correlations were often confounded by other differences in life-style.

Many controlled experiments in humans and animals have demonstrated that saturated fatty acids and cholesterol in the diet elevate serum cholesterol concentrations, and when saturated fatty acids were replaced with monounsaturated and polyunsaturated fatty acids, serum cholesterol concentrations were lowered (NRC, 1989a). A massive research project, the National Diet Heart Study, showed that serum cholesterol levels could be lowered in free-living populations by fat-modified diets. On the basis of early observations, AHA recommended reductions in dietary saturated fatty acids in 1957 (Page et al., 1957), and later it recommended reductions in dietary cholesterol intake (AHA, 1965). The Surgeon General's report (DHHS, 1988) and the NRC *Diet and Health* report (NRC, 1989a) reaffirmed these recommendations.

The concentration of cholesterol in plasma (or serum) has been considered a major risk factor for CHD. Fat and cholesterol, which are insoluble in an aqueous medium, are carried in the blood within particles stabilized by specialized proteins (apolipoproteins). There are several distinct classes of lipoproteins in plasma, each containing different proportions of cholesterol and other fats. Subsequent epidemiological studies disclosed that the concentration of low-density lipoprotein (LDL) cholesterol was positively associated with the risk of CHD (Medalie et al., 1973) and that the concentration of high-density lipoprotein (HDL) cholesterol was inversely associated with the risk of CHD (Gordon et al., 1977; Miller et al., 1977). These associations were confirmed in animal experiments and in postmortem human studies relating plasma lipoprotein cholesterol concentrations to atherosclerotic lesions (Solberg and Strong, 1983). Thus, it became important to distinguish between the effects of LDL and HDL cholesterol concentrations.

Evidence Regarding Saturated Fatty Acids   In 1952, two independent groups of investigators—in the United States (Kinsell et al., 1952) and in Europe (Groen et al., 1952)—discovered almost simultaneously that the saturation level of dietary fatty acids influenced plasma cholesterol concentrations. A large number of human and animal experiments subsequently confirmed that saturated fatty acids with chain lengths of 12 to 16 carbon atoms (lauric, myristic, and palmitic acids) were the most active in raising serum cholesterol concentrations, whereas fatty acids with chain lengths of 10 or fewer carbon atoms or 18 carbon atoms (stearic acid) had no effect. Investigators developed equations that consistently predicted (on average) the effects of changes in fatty acid intake on the plasma cholesterol concentration.

Monounsaturated fatty acids, represented mainly by oleic acid, had little or no effect on plasma cholesterol concentrations compared with the effects of equivalent calories such as those from carbohydrate and, therefore, were omitted from these predictive equations. The predictive power was also increased when stearic acid was omitted from the intake of saturated fatty acids. Recent experiments have reconfirmed the observation that, although stearic acid contributes calories, it does not raise plasma LDL or HDL cholesterol levels (Bonanome and Grundy, 1988).

When saturated fatty acids are replaced by polyunsaturated fatty acids, represented in the diet mainly by linoleic acid, serum cholesterol concentrations are reduced to as low as and possibly lower than the levels produced by equivalent calories such as those from carbohydrate (NRC, 1989a). Recent experiments have also reconfirmed that oleic acid maintains LDL cholesterol concentrations at about the same level that polyunsaturated fatty acids do and showed that it does not lower HDL cholesterol levels (Grundy, 1987). Thus, monounsaturated fatty acids might be included with polyunsaturated fatty acids in a computation of fatty acids that would be expected to produce more desirable plasma lipoprotein profiles.

Several epidemiological comparisons found a strong association between average intakes of saturated fatty acids and mortality from CHD (Keys, 1975). A low saturated fatty acid intake (less than 10 percent of total calories) is common to all populations with low CHD rates. The results of correlations based on individual intakes within a population have been less consistent and conclusive. This discrepancy is attributed to the low range of intakes within each population and to the misclassification of dietary intakes and endpoints. The effects of dietary fatty acids on plasma lipoproteins and atherosclerosis have generally been confirmed in animal experiments.

Another issue concerns the health effects of stearic acid, a saturated fatty acid. Unlike the other saturated fatty acids, it has been found that stearic acid does not elevate serum cholesterol levels. The results of early studies have been confirmed by recent experiments in humans; however, the controversy continues.

Evidence Regarding Omega-3 Fatty Acids   In early research on the effects of polyunsaturated fatty acids on lipoprotein metabolism, investigators noticed that some of the highly unsaturated oils from marine sources were as effective as vegetable oils in lowering serum cholesterol levels. Years later, it was reported that Eskimos who consumed large quantities of fish had low rates of atherosclerotic heart disease. Renewed investigations showed that the effects on lipoprotein metabolism were due to the high proportions of omega-3 polyunsaturated fatty acids in oils from marine mammals. When these fatty acids are included in the diet, they dramatically reduce plasma triglyceride levels but do not seem to reduce LDL cholesterol levels unless they are substituted for saturated fatty acids (Woodward and Carroll, 1988). They also affect the hemostatic system by altering platelet function and prostaglandin metabolism in ways that may reduce the risk of thrombosis (Herold and Kinsella, 1986). The potential beneficial effects of omega-3 fatty acids have led to some recommendations that individuals should increase their consumption of fish oils that contain these substances in order to prevent atherosclerosis and thrombosis. However, many studies have also found some adverse effects—for example, an increase in LDL cholesterol levels—and neither the beneficial effects nor the safety of high intakes of omega-3 fatty acids have been thoroughly documented. The Surgeon General's report (DHHS, 1988) and the NRC *Diet and Health* report (NRC, 1989a) did not recommend increased intakes of fish oils as a means of preventing CHD.

Fish oils and omega-3 fatty acids must be differentiated from fish as a food. Fish is widely recommended as an excellent source of protein that is low in fat, and in some epidemiological studies, fish consumption is inversely associated with cardiovascular disease (Kromhout et al., 1985).

Evidence Regarding Trans *Fatty Acids*   When vegetable oils are hydrogenated to make them more palatable as substitutes for animal fats, geometric isomers of the unsaturated fatty acids called *trans* fatty acids are formed. Because these isomers are not present in natural foods in the proportions that occur in hydrogenated fats, their effects on lipid and lipoprotein metabolism, plasma lipid levels, and atherosclerosis have been investigated intensively (NRC, 1989a). Although *trans* fatty acids lack any activity as essential fatty acids, no deleterious effects have been demonstrated in humans, and no deleterious effects have been found in animal experiments with levels of intake comparable to customary human intakes. There remains some possibility of a long-term effect of *trans* fatty acids on lipid metabolism, and this question should be reconsidered periodically as knowledge of lipid metabolism and the changes underlying chronic disease increases, but present knowledge provides no basis for limiting or reducing the current usual intake of *trans* fatty acids.

Evidence Regarding Dietary Cholesterol   Although the first evidence linking a dietary lipid with atherosclerosis came from experiments with rabbits in 1913, the discovery of the effects of saturated fatty acids on plasma cholesterol levels in 1952 overshadowed the potential effects of dietary cholesterol.

Most animal species, including guinea pigs, swine, and several nonhuman primates (notable exceptions are dogs and rats), have been found to be susceptible to the cholesterolemic effects of dietary cholesterol. Indeed, in animal models of diet-induced atherosclerosis, cholesterol seems to be more important than the type or amount of dietary fat. Epidemiological studies have almost invariably found strong correlations between dietary cholesterol intake, plasma cholesterol concentrations, and CHD (McGill, 1979). However, there were also strong correlations of saturated fatty acid intakes with CHD, and multivariate analyses of the data usually resulted in nonsignificant correlations of dietary cholesterol intake with CHD rates.

Cross-sectional dietary studies, designed to test individuals within a population for the association between dietary intakes and plasma cholesterol levels, usually found no association between dietary intakes of cholesterol and plasma cholesterol or lipoprotein concentrations. These negative results were considered inconclusive based on the limited range of dietary intakes found within population groups (in contrast to the wide ranges of mean intakes between population groups), and also because measurement error seriously degraded correlations based on individual values.

The independent effect of dietary cholesterol is an important issue, because one widely produced and consumed food, the egg, is rich in cholesterol but contains only moderate amounts of saturated fatty acids. Beginning in about 1960, a number of carefully controlled experiments in humans measured plasma cholesterol levels (and later, LDL and HDL cholesterol concentrations) in individuals fed diets containing varying amounts of cholesterol. Eventually, a consensus indicated that dietary cholesterol did affect plasma cholesterol levels, particularly LDL cholesterol levels, independent of total fat intake and type of fat. Furthermore, several long-term cohort studies of humans have recently reported that reliable estimates of dietary cholesterol intake, when expressed as milligrams per 1,000 kcal, were positively correlated with the incidence of CHD during subsequent years of follow-up (Shekelle et al., 1981; Stamler and Shekelle, 1988). The correlations were independent of the plasma cholesterol levels. These results suggest the possibility that dietary cholesterol might influence atherosclerosis or its clinical manifestations by some mechanism other than elevation of LDL cholesterol levels.

Cancer

There is less evidence linking total dietary fat and saturated fatty acids to cancer than to heart disease, but the accumulated epidemiological evidence does suggest that dietary fat intake is associated with the risk of colon, prostate, and ovarian cancers and, possibly, with breast cancer (NRC, 1982, 1989a). Animals fed high-fat diets are more likely to develop cancers of the breast, intestinal tract, and pancreas than are those fed low-fat diets. In animals, polyunsaturated fatty acids promote cancers more effectively than do saturated fatty acids, but high saturated fatty acid intakes also increase the probability of cancer in animals if the minimum requirement for polyunsaturated fatty acid intake is satisfied.

Although dietary cholesterol intake is highly correlated with saturated fatty acid intake in humans, there is no evidence that either high or low cholesterol intakes are associated with cancer at any site. Some reports that low plasma cholesterol levels were associated with a higher risk of cancer led to concern about the potential adverse effects of plasma cholesterol-lowering diets, but these associations were thought to be due, in part, to low plasma cholesterol levels in early cancers—that is, a result of the cancer rather than a precursor.

Gallbladder Disease

Most gallstones occurring in the U.S. population are the result of the presence of excess secretion of cholesterol into the bile by the liver. Because both dietary cholesterol and polyunsaturated fatty acids increase secretion of cholesterol by the liver, it has been hypothesized that these dietary components may be responsible for gallstones. Feeding of cholesterol to some species of rodents causes gallstones.

Obesity predisposes an individual to gallstone formation, presumably because it is associated with increased secretion of cholesterol into the bile. However, no epidemiological or experimental evidence in humans has directly implicated either dietary cholesterol or fat as a cause of gallstones. It is likely that some individuals who are genetically predisposed may be susceptible to the lithogenic effects of dietary fat or cholesterol, but these individuals cannot yet be identified (NRC, 1989a).

Current Provision of Desired Information

There are three locations on food labels that may provide useful information about fat and cholesterol, including the ingredient listing, the nutrition information panel, or descriptors of specific levels or types of fats and cholesterol on the principal display panel.

Ingredient Listing

Ingredients are required to be listed on a majority of packaged foods; this would provide information on food components that are fats and oils, whether derived from animal or plant sources (21 CFR § 101.4(b)(14); USDA, 1989). The common or usual names of fats and oils would reveal fat sources; however, the current ingredient listing rarely provides information about the saturated fatty acid or cholesterol content for consumers seeking this information. The use of weight as the criterion for listing ingredients may cause the consumer to overlook a more important measure, that is, the relative contribution of fats and oils to available calories in a food. For example, fats and oils provide more than twice the amount of calories per gram compared with protein and carbohydrate, but fats might not be listed first on the ingredient label because of their weight.

However, the actual fats and oils present in a product can be difficult to determine. Until 1971, all fats were allowed to be listed generically on ingredient labels as "vegetable shortening" by FDA and as "shortening" by USDA. When regulations that required listing of specific fats and oils by weight were proposed, a convincing case was made that product sources often change, depending on their availability and price. An individual listing was judged to be costly for manufacturers and, ultimately, for consumers, if labels had to be changed every time the source changed. The resulting compromise allows manufacturers to list fats and oils as they are contained in the product (by weight) or to list all those that might be used from time to time. Under this so-called "and/or" provision, any specific product would likely contain one or two of the oils listed.

The great disadvantage of "and/or" labeling of fats and oils is that many of the commonly used oils vary widely in fatty acid content. If coconut oil is the only oil used, over 80 percent of the fatty acid content of the product might be saturated; if rapeseed oil were chosen, the same product might have a fatty acid content that was less than 7 percent saturated fatty acids. Although fatty acid content varies among many of the commercial oils, functionality of the oil in many products such as baked goods limits the range of fatty acid content of oil that can be used. Nevertheless, the information that is clearly relevant to the product's composition and that many consumers consider important in planning their diets has often been unavailable.

Nutrition Information Panel

If a manufacturer chooses to or must provide nutrition labeling, the label must declare the amount of fat per serving in grams (21 CFR § 101.9(c)(6)). Only if a claim about the fatty acid content is made must the content of saturated and unsaturated fatty acids be declared on the nutrition information panel, using the terms *saturated fat* and *unsaturated fat*. In this case, the percentage of total calories contributed by fats is required; however, the cholesterol content is not (21 CFR § 101.25(c)). If a claim regarding cholesterol is made, the amount per serving must be given on the label, but no specific information about the fatty acids need be listed (21 CFR § 101.25(b)). As a result, foods rich in cholesterol but containing certain vegetable oils may describe their relatively low percentage of saturated fat without revealing the cholesterol content. For foods with a significant amount of vegetable fats, the fatty acid content may not be reported if there is a claim of the absence of cholesterol on the label.

For food labels that provide either fatty acid or cholesterol content, FDA requires that the label indicate that such information is given for individuals who, on the advice of a physician, are modifying their dietary intake of fat and/or cholesterol (21 CFR § 101.25(d)). Since the 1986 proposal to regulate cholesterol-related terms, this requirement has not been enforced but is an indication of the specific subpopulation on which the concept of a low-saturated-fat, low-cholesterol eating pattern was originally focused. Within the past 5 years, a national consensus on the efficacy of plasma cholesterol reduction in the prevention of CHD in the entire population has been reached that favors dietary modification as the first step in achieving a reduction in the risk of CHD.

In July 1990, FDA issued a tentative final rule that included revised quantitative fat declaration and definitions with criteria for their use (55 Fed. Reg. 29,456–29,473, July 19, 1990). The agency continued to use its existing rules on total fat content. When fatty acid or cholesterol content is declared, both are to be declared immediately following the statement of fat content and require the listing of polyunsaturated and saturated fatty acids and allow the voluntary listing of monounsaturated fatty acids. Cholesterol content is to be stated in milligrams per serving to the nearest 5-mg increment, except for a food that contains less than 2 mg/serving. In a food that contains less than 1 g of fat or fatty acids, a statement of "less than 1 g" is allowed in lieu of the specific amount.

No information is currently required on the nutrition information panel concerning the number of calories from fat in foods. Current dietary recommendations state that the percentage of calories from fat in the total diet should be 30 percent or less, with 10 percent or less each from saturated fatty acids and 10 percent or less each from monounsaturated and polyunsaturated fatty acids. Consumers must be encouraged to apply these guidelines in forming their dietary patterns over a total meal or in assessing a day's food rather than using them as standards for accepting or rejecting single products. For example, a single high-fat item can be perfectly acceptable as part of a generally low-fat meal. This concept suggests that fat should not ordinarily be expressed as a percentage of calories on individual food labels. To do so would tend to encourage consumers to apply fat intake recommendations to single foods.

With current information on total fat, a consumer needs to have some additional knowledge of the number of calories per gram of fat in order to make the calculation to determine the percentage of calories from fat in foods. No information is currently required concerning the saturated fatty acid content in foods without additional information. It can be assumed that the majority of consumers would be unable to determine the percentage of calories from total fat and saturated fatty acids in foods. At the same time it is important to avoid the apparent labeling of foods as good or bad based on a listing of the percentage of calories from fat on the package, since it is the percentage of calories from fat in the total diet, and not a specific food, that is the concept consumers need to understand.

Current regulations define polyunsaturated fatty acids to be *cis,cis*-methylene-interrupted polyunsaturated fatty acids, and saturated fatty acids to be the sum of lauric, myristic, palmitic, and stearic acids in foods (21 CFR § 101.25(c)(2)(ii)). The shorter-length saturated fatty acids (those with chain lengths of 10 or less) are excluded from the definition because decades ago they were determined to have no effect on serum cholesterol concentrations. Stearic acid was included in the definition because, presumably, the evidence did not support its exclusion at that time. Current recommendations concerning dietary fat advise that saturated fatty acid intake be reduced to 10 percent or less of calories, which at least implicitly accepts the existing regulatory definition of saturated fatty acids, which would include a few percentage points of stearic acid. However, the issue of retaining stearic acid in the regulatory definition of saturated fatty acids needs further examination. A definition for monounsaturated fatty acids as *cis*-monounsaturated fatty acids has been proposed in the recent FDA tentative final rule (55 Fed. Reg. 29,456–29,473, July 19, 1990).

Principal Display Panel Descriptors for Fat and Cholesterol

Descriptive words and phrases have been used by manufacturers on the principal display panel to describe the fat and cholesterol contents of their products; however, no specific descriptor definitions have been finalized for fatty acids or cholesterol. Statements that are demonstrably true, such as *cholesterol free* for products that are totally vegetable in origin, have been allowed. However, products bearing this label could be high in saturated fatty acids. For individuals who are attempting to lower their blood cholesterol levels, the claim could be confusing and is certainly not helpful on such products. Descriptors related to fat content, such as *lean, extra lean, low fat,* and *reduced* or *lower fat,* have been defined by USDA (1987). At present, FDA has only informal policy guidelines for several of these terms.

In 1986, FDA proposed a series of definitions, including those for *no cholesterol, low cholesterol,* and *cholesterol reduced* (51 Fed. Reg. 42,588–42,589, Nov. 25, 1986). However, these regulations were not finalized, in part because they failed to deal with the issue of fatty acids in conjunction with the cholesterol labeling terms. For labeling purposes, USDA has informally adopted FDA's 1986 proposed definitions.

In July 1990, FDA issued a tentative final rule that included revised quantitative fat declaration and definitions with criteria for their use (55 Fed. Reg. 29,456–29,473, July 19, 1990). In the tentative final rule, the agency defined the following terms by providing extensive criteria for their use: *cholesterol free, free of cholesterol, no cholesterol, low cholesterol, low in cholesterol, cholesterol reduced, reduced cholesterol, cholesterol free food,* and *low cholesterol food,* as well as comparative cholesterol statements. Statements such as "contains 100 percent vegetable oil" or "contains no animal fat" are allowed only if the nutrition label includes quantitative information on total fat, fatty acid, and cholesterol contents. Descriptors for cholesterol and saturated fat could be useful if well-founded definitions can be established. Their continued unqualified use on food products that are high in one component and low in another (e.g., high in saturated fat and low in cholesterol) is counterproductive.

Considerable discussion has surrounded the potential confusion created for many consumers when manufacturers use statements such as *95 percent fat free* on the principal display panel. For the manufacturer, this refers to a percentage of fat by weight. However, consumers normally would not consider the difference between the weight of fat and the calories from fat in a product. As a result, they would often misinterpret this reduction of fat by weight as a reduction of total calories from fat. For example, a frankfurter that is 80 percent fat free (by weight) may contribute over 70 percent of its total calories from fat. For consumers trying to follow current dietary recommendations to choose foods lower in total fat, such statements could create unnecessary confusion, leading to dietary practices that may actually increase the levels of fat in their diets. USDA Policy Memorandum 046 defines the requirements for such terms on product labels (USDA, 1982b). Percent fat free statements are acceptable on product labels if the label also bears a positive declaration of the product's fat content (e.g., along with the statement *95 percent fat free,* the label would have to also bear the declaration *contains 5 percent fat*). FDA does not have regulations for such statements.

Committee Recommendations

The Committee recommends that:

- FDA and USDA should require the disclosure of total fat, saturated fat, unsaturated fat, and cholesterol contents per serving in grams (milligrams for cholesterol) on the nutrition information panel, with saturated and unsaturated fat either indented or otherwise identified as subcategories of total fat.
- FDA and USDA should require the listing of calories per serving from total fat, saturated fat, and unsaturated fat on the nutrition information panel.
- FDA and USDA should allow, as an option, the disclosure of monounsaturated and polyunsaturated fatty acid content per serving in grams on the nutrition information panel.
- FDA and USDA should define descriptors for cholesterol content for use on the principal display panel.
- FDA and USDA should define descriptors for total fat and saturated, monounsaturated, polyunsaturated, and unsaturated fatty acid content on the principal display panel.
- FDA and USDA should require that when a manufacturer refers to "*x* percent fat free" (by weight) and other similar terms on a package, it should also be required to state "*x* percent calories from fat" in close proximity in the same type size and type face.
- FDA and USDA regulations should continue to permit "and/or" labeling of fats and oils in the ingredient listing on the conditions that the food carries full nutrition labeling and that the stated saturated fat content listed is the highest level that would be achieved with any mixture of the listed fats and oils.
- FDA and USDA should establish an entity to evaluate the issue of the cholesterolemic effects of stearic and other fatty acids (e.g., *trans* fatty acids) and related changes that may need to be made in redefining fatty acids for regulatory purposes.

CARBOHYDRATES

Health Relevance of Carbohydrates

The *Dietary Guidelines for Americans* recommended that Americans modify their intake of carbohydrates by eating foods containing adequate starch and fiber and avoiding too much sugar (USDA/DHHS, 1985). In the broadest sense, that report promoted a dietary pattern that emphasizes consumption of vegetables, fruits, and whole-grain products—foods that are rich in complex carbohydrates and fiber and relatively low in calories—and fish, poultry prepared without skin, lean meats, and low-fat dairy products selected to minimize consumption of total fat, saturated fatty acids, and cholesterol. More recently, the health relevance issues involving consumption of simple and digestible complex carbohydrates and dietary fiber were extensively evaluated in both the Surgeon General's report (DHHS, 1988) and the NRC *Diet and Health* report (NRC, 1989a). The recommendations from these reports serve as a cornerstone for the discussions presented below.

Complex Carbohydrates

Complex carbohydrates, or polysaccharides, are made up of long chains of glucose molecules. In typically consumed foods, this category is largely made up of starch. Some glycogen is also consumed, but it is a minor component of meats. Carbohydrates contribute about 45 percent of adult caloric intake (DHHS, 1988), more than half of which comes from complex carbohydrates (NRC, 1989a). Starches from cereals, tubers, beans, and certain legumes thus make up a significant proportion of human caloric intake. Most, but not all, starches in foods are digestible. Foods naturally high in complex digestible carbohydrates are invariably high in fiber as well. Thus, it is particularly difficult to divide the effects of these two component categories. Current dietary recommendations suggest that carbohydrate consumption be increased to more than 55 percent of calories. The *Diet and Health* report suggested that this increase from about 45 to 55 percent of calories be accomplished with complex carbohydrates, not sugars; however, the specific proportion of the 55 percent of total calories that should be from complex carbohydrates was not provided (NRC, 1989a).

In both the Surgeon General's and the NRC reports, there is a clear consensus on the beneficial health effects of eating foods containing high proportions of complex carbohydrates. *Diet and Health* recommended that the intake of starches and other complex carbohydrates be increased by eating six or more servings of a combination of breads, cereals, and legumes daily (NRC, 1989a). The Surgeon General's report stated, "The public would benefit from increased availability of foods and food products low in calories, total fat, saturated fat, cholesterol, sodium, and sugars, but high in a variety of natural forms of fiber and, perhaps, certain minerals and vitamins" (DHHS, 1988, p. 19). Selection of foods naturally high in starch is an excellent way to achieve this recommendation. They are readily available, generally inexpensive, and highly acceptable to the human palate.

Although there is no specific linkage between complex carbohydrate consumption and lowered chronic disease incidence, diets that exclude or that have low levels of whole-grain products, tubers, legumes, and vegetables are associated epidemiologically with a variety of chronic health problems, including obesity, cancer, heart disease, and diabetes mellitus. "Populations consuming high-carbohydrate diets . . . have a comparatively lower prevalence of noninsulin-dependent diabetes mellitus," according to *Diet and Health* (NRC, 1989a, p. 9).

An explanation for this observation may be that diets high in complex carbohydrates result in a lower prevalence of obesity, which is a risk factor for diabetes. Moreover, for individuals with diabetes mellitus, diets containing 50 to 60 percent of total calories as carbohydrates have been recommended by the Task Force on Nutrition and Exchange Lists of the American Diabetes Association (ADA, 1987). High-carbohydrate diets not only improve glucose tolerance and insulin sensitivity but are also generally low in fat. The ideal proportion of complex and simple carbohydrates in diets for individuals with diabetes is not yet resolved (DHHS, 1988). Health professionals generally recommend reliance upon foods containing complex digestible and indigestible carbohydrates and avoidance of simple sugars (especially sucrose) and fats.

In summary, foods containing high proportions of complex carbohydrates are highly desirable for overall good health, not necessarily because of their specific contribution to chronic disease prevention but because these foods are usually low in fat and calories and are high in fiber.

Simple Carbohydrates

The term *sugars* is used here generically to describe a group of mono- and disaccharides commonly found in foods. These simple carbohydrates include the monosaccharides glucose and fructose and the disaccharides sucrose, lactose, and maltose. Sucrose, or common table sugar, and two corn-based sweeteners, corn syrup (a cornstarch hydrolysate containing glucose, maltose, and longer-chained polymers of glucose) and high-fructose corn syrup (HFCS, which is made up of mixtures of fructose, glucose, and glucose polymers) are commonly added to processed foods for their sweetening and thickening properties.

Consumption patterns of carbohydrates have changed markedly in this century. Although Americans today consume fewer total carbohydrate calories due to a reduced intake of wheat flours, cereals, and potatoes, there have been increased intakes of simple sugars in the past 75 years. It is estimated that the per capita intake of total carbohydrates fell from 493 g/day during 1909–1913 to 413 g/day in 1985 (NRC, 1989a). During the period 1909–1913, 68 percent of total carbohydrate calories were from starch compared with a little over half today. In 1986, FDA estimated that Americans were obtaining 21 percent of their total calories from simple carbohydrates: 4 percent from fructose, 9 percent from sucrose, 5 percent from corn syrups, and 3 percent from other sugars. The most marked recent change in intake patterns is the displacement of sucrose with fructose. In the mid-1980s, HFCS began to replace sucrose in soft drinks and in a variety of other processed foods. Glinsmann et al. (1986) reported that in 1985, HFCS accounted for 30 percent of the total sugar used in foods.

The major shifts in simple carbohydrate intake patterns have led to a number of health concerns. The effects of sucrose, in particular, and simple sugars, in general, on the incidence of dental caries, CHD, diabetes mellitus, and even behavioral aberrations, such as hyperactivity and criminality, have been raised. Except for the unquestionable contribution of sugar to dental caries, nutrient dilution, and as a potential source of excess calories, none of the other concerns has been borne out.

Children and others vulnerable to dental caries should limit their consumption and frequency of use of foods high in sugars, according to the Surgeon General's report. "Caries-producing bacteria have a rather high need for a range of simple sugars (glucose, fructose, lactose, maltose, and sucrose) that they readily metabolize to acids that demineralize teeth" (DHHS, 1988, p. 15). Genetic, behavioral, and other factors also influence dental health.

At one time, there was concern whether sugar intake contributed to mortality from CHD (Yudkin, 1964). However, in 1986, a Sugars Task Force of FDA concluded that there was no conclusive evidence that dietary sugars are an independent risk factor for coronary artery disease in the general population (Glinsmann et al., 1986).

In individuals with diabetes mellitus, blood glucose and insulin respond differently to different types of simple and complex food carbohydrates (Crapo, 1984). The rise in blood sugar following ingestion of a food—commonly referred to as the glycemic index (Crapo, 1984)—varies with the type of sugar and starch, digestibility of the starch, food form, fiber type, and the cooking and preparation procedures (DHHS, 1988). Diets high in complex carbohydrates but low in sugars are generally recommended for people with diabetes mellitus. However, there is no scientific evidence that high-sugar diets cause or lead to non-insulin-dependent diabetes. The scientific data supporting beliefs that high-carbohydrate diets are associated with hypoglycemia, hyperactivity, or criminality are inadequate. Results of controlled clinical studies to test the carbohydrate-hypoglycemia-hyperactivity connection have been negative (NRC, 1989a).

Current Provision of Desired Information

Information on total, complex, and simple carbohydrate contents of foods may appear in the ingredient listing, the nutrition information panel, and the principal display panel. The ingredient list may provide useful information on the content of sugars and other carbohydrates in foods, provided that these components are added as ingredients to the food (21 CFR § 101.4). Quantitative information is indicated only by the order of ingredients listed on a food label. However, this format may be misleading if a consumer wants to know the relative amount of total simple sugars in the product. For example, a breakfast cereal may contain total simple sugars as a primary ingredient, but it may contain them at such levels that none of the individual sugars is the largest ingredient by weight in the food. Thus, one or more nonsugar ingredients (such as wheat flour) may be listed first on the ingredient list before any sugar is listed, although total sugars may be the major ingredient (by weight) of that cereal. Another issue is the increasing use of mild-flavored fruit juices or concentrated fruit juices stripped of their flavor to sweeten foods because consumers perceive sugars from fruit juices differently from other sugars (John Vanderveen, Center for Food Safety and Applied Nutrition, FDA, personal communication, 1990).

The nutrition information panel can be most helpful in providing quantitative carbohydrate information (21 CFR § 101.9(b)(5)). Carbohydrate content is listed in grams per serving, unless a serving contains less than 1 g. In that case, the statement "contains less than 1 g" or "less than 1 g" may be used as an alternative. Some manufacturers voluntarily subdivide total carbohydrate into total complex carbohydrate (containing more than 2 saccharide units) and total simple carbohydrates or sugars (mono- and disaccharides), although present regulations do not require or allow a listing of simple and/or complex carbohydrates on the nutrition information panel. This practice should be encouraged to aid consumers who desire such information.

Terms such as *sugar free, sugarless,* and *no sugar* may appear on the principal display panel (21 CFR § 101.66(f); USDA, 1982a), and brand names may imply some information regarding sugar content (for example, Sugar Smacks™). However, the principal display panel of most foods generally does not provide information about carbohydrate content.

Committee Recommendations

The Committee is concerned about the current provision of information about carbohydrates contained in foods, specifically, the fact that sugars contained in foods are dispersed throughout the ingredient listing based on the predominance by weight. A preferable approach would be to cluster them under the generic term *sugars,* and with individual sweeteners listed in descending order (by weight) in parentheses. For example, a wheat- and oat-flour-based cereal may have the following ingredient label: wheat flour, sugars (sucrose, corn syrup, and fructose), oats, etc.

Current FDA regulations allow the use of "and/or" labeling for fats and oils. The Committee believes that consideration should be given to allowing similar "and/or" labeling for sugars. By using the example given above, the ingredient list would read as follows: wheat flour, sugars (sucrose, corn syrup, and/or fructose), oats, etc. "And/or" labeling of sugars would give the manufacturer flexibility in the use of sweeteners and, presumably, could result in reduced costs for consumers.

The Committee recommends that:

- FDA and USDA should continue to require the disclosure of carbohydrate content per serving in grams on the nutrition information panel.
- FDA and USDA should allow, as an option, the listing of the content of complex carbohydrates (which are defined as digestible polysaccharides such as starch and glycogen) and sugars (which are defined as digestible mono- and disaccharides) per serving in grams on the nutrition information panel. The term *total carbohydrate* should be used when carbohydrate components are listed on the nutrition information panel, with these subgroups indented.
- FDA and USDA should allow, as an option, the listing of calories per serving from total carbohydrate, complex carbohydrate, and sugars on the nutrition information panel.
- The ingredient listing should group all sugars together under the term *sugars* with mono- and disaccharides (including glucose [dextrose], fructose, lactose, sucrose, invert sugar, and honey, as well as corn syrup, HFCS, and mild-flavored and "stripped" concentrated fruit juices) in a parenthetical listing, in descending order by weight under this term. Sugar alcohols, such as mannitol and sorbitol, would be listed separately and would not be grouped with sugars.
- FDA and USDA should consider allowing manufacturers to use "and/or" labeling for sugars.
- FDA and USDA should define descriptors that apply to terms used for carbohydrate and sugar content on foods labels.

DIETARY FIBER

Health Relevance of Dietary Fiber

The American public has been inundated with advice to increase consumption of dietary fiber. The *Dietary Guidelines for Americans* stated that Americans should eat foods containing adequate starch and fiber (USDA/DHHS, 1985). The Surgeon General's report and the NRC *Diet and Health* report advised consumers to increase consumption of whole-grain foods and cereals and vegetables and fruits in order to increase intakes of complex carbohydrate and fiber (DHHS, 1988; NRC, 1989a).

Unfortunately, trends in food intake patterns since the turn of the century indicate that Americans have been consuming fewer rather than greater numbers of foods that are rich in fiber. The National Cancer Institute's dietary guidelines suggested that adults consume 20 to 30 g of dietary fiber daily, with an upper limit of 35 g (Butrum et al., 1988). Lanza et al. (1987) estimated from the second National Health and Nutrition Examination Survey (NHANES II) that mean intake of fiber by adults (19 to 74 years) in the United States was 11.1 g/day (with women consuming an average of 9.4 g and men consuming 12.9 g), well below that recommended by the National Cancer Institute.

Dietary fiber is a term that refers to a heterogeneous group of plant food components that are resistant to digestion by enzymes produced by the human gastrointestinal tract (LSRO, FASEB, 1989). These components include cellulose, hemicelluloses, pectins, and lignins from plant cell walls and gums, algal polysaccharides, and mucilages from plant cells (NRC, 1989a).

There has been a great deal of interest in the specific effects of dietary fiber on several chronic diseases. The strongest argument for an increase in consumption of dietary fiber is the important contribution it makes to normal bowel function. Clear scientific associations of fiber intake with the incidence of heart disease, certain types of cancer, and diabetes mellitus have not been made. One reason may be the difficulty in designing appropriate experiments to specifically test for the effect of dietary fiber. Foods high in dietary fiber are also generally low in calories and total and saturated fatty acids and devoid of cholesterol; thus, determination of a specific fiber effect in a feeding study is difficult. Moreover, foods have a variety of fiber components, and each may have different actions. Chemically and physiologically, cellulose, lignin, hemicellulose, pectin, and alginates (all relatively purified fiber types) behave differently. Wheat bran, oat bran, and rice bran (all heterogeneous mixtures of fibers) are not similar in composition. It is also very difficult to analyze dietary fiber chemically, and thus it is hard to correlate the role of specific fiber components to health effects (NRC, 1989a).

Recently, there has been some effort to subclassify the possible health effects of soluble and insoluble dietary fiber. *Soluble* fiber includes pectins, gums, mucilages, and some hemicelluloses that are reasonably water soluble. *Insoluble* fiber includes cellulose, lignin, and most hemicelluloses. These subclasses of dietary fiber have physiologically different and potentially important effects on colon function. Wheat bran and other forms of insoluble fiber decrease transit time and increase dry and wet stool weight. Softer stools lead to easier elimination and lessen the chance of hemorrhoids. Higher-fiber diets may also increase satiety and, thus, may be beneficial for weight control (NRC, 1989a).

Some clinical studies have suggested that "water-soluble fiber from foods such as oat bran, beans, or certain fruits are associated with lower blood glucose and blood lipid levels," whereas there is "some evidence . . . that an overall increase in intake of foods high in fiber might decrease the risk of colon cancer" (DHHS, 1988, p. 12). However, *Diet and Health* concluded: "In general, the evidence for a protective role of dietary fiber per se in CHD, colon and rectal cancers, stomach cancer, female gynecologic cancers, diabetes, diverticulosis, hypertension, and gallstones is inconclusive. Even where the evidence is strongest, it has not been possible to adequately separate the effects of fiber from those of other components of the diet" (NRC, 1989a, p. 302). Appropriate studies are sorely needed to clarify the possible effects of fiber on health. For example, intervention studies in human populations could clarify the role of specific fiber components in health (NRC, 1989a).

Current Provision of Desired Information

Information on the dietary fiber content of a food may be stated in several places on food labels. No information would be readily available from the ingredient listing, unless a consumer was aware of the fiber sources among a product's ingredients.

The fiber content is allowed on a food product, although current regulations do not require its listing as part of the nutrition information panel. If the manufacturer chooses to list fiber content, it must follow the approved analytical method of the Association of Official Analytical Chemists (Prosky et al., 1985) to determine the total dietary fiber content of the product. The section on analytical considerations in Chapter 4 provides further discussion of difficulties associated with total dietary fiber analysis, and its subcomponents.

Descriptors such as *high in dietary fiber* have become increasingly common on the principal display panel. However, the agencies have not established formal rules or definitions for such terms. In a 1988 policy letter responding to a citizen petition, FDA proposed the following descriptor terms for dietary fiber: a *source* is 2 g, a *good source* is 5 g, and an *excellent source* is 8 g in a serving of food (Ronk, 1988). The terms *fair source* (10 percent of U.S. RDA), *good source* (25 percent), and *excellent source* (40 percent) were defined in a 1986 FDA policy letter, assuming that a minimum daily intake of 20 g of fiber daily was used in shelf labeling programs (Ronk, 1986). USDA does not currently have any official policy on declaring dietary fiber content on food labels.

Committee Recommendations

The Committee recommends that:

- FDA and USDA should require the disclosure of fiber content per serving in grams on the nutrition information panel under the term *total dietary fiber*.

- FDA and USDA should define the scope of foods from animal origin and other foods that contain little or no dietary fiber which should be exempted from this requirement.
- FDA and USDA should discourage labeling of soluble or insoluble fiber contents until methodologies approved by the agencies allow for the adequate and reproducible quantification of the soluble and insoluble fiber contents of a variety of foods.
- FDA and USDA should define descriptive terms allowed to be used for various source levels of dietary fiber on food labels.

PROTEIN

Health Relevance of Protein

The *Dietary Guidelines for Americans* stress that Americans should eat a variety of foods to have a healthful diet (USDA/DHHS, 1985). People need over 40 different nutrients to stay healthy. Although a certain amount of protein is needed for good health, the diets of the majority of Americans contain protein in excess of the Recommended Dietary Allowances (RDA) (NRC, 1989b). USDA surveys have consistently revealed that the average protein intake for all respondents ranging in age from infancy to over 75 years exceeds the RDA and represents approximately 11 to 16 percent of calories (NRC, 1989a).

Protein is an essential nutrient. Amino acids obtained from the digestion and absorption of dietary proteins are synthesized into enzymes, a variety of hormones, neurotransmitters, and carrier, structural, and binding proteins. The amino acid tryptophan can be converted to the vitamin niacin. Amino acids can also be used as a source of energy when energy is limiting, most can be made into glucose and stored as glycogen when carbohydrate is limiting, and all can be stored as fat. In mammals, 10 amino acids (histidine, isoleucine, leucine, lysine, methionine, phenylalanine, threonine, tryptophan, valine, histidine, and arginine [for premature infants and total parenteral nutrition-fed patients]) cannot be synthesized in sufficient amounts (Heird et al., 1972; NRC, 1989b). These essential amino acids must be supplied by the diet. The nonessential amino acids can be synthesized from dietary sources of utilizable carbon and nitrogen.

Protein intake has been associated with an increased risk for several chronic diseases. The data linking too much protein, specifically too much animal protein, with CHD risk in humans are primarily based on epidemiological evidence. Since animal protein and saturated fatty acid intakes are often highly correlated, it is difficult to establish a specific cause-and-effect relationship in population studies. However, some evidence in humans indicates that in cases where soy protein was substituted for animal protein, serum cholesterol was lowered. In addition, vegetarians tend to have serum cholesterol values lower than those of the general population (NRC, 1989a). This difference may also reflect, in part, other life-style differences.

The relationship between the amount and the type of dietary protein and cancer in humans is being actively studied. Epidemiological evidence suggests a possible relationship between high intakes of dietary protein and increased risk for certain cancers (NRC, 1982). Once again, this may be confounded by the high correlation between intakes of fat and protein in the Western diet (NRC, 1989a).

There is also some debate as to whether high intakes of dietary protein promote osteoporosis. A high dietary protein intake in the form of a purified isolated nutrient increases the amount of calcium excreted in the urine. However, there is little evidence that diets traditionally high in protein increase the risk for osteoporosis, especially if the phosphorus intake increases with protein intake, as it does in the United States (NRC, 1989a).

Finally, there are data linking high-protein diets with age-related progression of renal disease in humans and experimental animals (NRC, 1989a). More research is needed to clarify this relationship.

In summary, many of the studies linking high-protein diets with increased chronic disease in humans are epidemiological in nature, which does not prove that there is a cause-and-effect relationship. These associations also reflect the high correlations between the intakes of protein and other constituents such as fat and fiber. There is little or no evidence to indicate beneficial health effects from high protein intakes, as stated in the 1989 RDA report (NRC, 1989b).

Current Provision of Desired Information

Information on the protein content of packaged foods may be found in three areas on the food label, including the ingredient listing, the nutrition information panel, and the principal display panel. Although the ingredient listing includes food components in descending order of prominence by weight, it provides little useful information on protein content (21 CFR § 101.4). For example, milk-based formulated foods may contain various proteins in the form of nonfat dry milk, soy protein isolate, and yeast.

The current nutrition panel provides information about protein in two places: the amount of protein in grams per serving listed immediately after calories, and the percentage of the U.S. RDA, where protein is the first listed nutrient (21 CFR § 101.9(c)(4), (7)).

Terms such as *high protein* may appear on the principal display panel, although this term has not been officially defined. When used for shelf labeling, products must contain 18 g of high-quality protein (at 45 g/day) or 26 g of lower-quality protein (at 65 g/day) per serving to use the term *excellent source*.

Committee Recommendations

Although protein is an important nutrient, most Americans consume sufficient amounts. The Committee recommends that:

- FDA and USDA should continue to require the disclosure of protein content per serving in grams on the nutrition information panel. However, protein should be moved to a position of less prominence.
- The current requirement to list protein content as a percentage of the U.S. RDA should be eliminated.
- FDA and USDA should allow, as an option, the listing of total calories per serving from protein.
- FDA and USDA should define descriptors that apply to terms used for protein content on food labels.

SODIUM

Health Relevance of Sodium

Recent dietary recommendations have advised Americans to reduce their intake of sodium. The *Dietary Guidelines for Americans* recommended avoiding too much sodium (USDA/DHHS, 1985). The Surgeon General's report (DHHS, 1988) recommended that consumers reduce their intake of sodium by choosing foods relatively low in sodium and limiting the amount of salt added during food preparation and at the table. *Diet and Health* (NRC, 1989a) recommended that Americans limit their total daily intake of salt (sodium chloride) to 6 g or less by limiting the use of salt during cooking, by avoiding the addition of salt to food at the table, and by greatly limiting the consumption of salty, highly processed salty, salt-preserved, and salt-pickled foods.

Sodium is one of the most common, yet most important, minerals. It is found in most plant and animal tissues and fluids and is essential to life. In humans, sodium is the major cation in extracellular fluids (blood, lymph, and interstitial fluid), and its concentration is a major determinant of intra- and extracellular fluid volumes. Along with potassium, the major cation of intracellular fluid, sodium controls the passage of water in and out of the cells. It is a major electrolyte in the body and, along with a few other ions, controls the electrical properties of cells (NRC, 1989a).

The sodium concentration in extracellular fluids, and thus extracellular fluid volume, is maintained primarily by the kidneys, interacting with the endocrine and nervous systems. Too little sodium in extracellular fluid (hyponatremia) can result from abnormally high sodium excretion by individuals with certain kidney diseases. In normal humans, salt ingested in excess of that needed to maintain normal serum levels is excreted in urine and sweat. If renal function is impaired, the sodium concentration in extracellular fluid can increase and, through its osmotic pressure, draw fluid from cells into the extracellular fluids (including blood), thus causing susceptible individuals to develop edema and heart failure.

Beyond its physiological properties, salt has always been prized for its value as a preservative and a flavor in the majority of foods. In recent decades, Americans have developed a strong taste for salt and now consume it in amounts far in excess of normal physiological requirements. Salt, or sodium chloride, is 40 percent sodium by weight.

Most sodium is ingested as sodium chloride in solid foods, but other sources of dietary sodium can be important. Most municipal water supplies contain less than 20 mg of sodium per liter, but some contain naturally as much as 1,000 mg/liter. Sources of dietary sodium, in addition to sodium chloride, are other salts (e.g., sodium bicarbonate) and sodium-containing preservatives and flavor enhancers that are added during food manufacturing or processing.

The majority of dietary salt is added to food during processing. Results of studies vary, but estimates are that 10 to 35 percent of dietary salt occurs naturally in the food, 35 to 75 percent is added during manufacturing and processing, and 15 to 35 percent is added by the consumer at mealtime (NRC, 1989a; Shank et al., 1983).

The sodium intake of Americans has increased markedly since World War II, along with the consumption of foods manufactured and/or prepared outside the home. The sodium content of some prepared foods can be quite high. At limited-menu restaurants, sandwiches frequently contain more than 900 mg of sodium; a meal of a hamburger, fries, ketchup, and a milkshake can provide more than 1,000 mg of sodium; a triple cheeseburger can contain over 1,800 mg of sodium (Massachusetts Medical Society, 1989).

Physicians have been concerned about the adverse health effects of sodium ingestion since the early 1900s. The principal concerns have been the role of sodium in causing high blood pressure (hypertension), heart failure, and edema. Dietary restriction of sodium can be lifesaving for certain individuals with severe renal or heart failure and for those who retain sodium and/or water, thus building up their extracellular fluid volume. Lowering of sodium intake helps to reduce blood volume and edema; at times, an extremely low sodium intake is mandatory to preserve life. Sodium's role in increasing blood volume and edema is generally well understood. Much less well understood is the role that sodium plays as a causative factor in high blood pressure (hypertension).

Hypertension, generally uncommon in populations with low sodium intakes, is a common cause of morbidity and mortality in the United States. It is estimated that as many as 60 million people in the United States are hypertensive, as defined by the National Heart, Lung, and Blood Institute (NHLBI). Hypertension is a major risk factor for some of the most common causes of death in the United States: coronary artery disease, hypertensive heart disease, arteriosclerosis, and stroke. In addition, hypertension is a major cause of renal failure. It is often familial; individuals can have a genetic predisposition to hypertension, but there is no known genetic marker (NRC, 1989a). Perhaps 10 to 30 percent of the U.S. population is genetically predisposed to hypertension and has a higher risk of developing hypertension as a result of sodium ingestion. The incidence of hypertension increases with age; it has been estimated that 65 percent of Americans will develop hypertension by the time they are age 65 to 74. It is much more common among black Americans than among whites, suggesting a genetic predisposition of blacks to develop the disease.

Although the etiology of some types of hypertension is known (e.g., renovascular hypertension), the cause of the most common form—essential hypertension—is not known. Sodium plays an important role in the development of hypertension in at least some populations, along with other factors (age, obesity, alcohol consumption, stress, and other nutrients, such as potassium and chloride). It is clear that reductions of dietary sodium can achieve a modest amelioration of hypertension in at least some population subgroups. It would therefore seem reasonable, given the high incidence of hypertension in Americans, for the U.S. population to reduce its sodium consumption.

The above statements are generally undisputed within the medical and scientific communities. What is disputed is the precise role that sodium plays in the etiology of hypertension. Most authorities agree that sodium is an important factor in the development of hypertension in susceptible individuals and that excess sodium can exacerbate hypertension.

The most telling information comes from epidemiological studies, many of which show a relationship between sodium intake and the incidence of hypertension. Although studies of some societies whose populations ingest relatively large amounts of sodium did not find an increased incidence of hypertension, studies of other cultures did, giving credence to the role of genes in causing hypertension (NRC, 1989a).

Conversely, certain societies with traditionally low levels of dietary sodium have a low incidence of hypertension. It is difficult to control studies of large populations for other factors known to influence blood pressure, such as body weight, exercise, and stress levels. Nevertheless, experts agree that there is a positive correlation between dietary sodium and blood pressure in large populations (DHHS, 1988; NRC, 1989a).

Finally, a reduction of sodium intake does not have a significant effect on the blood pressure of all hypertensive individuals, but it does benefit certain individuals. It has been estimated that about half of all hypertensive individuals in the U.S. population are sensitive to salt. At present, the only way to determine whether an individual's blood pressure is related to salt intake is through a lengthy dietary trial during which salt intake is varied. It is hoped that, in the future, some simple test performed early in life could make that determination.

The overwhelming consensus of medical experts who have considered the health effects of sodium is that Americans should reduce the amount of sodium they consume. The reasons are that the average American diet contains an amount of sodium far in excess of that required for good health, high sodium intake correlates positively with the development of hypertension in a large number of individuals, and hypertension and its sequelae are major health problems in the United States. It can reasonably be expected that a lowering of sodium intakes in the United States will lower both the incidence and the severity of hypertension. Americans are now concerned about the amount of sodium they consume and its role in disease. Through the success of public information campaigns such as those by FDA, NHLBI, and the AHA, the majority of Americans now know that excess salt or sodium ingestion is associated with poor health.

Current Provision of Desired Information

Information on the sodium content of packaged foods may be found in the ingredient listing, the nutrition information panel, and the principal display panel. The ingredient listing provides information about salt and sodium-containing compounds added to foods (21 CFR § 101.4)

FDA's original nutrition labeling regulations did not require that sodium be listed unless a sodium or salt claim was made. If sodium was declared voluntarily, the label had to state the amount of sodium in milligrams per serving. Sodium content was to be listed when the serving contained more than 10 mg of sodium, and was to appear in 5-mg increments.

The voluntary listing of the sodium content of ordinary foods did not trigger full nutrition labeling. If a food's label claimed that it was useful in regulating sodium or salt intake (food for special dietary use), however, the label had to declare the food's sodium content both as sodium per serving and the amount of sodium per 100 g of food.

Because of a growing national concern over the deleterious health effects of excessive dietary sodium, FDA made the quantitative listing of sodium a required part of nutrition labeling effective in 1986. Sodium content was to be listed when the serving contained more than 5 mg per serving, and was to appear in 5-mg increments up to 140 mg of sodium per serving. Above that level, it was to be given in 10-mg increments (21 CFR § 101.9(c)(8)(i)). The same regulations defined the descriptive terms *sodium free, low sodium, very low sodium,* and *reduced sodium,* and provided for the proper use of those terms on the principal display panel. They also defined the terms *without added salt, unsalted,* and *no salt added* (21 CFR § 101.13).

Thus, only for the past few years has the quantitative labeling of sodium been required as part of nutrition labeling whenever it is used or when a specific claim is made that the food is useful in regulating sodium or salt intake. On foods for special dietary use, the previously mandated dual listing of milligrams of sodium per serving and milligrams per 100 g of food is no longer required; sodium is to be listed only in milligrams per serving.

USDA requirements for listing the sodium content of foods are essentially identical to those of FDA. Unless a sodium claim is made, the listing of sodium content is voluntary and the listing of sodium content per serving alone does not trigger full nutrition labeling. When provided or required, sodium content must be expressed in milligrams per serving. One difference from FDA's requirements is that in the absence of a sodium claim, sodium content is not a required component of nutrition labeling. USDA's definitions for descriptors of sodium content on the principal display panel are identical to FDA's, but USDA also permits use of the term *salt free*, following the same criteria for *sodium free* (USDA, 1984a).

Committee Recommendations

Current regulations for the provision of information on the sodium content of foods are faulty only in that sodium content is not required to be declared on all foods. Therefore, the following recommendations are similar to current FDA regulations and USDA policy. The Committee recommends that:

- FDA and USDA should continue to require the disclosure of sodium content per serving in milligrams, regardless of source (whether natural or added), on the nutrition information panel.
- Descriptors for sodium content on the principal display panel, as currently defined by FDA and USDA, should be continued.

POTASSIUM

Health Relevance of Potassium

Potassium was accorded status as a potential public health issue by the recent report on nutrition monitoring (LSRO, FASEB, 1989). No specific recommendation was made in either the Surgeon General's or the NRC reports.

Potassium is closely related to sodium in many ways. It is the major cation in intracellular fluid, and so its concentration is a primary determinant of intracellular fluid volume. Along with sodium, potassium controls the passage of water in and out of cells and the electrical properties of cellular membranes.

Because of its importance in maintaining the function of all cellular membranes in the body, marked derangements of intracellular potassium concentrations, either high or low, can cause serious illness and death. Generally, the body's homeostatic mechanisms are quite efficient in maintaining normal potassium levels, and healthy individuals who are not taking diuretics rarely suffer from potassium imbalance. Severe alterations are relatively rare, and they are almost always associated with other serious, symptomatic disease.

Most severe potassium losses from the body are associated with losses of body fluids. Copious vomiting or diarrhea can cause low serum potassium levels. Relatively large amounts of potassium can be excreted in urine through the prolonged use of diuretics. The development of kidney disease leads to an imbalance of potassium that needs to be controlled by therapeutic means. The importance of potassium to normal body function means that serious potassium depletion is associated with marked clinical symptoms of disease.

The observation that increased potassium and reduced sodium intakes can lower blood pressure was first made decades ago, but the significance of this finding is still being debated (HPTRG, 1990; LSRO, FASEB, 1989; NRC, 1989a). Because of the frequency of use of diuretics for the treatment of heart failure and hypertension, many consumers are aware of the possibility that diuretic agents may lower serum potassium levels in individuals with these diseases. The general public is relatively unaware of the possible role of potassium in lowering blood pressure.

Current Provision of Desired Information

Under current FDA regulations and USDA policy governing nutrition labeling, the declaration of potassium is voluntary. If potassium is declared, the amount must immediately follow the sodium content and include the number of milligrams of potassium in a specified serving (portion) of food. As with sodium, the content can be zero when the serving contains less than 5 mg of potassium, and must be given in 5-mg increments up to 140 mg of potassium per serving. Above that level, it must be given in 10-mg increments (21 CFR § 101.9(c)(8)(ii); USDA, 1984b).

Committee Recommendations

Neither an excess nor a deficit of dietary potassium is a public health problem for Americans. A relatively small number of individuals who excrete high amounts of potassium (e.g., those on certain diuretics) need potassium-rich diets or potassium supplementation of their diets. Thus, the quantitative listing of this mineral should be permitted for foods that are rich in potassium and required on foods when a claim is made that the food is useful in providing dietary potassium.

Existing FDA regulations and USDA policy are satisfactory. Therefore, the Committee recommends that:

- Disclosure of potassium content on the nutrition information panel should remain voluntary, unless a potassium claim is made.

- If disclosed on the label, potassium content per serving should be listed in milligrams.

VITAMINS AND MINERALS

The following discussion includes a review of the micronutrients currently required on the nutrition panel (vitamins A and C, thiamin, niacin, riboflavin, calcium, and iron) and several additional ones (vitamin B_6, fluoride, folate, potassium, and zinc), for which current public health concerns have been raised (LSRO, FASEB, 1989; NRC, 1989a). Other micronutrients, many of which are currently allowed on an optional basis on the nutrition label, that were discussed in recent reports were not judged in those documents to be current or potential public health problems, nor were specific recommendations made concerning their consumption; therefore, they are not considered for food labeling.

Health Relevance of Nutrition Labeling Recommendations

Calcium

Recent dietary recommendations have advised Americans to increase their intake of calcium. The Surgeon General's report recommended that adolescent girls and adult women should increase their consumption of foods high in calcium, including low-fat dairy products (DHHS, 1988). The *Diet and Health* report advised that consumers maintain adequate calcium intake (NRC, 1989a). The 1989 report, *Nutrition Monitoring in the United States,* advised that calcium merited priority monitoring due to the low dietary intakes by women and the possible association with age-related osteoporosis (LSRO, FASEB, 1989).

In the body, 99 percent of the calcium is stored in the bones and teeth, where it contributes to the formation and maintenance of these tissues. The rest is in fluids and soft tissue, playing a role in nerve conductivity, muscle contraction, and blood clotting. Throughout life, skeletal calcium is continuously turned over through resorption and formation. Calcium absorption is influenced by dietary calcium intake, the interaction of calcium with other dietary substances in the small intestine, and the level of activity of the transport systems that moves calcium into the body.

The 1989 RDA subcommittee judged that adequate calcium during the formative years was the way to reduce the risk of osteoporosis (NRC, 1989b). Peak bone mass is determined by a number of factors, including hormonal status, genetics, and various dietary components during the years of bone mineralization. Evidence of the role of dietary calcium in peak bone mass is still unclear, inconsistent, and incomplete. Further research is needed to determine the exact mechanism of skeletal formation and other factors that influence skeletal health. However, the efficiency of absorption is increased during periods of high physiological requirements, such as during pregnancy and in children during growth periods.

Conversely, calcium absorption in elderly individuals and other population subgroups is impaired. The presence of various other dietary factors, notably protein and vitamin D, affect calcium absorption. For women who are in the postmenopausal stage of life, the rate of decline in bone mineral is strongly dependent on estrogen status. At present, results of studies of the effect of calcium supplementation on age-related bone loss are inconclusive, but supplementation combined with estrogen treatment has been reported to be as successful as estrogen alone in slowing the rate of bone loss. Factors other than calcium intake (genetics, age, sex, body weight, hormonal status, and physical activity) are related to osteoporosis (NRC, 1989a). Some studies have suggested that a high calcium intake has been associated with lowering blood pressure.

The Surgeon General's report indicated that men and children had estimated mean intakes of 105 and 115 percent, respectively, of the RDA for calcium, whereas women had estimated mean intakes that were 78 percent of the RDA (DHHS, 1988). The 1989 RDA included a higher recommendation for calcium (1,200 mg) for males and females aged 11 to 24 in order to permit full mineral deposition (NRC, 1989b). The same level is set for pregnant and lactating women. For people in older age groups, the 1980 level of 800 mg was retained. A level of 250 mg/day is recommended for newborns. Assessment of calcium status in survey populations has not been done.

Iron

The Surgeon General's report recommended that because dietary iron deficiency is responsible for the most prevalent form of anemia in the United States, children, adolescents, and women of childbearing age should be sure to consume foods that are good sources of iron (DHHS, 1988). The report indicated that this was of special concern for low-income families. The recent nutrition monitoring report concluded that high monitoring priority should be accorded to iron because it is a current public health issue (LSRO, FASEB, 1989).

Iron is a constituent of blood, most notably hemoglobin, in tissues such as myoglobin and in a variety of cytochromes and enzymes, all of which make it essential for life. It is also stored in several body organs. The main physiological role of iron is to carry oxygen to the body tissues. The body's iron content is regulated by the amount of iron absorbed by the intestinal mucosa. Absorption is influenced by body stores, the amount and form of dietary intake, and the dietary components with which it is ingested.

Inadequate intakes of dietary iron can ultimately lead to anemia. Currently, there is no single biochemical indicator available to assess iron inadequacy in the general population in a reliable manner; however, operational definitions of anemia have been set by the World Health Organization and proposed by the Centers for Disease Control. The consequences of iron deficiency ascribed to the resulting anemia can occur before reduced hemoglobin levels are apparent. Decreased work capacity, reduced physical performance, and impaired immune function have been reported to be associated with low hemoglobin levels in adults. In children, iron deficiency has been associated with apathy, short attention span, irritability, and a reduced ability to learn (NRC, 1989b).

In the United States, iron deficiency is primarily observed during four specific periods in life (NRC, 1989b). The first is from 6 to 48 months of age and is due to the low iron content of milk, rapid body growth, and limited iron stores in the body. The second period is during adolescence, another time of rapid body growth and expanding red blood cell mass. The third is the female reproductive period and is due to menstrual iron losses. Finally, the fourth period is during the female reproductive process, when the mother's blood volume expands, there are increased demands due to fetus and placenta, and there are blood losses during childbirth.

Heme iron, primarily obtained from animal sources, is a highly absorbable form and seems to represent a significant source in many individuals. Absorption of non-heme iron, primarily obtained from plant sources, is believed to be enhanced by consumption with foods containing vitamin C, which is present in high amounts in the diets of most age groups. Other dietary substances can substantially decrease the absorption of nonheme iron. The recent trend of reduced meat intake may decrease iron intake in the population, because red meats are an important source of dietary iron. The Surgeon General's report indicated that the estimated mean intakes by women and children were 61 and 88 percent of the 1980 RDA, respectively, whereas estimated mean intakes by men were 159 percent of the RDA (DHHS, 1988).

The 1989 RDA for iron was set at 15 mg/day for adult women in the United States, a level believed to provide a sufficient margin of safety. This level was a reduction from the 18-mg/day level set in 1980, since the prevalence of iron deficiency anemia in that age group is low. Available data suggest that 10 to 11 mg of iron per day in a typical American's diet is sufficient for most women. The RDA level of 10 mg/day for males aged 19 to 60 remained unchanged. With little evidence of iron deficiency among the elderly, the RDA for this group is set at 10 mg/day. On average, an additional 15 mg/day is needed throughout pregnancy; however, this is usually obtained through the use of iron supplements. Infants aged 3 months to 3 years need 1 mg/day if they are bottle-fed. For children aged 6 to 36 months, the RDA is set at 10 mg/day. Adolescent males need 12 mg/day, whereas the level for adolescent females is 15 mg/day.

Vitamin A

Vitamin A and carotenes were accorded the status of a potential public health issue by the Expert Panel on Nutrition Monitoring (LSRO, FASEB, 1989). No specific recommendation was made in either the Surgeon General's or NRC reports.

Vitamin A represents a group of compounds that are critical for vision, growth, cellular differentiation and proliferation, reproduction, and the immune system. The body's need for vitamin A can be met by dietary intake of preformed retinoids with vitamin A activity, generally from animal products, or by consumption of carotenoid precursors of vitamin A. Carotenoid precursors are found in plants, the best known being beta-carotene. Carotenoid-rich food consumption is inversely associated with lung cancer risk, though such foods are not protective against lung cancer for smokers (NRC, 1989a).

Preformed vitamin A, mainly retinyl esters, is efficiently absorbed. Most carotenoids are not well absorbed, unless they are present in oil. Retinol and a portion of the active carotenoids are absorbed and transferred to the liver which contains about 90 percent of the total body stores of the vitamin. Carotenoids that are not otherwise converted are generally deposited in adipose tissue or the adrenal glands. The absorption and utilization of carotenoids and vitamin A are enhanced by dietary fat, protein, and vitamin E. Absorption is depressed by diets that are very low in fat and when either peroxidized fat and other oxidizing agents are present or when deficiencies exist for protein, vitamin E, iron, or zinc.

Inadequate dietary intake of vitamin A is found most commonly in children under age 5. Deficiency can also occur in situations of chronic fat malabsorption. Clinical signs range from night blindness to total blindness. Other signs of deficiency include loss of appetite, hyperkeratosis, and increased susceptibility to infections.

The estimated mean intakes of vitamin A by men, women, and children are reported to be close to or above the RDA for vitamin A (DHHS, 1988). The RDA for adults is set at 1,000 retinol equivalents (RE) for men and 800 RE for women (NRC, 1989b). No increment of vitamin A intake is necessary during pregnancy; however, a daily increment of 400 to 500 RE is needed during lactation. For an infant consuming 3 cups of milk daily, the RDA of 375 mg will be met. Because of the demands of rapid growth, the RDA for vitamin A is set at 400, 500, and 700 RE daily for the age groups 1 to 3, 4 to 6, and 7 to 10, respectively. Beyond age 11, the sexes have separate RDAs that are the same as those for adults.

Vitamin C

Ascorbic acid was accorded the status of a potential public health issue by the Expert Panel on Nutrition Monitoring (LSRO, FASEB, 1989). No specific recommendation was made in either the Surgeon General's or NRC reports.

The primary function of vitamin C (ascorbic acid) is its role as a cofactor in hydroxylation reactions requiring molecular oxygen and reactions with other dietary factors. It also affects the function of leukocytes and macrophages, immune response, wound healing, and allergic reactions. Ascorbic acid is well absorbed in the intestines and increases the absorption of inorganic iron when the two nutrients are ingested together. Epidemiological studies suggest some possible protection against cancer by vitamin C-containing foods and vitamin C itself, but the effect of vitamin C on cancer in experimental studies in animals is far less clear.

Dietary deficiency of vitamin C can eventually lead to scurvy, characterized by weakening of collagenous structures that result in widespread capillary hemorrhaging. In the United States, scurvy is rare but can occur in infants fed diets consisting exclusively of cow's milk and in elderly individuals on inadequate diets.

The calculated amount of vitamin C intake can vary due to destruction during storage and preparation, use of supplements (which are ingested by 35 percent of the population), limitations of food composition tables, and the addition of ascorbic acid to processed foods for its properties as an antioxidant. The average dietary vitamin C intake by adult men is 109 mg; for adult women and children the average intakes were 77 mg and 84 mg, respectively (DHHS, 1988). The RDA for adults and elderly individuals is set at 60 mg/day, which is usually provided in mixed diets (NRC, 1989b). The recommendation for vitamin C intake by smokers is set at 100 mg/day, due to the increased requirements in this group. The increment for pregnant women is 10 mg/day and for lactating women it is 35 mg/day for the first 6 months of lactation and 30 mg/day for the second 6 months of lactation. The RDA for infants is set at 30 mg/day, which increases gradually for children to the adult levels by age 15.

Thiamin

In *Nutrition Monitoring in the United States* (LSRO, FASEB, 1989), thiamin was not considered to be a current public health issue. No specific recommendation concerning thiamin was given in either the Surgeon General's or NRC reports.

Thiamin is used in the body as the coenzyme thiamin pyrophosphate for the oxidative decarboxylation of alpha-keto acids and the activity of transketolase in the pentose phosphate pathway. It is rapidly absorbed in the small intestine.

Thiamin deficiency primarily occurs in situations in which the enrichment of white rice and white flour has not been implemented or low levels of dietary thiamin are associated with consumption of raw fish, whose intestinal microbes contain thiaminase. In the United States, thiamin deficiency is unlikely in healthy individuals but has been observed in individuals whose health is otherwise compromised by such conditions as alcoholism, renal disease, chronic febrile infections, chronic intravenous feeding, or inborn errors in metabolism. Deficiency is associated with abnormalities of carbohydrate metabolism related to decreased oxidative decarboxylations. The clinical condition associated with a prolonged deficient intake is beriberi, which is characterized by mental confusion, anorexia, muscle weakness, ataxia, peripheral paralysis, edema or muscle wasting (depending on the type of beriberi), tachycardia, and enlarged heart.

The average thiamin daily intake is reported to be 1.75 mg by adult men, 1.05 mg by adult women, and 1.12 mg by children aged 1 to 5 (NRC, 1989b). A minimum of 1.0 mg/day is the recommended level for all adults (NRC, 1989b). An additional 0.4 mg/day is recommended throughout pregnancy for maternal and fetal growth as well as increased maternal caloric intake. An increment of 0.5 mg/day is recommended throughout lactation. The 1989 RDA allowance for infants is 0.4 mg/1,000 kcal; this increases to 0.5 mg/1,000 kcal for children and adolescents.

Riboflavin

In *Nutrition Monitoring in the United States* (LSRO, FASEB, 1989), riboflavin was not considered to be a current public health issue. No specific recommendation concerning riboflavin was given in either the Surgeon General's or NRC reports.

This B vitamin functions primarily as a part of two flavin coenzymes (flavin mononucleotide and flavin adenine dinucleotide) that catalyze many oxidation-reduction reactions. Riboflavin is essential in the function of vitamin B_6 and niacin. Riboflavin is readily absorbed in the small intestine. Deficiency is rare in the United States, but symptoms include oral-buccal cavity lesions, a generalized seborrheic dermatitis, and normocytic anemia.

Average reported intakes are 2.08 mg/day by men, 1.34 mg/day by women, and 1.57 mg/day by children ages 1 to 5 (NRC, 1989b). A minimum intake of 1.2 mg/day is recommended for adults (NRC, 1989b). An additional intake of 0.3 mg/day is recommended during pregnancy; and 0.5 mg and 0.4 mg/day are recommended for the first 6 months and thereafter, respectively, for lactation. Because of the possibility of growth inhibition with inadequate intakes by children, the allowance is set at 0.6 mg/100 kcal for infants and approximately 1 mg/day for children.

Niacin

In *Nutrition Monitoring in the United States* (LSRO, FASEB, 1989), niacin was not considered to be a current public health issue. No specific recommendation concerning niacin was given in either the Surgeon General's or NRC reports.

This nutrient functions in the body as part of two coenzymes—nicotinamide adenine dinucleotide and nicotinamide adenine dinucleotide phosphate. These coenzymes are present in all cells and function as part of the metabolic processes of glycolysis, fatty acid metabolism, and tissue respiration. Pellagra is a deficiency disease characterized by dermatitis, diarrhea, inflammation of the mucous membranes, and ultimately, dementia. Pellagra was once a common nutritional disease in the United States but it is no longer a public health issue.

Niacin occurs in the diet in high concentrations in meats. Conversion of tryptophan to niacin contributes to the dietary source pool for niacin. The conversion factor is 60:1 tryptophan to niacin. As a result, milk and eggs are considerable sources of tryptophan because it is converted to niacin. Niacin in processed cereal grains is biologically unavailable. However, fully synthetic niacin is added to fortified milled grain products, making them good sources.

The calculated daily intakes of total niacin equivalents are 27 mg by women and 41 mg by men (NRC, 1989b). The RDA for niacin is 15 mg/day for adult women and 19 mg/day for adult men. During pregnancy and lactation, the increments are 2 mg/day and 3 mg/day, respectively. For infants under age 6 months, the RDA for niacin is 5 mg/day and increases to 6 mg/day until age 1. For children the niacin RDA climbs gradually to the adult levels.

Vitamin B_6

In *Nutrition Monitoring in the United States* (LSRO, FASEB, 1989), vitamin B_6 was considered to be a potential public health issue. No specific recommendation concerning vitamin B_6 was given in either the Surgeon General's or NRC reports.

Vitamin B_6 is comprised of various dietary compounds—pyridoxine, pyridoxal, pyridoxamine, their phosphate esters, and glycosylated forms of pyridoxine. The various dietary forms are all absorbed by intestinal mucosal cells. In the liver, erythrocytes, and other tissues, these forms are converted to pyridoxal phosphate and pyridoxamine phosphate, which serve as coenzymes in transamination and numerous other reactions. Deficiency rarely occurs alone, but rather is seen in individuals who are deficient in several B-complex vitamins. Characteristics of severe deficiency include epileptiform convulsions, dermatitis, and anemia. Infants experience a variety of neurological symptoms and abdominal distress. Biochemically detected marginal vitamin B_6 nutriture has been observed in certain subgroups of the U.S. population.

Although present in a number of foods, considerable losses of the vitamin occur during processing. Bioavailability varies widely and is influenced by food composition and certain drug interactions. The requirement for vitamin B_6 increases as the intake of protein increases.

Average vitamin B_6 intake was 1.87 mg/day by adult males, 1.16 mg/day by adult females, and 1.22 mg/day for children aged 1 to 5 (NRC, 1989b). The RDA for vitamin B_6 is 2.0 mg/day for men and 1.6 mg/day for women, with an average protein intake of 100 g/day and 60 gm/day, respectively (NRC, 1989b). However, the RDA would not be sufficient for individuals whose habitual protein intake is above the 90th percentile. During pregnancy an increase of 0.6 mg/day is needed, and during lactation an additional allowance of 0.5 mg/day is needed to compensate for additional protein requirements. During the first 6 months of life, 0.3 mg/day is recommended and 0.6 mg/day is recommended for older infants. The recommendation is 1.0 mg/day for children aged 1 to 3, 1.1 mg/day for children aged 4 to 6, and 1.4 mg/day for children aged 7 to 10. Toxicity of vitamin B_6 supplements has been reported at doses greater than 100 mg/day.

Folate

In *Nutrition Monitoring in the United States* (LSRO, FASEB, 1989), folate was considered to be a potential public health issue. No specific recommendation concerning folate was given in either the Surgeon General's or NRC reports.

Folate functions metabolically as a coenzyme in the transport of single-carbon fragments from one compound to another in amino acid metabolism and nucleic acid synthesis. Deficiency of folate leads to impaired cell division and altered protein synthesis. Late consequences lead to overt megaloblastic bone marrow and macrocytic anemia.

Folate is widely distributed in the food supply, being particularly rich in liver, yeast, leafy vegetables, legumes, and some fruits. However, up to 50 percent of food folate can be destroyed during food preparation, processing, and storage. Bioavailability is variable, depending on the physical form, and the presence of inhibitors, binders, or other factors in foods. The average daily intake is generally from 280 to 300 µg in the United States. The RDA for folate is 200 µg/day for adult males and 180 µg/day for adult females (NRC, 1989b). These levels appear to provide normal tissue stores and other indicators of folate status. Due to the problems of absorbability, the RDA during pregnancy is set at 400 µg/day to accommodate increased requirements. During lactation the RDA is set at 280 µg/day for the first 6 months of pregnancy and 260 µg/day up to 1 year. For the first 6 months of life, the RDA is set at 25 µg/day and at 35 µg/day up to age 1. For children, the RDA increases incrementally to the adult level.

Fluoride

The Surgeon General's report (1988) recommended that community water systems should provide fluoride at optimal levels for the prevention of dental caries. *Diet and Health* (NRC, 1989a) advised that it is necessary to maintain an optimal fluoride intake, primarily during the years of tooth formation and growth. In *Nutrition Monitoring in the United States* (LSRO, FASEB, 1989), fluoride was considered to be a potential public health issue.

This mineral is incorporated into bone and tooth enamel in the human body and is believed to be beneficial, if not essential, to dental health. The negative correlation between tooth decay in children and fluoride concentrations in drinking water was demonstrated nearly 50 years ago. Subsequent studies have confirmed that fluoridation of public water supplies is an effective and practical means of reducing dental caries. The protective effect against caries is greatest during maximal tooth formation in the first 8 years of life. Evidence sugggests, however, that adults can benefit from continued consumption of fluoridated water.

The richest dietary sources of fluoride are tea and marine fish consumed with their bones. Much of the fluoride intake depends on the effects of the water supply on beverages and food preparation where fluoridation is used. Absorption of fluoride is variable, creating difficulties in establishing dietary recommendations.

Although no RDA has been established for fluoride, the estimated safe and adequate daily dietary intake ranges from 1.5 to 4 mg/day for adults (NRC, 1989b). For those in younger age groups, the range is set to a maximum level of 2.5 mg/day. Ranges of 0.1 to 1 mg/day are set for birth to 12 months, and 0.5 to 1.5 mg/day for ages 12 to 36 months.

Zinc

In *Nutrition Monitoring in the United States* (LSRO, FASEB, 1989), zinc was considered to be a potential public health issue. No specific recommendation concerning zinc was given in either the Surgeon General's or NRC reports.

Zinc is an essential mineral and is a constituent of several hundred enzymes that are involved in numerous metabolic pathways. Zinc status is subject to strong homeostatic regulation. Although large amounts are deposited in bone and muscle, the body pool of readily available zinc is small and has a rapid turnover rate. As a result, there is evidence that zinc deficiency has a rapid effect on cell growth and repair. The general signs of dietary zinc deficiency include loss of appetite, growth retardation, skin changes, and immunological abnormalities. Pronounced deficiency results in hypogonadism and dwarfism. Signs of marginal deficiency are manifested as slowed wound healing, hair loss, and impaired taste and smell acuity.

The bioavailability of zinc from foods varies widely; animal products are good sources, whereas whole-grain products contain less available forms of the mineral. The interaction of zinc with dietary protein, phytic acid, and copper may have practical significance in Americans' diets.

The zinc content of typical diets of adults furnishes 10 to 15 mg/day (NRC, 1989b). Dietary intakes are lower than recommended levels in some groups (LSRO, FASEB, 1989). Infants and young children consume diets containing about 5.5 to 8.5 mg of zinc per day. Elderly individuals generally consume from 7 to 10 mg of zinc per day. The RDAs for zinc for adult men and women are 15 mg/day and 12 mg/day, respectively (NRC, 1989b). A zinc intake of 15 mg/day is recommended during pregnancy; during lactation, an additional zinc intake of 7 mg/day is recommended for the first 6 months and an additional 4 mg/day is recommended for the second 6 months. A recommendation of 5 mg/day is set for formula-fed babies. For adolescent children, the recommendation is set at 10 mg/day.

Current Provision of Desired Information

Current food labels provide information on the vitamin and mineral content in the ingredient listing, the nutrition information panel, and the principal display panel. The ingredient listing provides information about any individual vitamins and minerals that have been added to foods during the manufacturing process (21 CFR § 101.4). No information is available about the micronutrient composition of other ingredients of foods in the ingredient listing.

The nutrition information panel lists the micronutrients currently required when nutrition labeling is used in the following order: vitamins A and C, thiamin, riboflavin, niacin, calcium, and iron (21 CFR § 101.9(c)(7)). Other optional vitamins and minerals, when they are added or naturally occurring, must be listed following the required micronutrients. Each micronutrient is listed as a percentage of the U.S. RDA contained in the food. The U.S. RDAs are standards based on the 1968 RDA, and a more extensive discussion is provided in Chapter 7. The percentages are expressed in 2 percent increments up to the 10 percent level, in 5 percent increments up to the 50 percent level, and in 10 percent increments above the 50 percent level. Nutrients present in amounts less than 2 percent of the U.S. RDA may be indicated by a zero or an asterisk referring to a footnote at the bottom of the table: "contains less than 2 percent of the U.S. RDA of this (these) nutrient (nutrients)" (21 CFR § 101.9(c)(7)(i)). When a product contains less than 2 percent of the U.S. RDA for at least five of the required nutrients, the manufacturer may choose to declare no more than three of those nutrients, with an appropriate accompanying statement.

The principal display panel frequently carries terms describing the content of vitamins and minerals that manufacturers wish to highlight in promoting a food. FDA regulations provide that a claim may be made that a food is a significant source of a vitamin or mineral if that micronutrient is present in a food at a level equal to or in excess of 10 percent of the U.S. RDA in a serving (21 CFR § 101.9(c)(7)(v)). Other examples of micronutrient descriptors include *high in vitamin C, iron fortified,* or *high in calcium.* However, currently there are no official definitions for such terms for specific micronutrients.

Committee Recommendations

On the basis of recent dietary recommendations, current public health issues, and the consumption patterns of Americans, the Committee considered the current requirements for and potential changes in the listing of micronutrients on the nutrition information panel and acknowledges that the current selection of micronutrients required to be listed is dated. The Committee's recommendations for change are based on current consumer interest, scientific evidence to support consensus on health benefit, conclusions drawn by reports of expert panels, and knowledge of essential nutrients. Although a more comprehensive listing could be recommended, the limitation of space on labels for nutrition information and the lack of scientific evidence demonstrating general public health problems led the Committee to focus its attention on micronutrients reported to be current public health issues (see Table 6-1). The Committee based its decision primarily

TABLE 6-1   Priority Status as a Public Health Issue of Food Components

Current Public Health Issue	Potential Public Health Issue, Further Study Needed	Not Currently Public Health Issue
Food energy	Dietary fiber	Protein
Fat	Vitamin A	Carbohydrates
Saturated fat	Carotenes	Vitamin E
Cholesterol	Folacin	Thiamin
Alcohol	Vitamin B_6	Riboflavin
Iron	Vitamin C	Niacin
Calcium	Potassium	Vitamin B_{12}
Sodium	Zinc	Magnesium
	Fluoride	Copper
		Phosphorus

SOURCE: Adapted from LSRO, FASEB (Life Sciences Research Office, Federation of American Societies for Experimental Biology). 1989. Nutrition Monitoring in the United States: An Update Report on Nutrition Monitoring. Prepared for the U.S. Department of Agriculture and U.S. Department of Health and Human Services. Government Printing Office, Washington, D.C. 408 pp.

on the attention given to them by reports from the Surgeon General, the Expert Panel on Nutrition Monitoring, and NRC (DHHS, 1988; LSRO, FASEB, 1989; NRC, 1989a).

As indicated several times in this report, the Committee put primary emphasis on the importance of consuming a diet consisting of a variety of foods. The decision to limit the number of micronutrients to be listed engendered concern, and therefore led the Committee to add the following words of caution on important dietary sources of nutrients. Labeling dairy products as particularly good sources of calcium might lead to the consumption of foods also rich in animal protein, which has been shown to enhance urinary calcium excretion, thereby compromising calcium status and perhaps even exacerbating the risk of osteoporosis (NRC, 1989b). Emphasizing iron richness may bring particular attention to foods for which the bioavailability of iron is said to be high, such as meats that contain the heme forms of iron, whereas recent reports (such as the Surgeon General's, *Diet and Health,* and the Dietary Guidelines) have urged moderation in the consumption of these foods (DHHS, 1988; NRC, 1989; USDA/DHHS, 1985). On balance, however, the Committee acknowledges the considerable consumer interest generated in these nutrients, in part, by these recent reports and recognizes that there are other sources of calcium and iron that possess considerable nutritional benefit and that need to be identified for the consumer.

For vitamins A and C, there is little evidence of a public health problem in the U.S. population. If food sources rich in vitamin A were to be listed, it is unlikely that the nutritional value of provitamin A-type compounds (carotenoids) would be distinguished from preformed vitamin A (retinoids). Not only are there likely to be important biological differences in the ability of these compounds to inhibit chronic degenerative diseases but also carotenoids are found in foods (plants) whose consumption is encouraged, and retinoids are found in foods (animal products such as liver) whose consumption is not encouraged. Listing of vitamin C would provide information on good sources of this nutrient (e.g., fruits and vegetables), but those sources also provide a variety of other important micronutrients. For zinc and folate, there was even less evidence demonstrating the need to emphasize consumption of foods rich in these nutrients.

Consumers should likewise assess their intake of vitamins and minerals in terms of total diet rather than the contribution of individual foods. The current listing on the food label of micronutrients as a percentage of the U.S. RDA encourages manufacturers of some food products to fortify each micronutrient to 100 percent. Treatment of vitamins and minerals in qualitative rather than quantitative terms would help to reduce the incentives for overfortification of foods. Furthermore, the current listing implies more precision and accuracy than really exists due to the inaccuracy in measuring at least some of the nutrients in this group.

The Committee recommends that:

- FDA and USDA should continue to require disclosure of calcium and iron content per serving, but use the source definitions described in Chapter 7 (i.e., *very good source of, source of,* and *contains*).
- FDA and USDA should allow, as an option, disclosure of the content of all other micronutrients for which RDAs exist.
- FDA and USDA should establish standardized definitions for the terms used to describe the micronutrient content of foods on the principal display panel and these definitions should be the same as those used on the nutrition information panel (see Chapter 7).

REFERENCES

ADA (American Diabetes Association), Task Force on Nutrition and Exchange Lists. 1987. Nutritional recommendations and principles for individuals with diabetes mellitus. Diabetes Care 10:126–132.

AHA (American Heart Association), Committee on Nutrition. 1965. Diet and Heart Disease. American Heart Association, New York.

AHA (American Heart Association), Committee on Nutrition. 1986. Dietary guidelines for healthy American adults. Circulation 74:1465A–1468A.

Bonanome, A., and S.M. Grundy. 1988. Effect of dietary stearic acid on plasma cholesterol and lipoprotein levels. N. Engl. J. Med. 318:1244–1248.

Butrum, R.R., C.K. Clifford, and E. Lanza. 1988. NCI dietary guidelines. Rationale. Am. J. Clin. Nutr. 48:Suppl.

CCC (Calorie Control Council). 1985. Sweet Choices—questions and answers about sweeteners in low-calorie foods and beverages. CCC, Atlanta. 6 pp.

Crapo, P.A. 1984. Theory vs. fact: The glycemic response to foods. Nutr. Today 19:6–11.

DHHS (U.S. Department of Health and Human Services). 1988. The Surgeon General's Report on Nutrition and Health. Government Printing Office, Washington, D.C. 727 pp.

Glinsmann, W.H., H. Irausquin, and Y.K. Park. 1986. Evaluation of health aspects of sugars contained in carbohydrate sweeteners: Report of Sugars Task Force. J. Nutr. 116:S1–S216.

Gordon, T., W.B. Castelli, M.C. Hjortland, W.B. Kannel, and T.R. Dawber. 1977. High density lipoprotein as a protective factor against coronary heart disease. The Framingham Study. Am. J. Med. 62:707–714.

Groen, J., B.K. Tjiong, C.E. Kamminga, and A.F. Willebrands. 1952. The influence of nutrition, individuality and some other factors, including various forms of stress, on the serum cholesterol; an experiment of nine months duration in 60 normal human volunteers. Voeding 13:556–587.

Grundy, S.M. 1987. Monounsaturated fatty acids, plasma cholesterol, and coronary heart disease. Am. J. Clin. Nutr. 45:1168–1175.

Heird, W.C., J.F. Nicholson, J.M. Driscoll, Jr., N.J. Schullinger, and R.W. Winters.

1972. Hyperammonemia resulting from intravenous alimentation using a mixture of synthetic l-amino acids: A preliminary report. J. Pediatr. 81:162–165.

Herold, P.M., and J.E. Kinsella. 1986. Fish oil consumption and decreased risk of cardiovascular disease: A comparison of findings from animal and human feeding trials. Am. J. Clin. Nutr. 43:566–598.

HPTRG (Hypertension Prevention Trial Research Group). 1990. The hypertension prevention trial: Three-year effects of dietary changes on blood pressure. Arch. Intern. Med. 150:153–162.

Kayman S., W. Bruvold, and J.S. Stern. 1990. Maintenance and relapse after weight loss in women: Behavioral aspects. Am. J. Clin. Nutr. In press.

Keys, A. 1975. Coronary heart disease—the global picture. Atherosclerosis 22:149–192.

Kinsell, L.W., J. Partridge, L. Boling, S. Margen, and G. Michaels. 1952. Dietary modification of serum cholesterol and phospholipid levels. J. Clin. Endocrinol. 12:909–913.

Kromhout, D., E.B. Bosschieter, and C. de Lezenne Coulander. 1985. The inverse relation between fish consumption and 20-year mortality from coronary heart disease. N. Engl. J. Med. 312:1205–1209.

Lanza, E., D.Y. Jones, G. Block, and L. Kessler. 1987. Dietary fiber intake in the U.S. population. Am. J. Clin. Nutr. 46:790–797.

LSRO, FASEB (Life Sciences Research Office, Federation of American Societies for Experimental Biology). 1989. Nutrition Monitoring in the United States: An Update Report on Nutrition Monitoring. Prepared for the U.S. Department of Agriculture and the U.S. Department of Health and Human Services. Government Printing Office, Washington, D.C. 408 pp.

Massachusetts Medical Society, Committee on Nutrition. 1989. Fast Food Fare: Consumer Guidelines. Prepared by Connie Roberts. N. Engl. J. Med. 321:752–756.

McGill, H.C., Jr. 1979. The relationship of dietary cholesterol to serum cholesterol concentration and to atherosclerosis in man. Am. J. Clin. Nutr. 32:2664-2702.

Medalie, J.H., H.A. Kahn, H.N. Neufeld, E. Riss, and U. Goldbourt. 1973. Five-year myocardial infarction incidence. II. Association of single variables to age and birthplace. J. Chronic Dis. 26:325–349.

Miller, N.E., D.S. Thelle, O.H. Forde, and O.D. Mjos. 1977. The Tromso Heart Study. High-density lipoprotein and coronary heart-disease: A prospective case-control study. Lancet 1:965–968.

NCEP (National Cholesterol Education Program). 1990. Report of the Expert Panel on Population Strategies for Blood Cholesterol Reduction, National Institutes of Health. Government Printing Office, Washington, D.C. 140 pp.

NRC (National Research Council). 1982. Diet, Nutrition, and Cancer. Committee on Diet, Nutrition and Cancer, Food and Nutrition Board, Commission on Life Sciences. National Academy Press, Washington, D.C. 478 pp.

NRC (National Research Council). 1988. Designing Foods: Animal Product Options in the Marketplace. Report of the Committee on Technological Options to Improve the Nutritional Attributes of Animal Products, Board on Agriculture. National Academy Press, Washington, D.C. 367 pp.

NRC (National Research Council). 1989a. Diet and Health: Implications for Reducing Chronic Disease Risk. Report of the Committee on Diet and Health, Food and Nutrition Board, Commission on Life Sciences. National Academy Press, Washington, D.C. 749 pp.

NRC (National Research Council). 1989b. Recommended Dietary Allowances, 10th ed. Committee on the 10th Edition of the Recommended Dietary Allowances, Food and Nutrition Board, Commission on Life Sciences. National Academy Press, Washington, D.C. 285 pp.

Page, I.H., F.J. Stare, A.C. Corcoran, H. Pollack, and C.F. Wilkinson. 1957. Atherosclerosis and the fat content of the diet. Circulation 16:163–178.

Prosky, L., N.G. Asp, I. Furda, J.W. DeVries, T.F. Schweizer, and B.F. Harland. 1985. Determination of total dietary fiber in foods and food products: Collaborative study. J. Assoc. Off. Anal. Chem. 68:677–679.

Ronk, R.J. 1986. Policy letter of June 24, 1986, to Giant Food, Inc., Washington, D.C. Center for Food Safety and Applied Nutrition, Food and Drug Administration, Washington, D.C.

Ronk, R.J. 1988. Policy letter of August 26, 1988, to J.S. Kahan and B.L. Rubin, Hogan and Hartson, Washington, D.C. Center for Food Safety and Applied Nutrition, Food and Drug Administration, Washington, D.C.

Schemmel, R., O. Mickelson, and J.L. Gill. 1970. Dietary obesity in rats: Body weight and body fat accretion in seven strains of rats. J. Nutr. 100:1041–1048.

Shank, F.R., L. Larsen, F.E. Scarbrough, J.E. Vanderveen, and A.L. Forbes. 1983. FDA perspective on sodium. Food Technol. 37:73–77.

Shekelle, R.B., A.M. Shryock, O. Paul, M. Lepper, J. Stamler, S. Liu, and W.J. Raynor, Jr. 1981. Diet, serum cholesterol, and death from coronary heart disease. The Western Electric Study. N. Engl. J. Med. 304:65–70.

Solberg, L.A., and J.P. Strong. 1983. Risk factors and atherosclerotic lesions. A review of autopsy studies. Arteriosclerosis 3:187–198.

Stamler, J., and R. Shekelle. 1988. Dietary cholesterol and human coronary heart disease: The epidemiologic evidence. Arch. Pathol. Lab. Med. 112:1032–1040.

USDA (U.S. Department of Agriculture). 1982a. FSIS Policy Memorandum 039. Food Safety and Inspection Service, Washington, D.C.

USDA (U.S. Department of Agriculture). 1982b. FSIS Policy Memorandum 046. Food Safety and Inspection Service, Washington, D.C.

USDA (U.S. Department of Agriculture). 1984a. FSIS Policy Memorandum 049C. Food Safety and Inspection Service, Washington, D.C.

USDA (U.S. Department of Agriculture). 1984b. FSIS Policy Memorandum 078. Food Safety and Inspection Service, Washington, D.C.

USDA (U.S. Department of Agriculture). 1987. FSIS Policy Memorandum 070B. Food Safety and Inspection Service, Washington, D.C.

USDA (U.S. Department of Agriculture). 1989. FSIS Standards and Labeling Policy Book. Food Safety and Inspection Service, Washington, D.C.

USDA (U.S. Department of Agriculture). 1990. Report of the Dietary Guidelines Advisory Committee on the Dietary Guidelines for Americans, 1990. Government Printing Office, Washington, D.C. 48 pp.

USDA/DHHS (U.S. Department of Agriculture and U.S. Department of Health and Human Services). 1985. Nutrition and Your Health: Dietary Guidelines for Americans, 2nd ed. Government Printing Office, Washington, D.C. 24 pp.

Woodward, C.J.H., and K.K. Carroll. 1988. Nutrition and human health aspects of marine oils and lipids. Pp. 2–28 in Marine Biogenic Fats and Oils, R.G. Ackman, ed. CRC Press, Boca Raton, Fla.

Yudkin, J. 1964. Dietary fat and dietary sugar in relation to ischemic heart disease and diabetes. Lancet 2:4–5.

7

Presentation of Nutrition Information on Food Labels

CRITERIA FOR PRESENTING INFORMATION

To assure that the nutrition information provided on a food label is conveyed in a manner that will allow the majority of consumers to use it successfully, a number of criteria need to be considered, including literacy of users, computational abilities, knowledge of English, and knowledge of the specialized vocabulary of nutrition labeling. The actual label presentation scheme needs to make it possible for consumers to understand the nutrition contents of individual food products, compare nutrition contents across product categories, and choose among relevant food alternatives.

REFERENCE UNITS FOR DECLARING NUTRIENT CONTENT (SERVING SIZE)

In assessing the adequacy of current food labels, the element of serving size affects the usability of all other label components. Over a decade ago, the Food and Drug Administration (FDA) indicated that, "serving size has been one of the issues that has most concerned consumers and manufacturers alike" (DHEW/USDA/FTC, 1979, p. 77).

Concept of Serving

Originally, the concept of serving was geared to the actual amount likely to be consumed at a single sitting. However, the concept of serving size is currently used to provide a reference point for information about the nutritional and other qualities of the food product. Once serving size is regarded as a standard unit rather than as an estimate of likely consumption, it is possible to visualize varying amounts for similar products, such as a 2-oz serving size for canned tuna and a 3.5-oz serving size for salmon. For maximum usefulness and understanding, however, labeled serving size should not depart widely from the amount normally consumed at one time.

Nutrient information on food labels under FDA and U.S. Department of Agriculture (USDA) jurisdiction is declared in relation to the average or usual serving, or, when the food is customarily used as an ingredient, in relation to the average or usual portion. The *FSIS Standards and Labeling Policy Book* and policy memoranda simply stipulate that "when a label contains a statement or claims identification of the number of servings, it must be qualified to identify the size of the servings, e.g. 3, 2 oz servings—or, 1-6 oz serving—or, 3 portions, 2 oz each" (USDA, 1989b, p. 139).

In the dietary assessment literature, serving size is typically regarded as a term for a standardized or commonly ingested portion of food. In contrast, portion size refers to that amount of food reported to be ingested at an eating occasion.

Definitions

There is considerable confusion among three terms: *serving, portion,* and *helping.* The term *serving* was defined by FDA as a reasonable quantity of food suited for or practicable of consumption as a part of a meal by an adult male engaged in light physical activity, or by an infant or child under age 4 when the article purports or is represented to be for consumption by an infant or child under age 4 (21 CFR § 101.9(b)(1)). In contrast, FDA defined the term *portion* as the amount of food customarily used only as an ingredient in the preparation of a meal component, e.g., $\frac{1}{2}$ tablespoon of cooking oil or $\frac{1}{4}$ cup of tomato paste. FDA has further specified that servings and portions must be expressed in terms of common household measuring units or other easily identifiable units such as cups, tablespoons, ounces, or slices.

Disparities in Serving Sizes

Serving size is provided as a tool for consumers and users of dietary guidance information, nutrient composition data bases, food consumption research, and on food labels. There are great variations and wide disparities in the information presented to consumers in each of these domains for the same foods or for items in the same product categories. A comparison of the serving sizes specified by various dietary guidance plans, used in food composition data bases, amounts actually consumed, and the range currently shown on food labels is presented in Table 7-1.

Serving Size Information as Portrayed in Dietary Guidance Materials

Dietary guidance systems provide information to consumers about the individual foods they are advised to consume. The common approach has been to recommend a number of daily servings of each of several food groups. In some, but not all, cases the sizes of servings are specified.

In 1958 the *Basic Four* food guide, officially known as *Food for Fitness: A Daily Food Guide*, was developed by USDA nutritionists (USDA, 1958). That guide recommended "some milk for everyone," with servings from the milk group of 2 or more cups a day for adults to 4 or more cups a day for teenagers. However, no sizes were specified for the number of servings of food from the meat, vegetable and fruit, or bread and cereal groups.

In 1980 and 1985, dietary guidance information was presented to consumers in *Nutrition and Your Health: Dietary Guidelines for Americans,* but these advisory statements made no specific quantitative recommendations. Instead, they offered seven qualitative, directional statements, such as "eat a variety of foods," "eat foods with adequate starch and fiber," and "avoid too much . . ." (USDA/DHHS, 1980, 1985). The third edition is expected to provide essentially the same type of directives (USDA, 1990).

In the late 1980s, USDA developed and published a food guidance system, using both a menu planning strategy and commonly used food guides that did specify serving sizes (Cronin et al., 1987). The pattern for daily food choices recommended consumption of 6 to 11 servings of grains, breads, and cereals; 2 servings of milk, cheese, and yogurt; 2 to 3 servings of meat, poultry, fish, and eggs; 3 to 5 servings of vegetables; 2 to 4 servings of fruits; and moderate amounts of fats, sweets, and alcohol. In general, amounts of food that counted as a serving were based on typical serving sizes reported by individuals in the 1977–1979 Nationwide Food Consumption Survey conducted by USDA. A typical serving of food was defined as "the median amount of food consumed at a single eating occasion." The amounts of typical servings were specified for food groups and are shown in Table 7-1.

The National Research Council (NRC) report, *Diet and Health: Implications for Reducing Chronic Disease Risk* (NRC, 1989a), advised that consumers should "every day eat five or more servings of a combination of vegetables and fruits" and should "increase intake of starches and other complex carbohydrates by eating six or more daily servings of a combination of breads, cereals, and legumes." The *average serving* of these foods was defined as "equal to a half cup for most fresh or cooked vegetables, fruits, dry or cooked cereals and legumes, one medium piece of fresh fruit, one slice of bread, or one roll or muffin" (NRC, 1989a, p. 15).

For the most part, the various sources of authoritative dietary advice offer fairly consistent messages about recommended serving sizes for products in the same categories (Table 7-1). However, it remains to be determined whether

TABLE 7-1 Serving Sizes as Depicted by Several Means for Selected Food

Food Item	Diet and Health[a]	Dietary Guidance Recommendations		
		Diabetic Exchange Lists[b]	Basic Four Food Groups	USDA Food Guidance System[c]
Grains				
Bread	1 slice	1 slice	—[e]	1 slice
Muffin, bagel	1	1	—	1 small
Cereals, pasta, rice	½ c	½ c, ckd ¾ c, dry	—	½ c, ckd
Legumes, beans	½ c	⅓ c	—	—
Dairy				
Milk, fluid	—	1 c	1 c	1 c
Cheese	—	1 oz, low-fat	—	1½ oz natural, 2 oz processed
Yogurt	—	8-oz carton	—	8 fl oz
Fruit				
Fresh	½ c	1 piece	—	Average piece
Juice	—	½ c	—	6 oz
Vegetable				
Cooked	½ c	½ c	—	½ c
Raw	—	1 c	—	1 c raw 1 c leafy raw
Meat				
Ground beef	—	1 sm. hamburger	—	Total of
Poultry	—	½ chicken breast	—	5 to 7 oz Lean
Tuna (canned)	—	½ c	—	daily
Peanut butter	—	1 T	—	
Condiments				
Butter, margarine	—	1 t	—	—
Catsup	—	—	—	—

[a] NRC (National Research Council). 1989. Diet and Health: Recommmendations for Reducing National Research Council. National Academy Press, Washington, D.C. 749 pp.

[b] American Diabetes Association and The American Dietetic Association. 1989. Exchange Alexandria, Va. 32 pp.

[c] Cronin, F. et al. 1987. Developing a food guidance system to implement the Dietary

[d] Krebs-Smith, S.M., and H. Smiciklas-Wright. 1985. Typical serving sizes: Implications for

[e] Not specified.

[f] Sandwich steaks.

Products

As Consumed[d]	Food Composition Data Bases		Giant Food, Inc., Food Guide (average)	Food Labels (ranges for selected products)
	USDA Handbook 8	USDA Home & Gdn. Bltn. 72		
2 slices	100 g	1 slice	2 slices	1–2 slices
—	"	1	1	1
1 c, ckd rice	"	1 c	1 c (approx)	1 oz (dry wt)
—	"	1 c	½ c	½ c
1 c	"	1 c	8 fl oz	1 c
1 ½ oz (males)	"	1 oz	1 oz	1 oz
1 oz (females)	"			
	"	8 oz container	6 oz	6 oz
1 med. piece	"	1 unit	1 piece	
¾ c	"	1 c	6 fl oz	6 fl oz
½ c	"	1 c	½ c	½ c
2 leaves (males)	"	1 c	⅔ c lettuce	
½ c (females)				
	"	3 oz ckd	2 oz[f]	
6 oz daily (males),	"	3 oz	1 oz	
4 oz daily (females)	"	3 oz	3 oz	2 oz
	"	1 T	2 T	2 T
—	"	1 T	1 T	1 T
—	"	1 T	1 T	—

Chronic Disease Risk. Report of the Committee on Diet and Health, Food and Nutrition Board,

Lists for Menu Planning. American Diabetes Association and The American Dietetic Association,

Guidelines. J. Nutr. Ed. 19(6):281–302.
food guidance. J. Am. Diet. Assoc. 85:1139—1141.

consumers visualize or consume portions in the same sizes and dimensions as recommended.

Serving Size in Nutrient Composition Data Bases

The USDA Agriculture Handbook No. 8 series, *Composition of Foods,* comprise a group of technical publications that provide nutrient composition information for an extensive list of raw, processed, and prepared foods. It is now frequently updated and will consist of 22 sections when fully completed. This series of publications provides nutrient composition information based on 100-g portions of foods (USDA, 1976).

In an effort to compile a document that would be more useful to professional and technical personnel as well as researchers, USDA issued *Nutritive Value of American Foods in Common Units* (USDA, 1975). In that publication, nutrient composition information was presented for approximately 1,500 foods in frequently used household measures and market units of food. The measurements for specific quantities listed are the customary units now in use for the edible portion of the food item. For example, information for breads is presented both by the loaf and by the slice; for juices, cereals, and fluid milk, by 1 cup; for vegetables and fruits, by the piece or 1-cup portions; and for meats, by 1-pound or 1-cup portions or by the piece.

A more concise document for consumer use is *Nutritive Value of Foods,* Home and Garden Bulletin No. 72, first published in 1960 and last revised in 1981 (USDA, 1981). It provided a table of nutritive values for household measures of 908 commonly used foods grouped under 15 different main headings. Most foods were listed in ready-to-eat form, but some were basic products widely used in food preparation, such as flour, fat, and cornmeal. The Bulletin was careful to point out that:

> The approximate measure shown for each food is in cups, ounces, pounds, some other well-known unit, or a piece of a certain size. The measures shown do not necessarily represent a serving, but the unit given may be used to calculate a variety of serving sizes. For example, values are given for 1 cup of applesauce. If a serving is ½ cup, divide the values by 2 or multiply by 0.5; for a ⅔ cup serving multiply values by 0.67 (USDA, 1981, p. 4).

Serving Size Reported by Consumers

Data bases containing food consumption data taken from national surveys are another source of typical serving sizes. Pao et al. (1982) used 3-day reports from a weighted sample of about 38,000 individuals to determine the weights (in grams) of various foods eaten per meal or snack.

Krebs-Smith and Smiciklas-Wright (1985) converted the amounts reported by Pao and fellow researchers to common household measures for several age and sex groups and used these amounts to determine the most common serving size for different foods. They showed that, for many food items, typically reported servings deviate considerably from the amount accepted as standard servings. Fruit juices, breads, and cereals were frequently consumed in larger amounts than expected, whereas quantities of raw vegetables, meat, fish, and poultry varied widely. Typical serving sizes of breads and cereals were usually twice the size found in earlier recommendations (2 slices versus 1 slice).

The study by Hunter et al. (1988) of 194 women to determine the serving sizes of 68 foods found that for most foods there was no usual serving size even for foods that are in well-defined units, such as crackers. Guthrie (1984) reported that food portions self-served by young adults deviated by more than 25 percent from the generally accepted serving size for 28 to 80 percent of the serving selections.

Recently, FDA conducted a survey of the amount of food consumed per eating occasion from USDA's 1977–1978 Nationwide Food Consumption Survey and foods in the marketplace. The data were used to determine the standard serving sizes for 159 food product categories and to define single-serving containers for its proposed rule on serving size (55 Fed. Reg. 29,476–29,533, July 19, 1990).

Research on Portion Size Estimation

Dietary assessment research has examined the issue of whether consumers are able to provide realistic, valid estimates of the amount of food they consume. A number of the studies that have addressed this topic have documented that a large proportion of respondents cannot accurately judge the amounts of foods and beverages they consume. Both Madden et al. (1976) and Gersovitz et al. (1978) observed overreporting of low intakes and underreporting of high intakes in the subjects they studied—a phenomenon commonly referred to as "regression to the mean."

The conclusions from various studies on portion size estimation indicate that people do not give accurate estimates of the amounts of foods they consume. In general, there is a greater tendency to overestimate than to underestimate portion sizes, with the magnitude of the error varying with the specific food item (Guthrie, 1984; Lansky and Brownell, 1982; Lewis et al. 1988; Webb and Yuhas, 1988). Some studies have suggested that food preparation experience seems to help subjects better estimate the amounts of foods they consume, which may explain why women are better than men at estimating quantities of foods. Training and the use of measuring utensils or food models have been shown to improve some estimates of sizes, but the results are not consistently reliable across all types of foods or memory aides used (Yuhas et al., 1989).

Serving Sizes on Food Labels

There is tremendous variability in the serving sizes currently declared as the reference standard on food labels in different product categories, among foods, and between foods in the same product category as shown in Table 7-2. Ready-to-eat breakfast cereals, perhaps, show the greatest variability, with serving sizes usually designated as 1 oz, regardless of the volume of the product; 1-oz volumes range from 2½ tablespoons to 1 cup. Not only are the actual quantities not the same for serving sizes for foods in the same product categories but the units of measurement also vary. For example, serving sizes may be expressed in ounces, units (such as pieces or sticks), cups, tablespoons, or teaspoons.

When nutrition labeling was first introduced in 1973, it was left to industry to adopt reasonable serving sizes (21 CFR § 101.9(b)(1)). After the nutrition

TABLE 7-2   Serving Sizes Currently Used on Food Labels (Selected sample of commonly used products)[a]

Food Item	Serving Size	Servings/Package or Container
Breads		
Bread, white	2 slices (2 oz)	12
Bread, whole wheat	2 slices (1.7 oz)	9.5
Bread, cinnamon (Pepperidge Farm)	1 slice	16
Bagel (Lenders)	1	4
English muffin (Thomas')	1	6
Cereals		
100% Bran (Nabisco)	1 oz (½ c)	17
All Bran (Kellogg)	1 oz (⅓ c)	13
Cream of Wheat (Nabisco)	1 oz (2½ T dry)	—[b]
Crispix (Kellogg)	1 oz (1 c)	12
Frosted Mini Wheats (Kellogg)	1 oz (½ c)	17
Fruit and Fibre (Post)	1.25 oz (⅔ c)	12
Fiber One (General Mills)	1 oz (½ c)	13.5
Golden Grahams (General Mills)	1 oz (¾ c)	18
Grape Nuts (Post)	1 oz (¼ c)	16
Instant Oatmeal (General Mills)	1 pkt (1.6 oz)	8
Instant Oatmeal (Quaker)	1 pkt (1¼ oz)	10
Quaker Oat Squares (Quaker)	1 oz (½ c)	—
Meat, poultry, fish		
Frankfurters	1	10
Luncheon meat	1 slice	8
Sausage	1 cooked patty (33 g)	10
Fish sticks, frozen	4 sticks	8
Salmon, canned	½ c	4
Tuna, canned	2 oz	3.3

TABLE 7-2—Continued

Food Item	Serving Size	Servings/Package or Container
Beverages		
Diet soda	6 fl oz	2
Orange juice, prepared from frozen conc.	6 fl oz	8
Hawaiian Punch (drink box)	6 fl oz	1.4
Hot chocolate mix	1 pkt (6 fl oz)	10
Pink grapefruit juice cocktail	6 fl oz	1.4
Dairy		
Cream cheese	1 oz	8
Ice cream	½ c	—
Milk	1 c (8 fl oz)	Varies
Sour cream	2 T	
Spreads		
Butter	1 T	—
Margarine	1 T	—
Mayonnaise	1 T	64
Fruits and vegetables		
Blueberries, frozen	4 oz	4
Fruit cocktail, canned	½ c	7
Peas, canned	½ c	4
Peas, frozen	½ c	6
Tomatoes, canned	½ c	4
Other		
Macaroni and cheese dinner, box	¾ c (as prepared)	4
Noodles Alfredo, box	½ c (as prepared)	4
Peanut butter, jar	2 T (32 g)	10
Pork and beans, canned	½ c (130 g)	3.5
Potato chips, bag	15 chips (1 oz)	7
Soup, canned, condensed	8 oz (as prepared)	2.5
Soup, canned, single serving	10¾ oz	1
Spaghetti sauce, jar	4 oz	12

[a] Information compiled from visits to local Washington, D.C., area supermarkets by L.S. Sims, 1990.

[b] Not specified.

labeling regulations were implemented, FDA conducted an informal survey of product labels that provided nutrition information. The results of that survey indicated that, in many cases, serving sizes were not reasonable or uniform within a product class (39 Fed. Reg. 20,878–20,887, June 14, 1974).

In 1974, FDA published proposed serving sizes for several foods, including fluid milk beverages, noncarbonated breakfast beverage products, hot and ready-to-eat cereals, and formulated meal replacements (39 Fed. Reg. 20,895–20,900, June 14, 1974). Since then, a serving size has been proposed for soft drinks (40

Fed. Reg. 4315–4316, Jan. 29, 1975), and petitions have been received seeking to establish a portion size for flour and serving sizes for bread and peanut butter. However, the agency has taken no further action on either the proposed serving sizes or amending the portion size definition.

As a result, FDA (and, consequently, USDA as well) does not specify serving sizes for any of the thousands of food products on the market. Rather, the manufacturer decides the serving size to be designated, subject only to the loose requirements that the serving size must be (1) a "reasonable quantity of food suited for or practicable of consumption as part of a meal by an adult male engaged in light physical activity" (or by a child, for foods intended for children) (21 CFR § 101.9(b)(1)), and (2) it must be expressed "in terms of a convenient unit of such food or a convenient unit of measure that can be easily identified as an average or usual serving and can be readily understood by purchasers of such food" (Heimbach et al., 1990).

Over time, a hybrid system for serving size has evolved. For most foods, the declared serving size is neither an arbitrarily fixed amount that is uniform for similar products nor an average or usual serving, but rather is something in between—a standard unit—which is set by food manufacturers rather than by the federal government and is unique to each product type. FDA believed that declaration of the nutrition content in terms of a usual serving of each different food product would be more flexible and more meaningful to consumers so that they could relate the label information to individual intakes. This rationale may still be valid, but it has allowed manufacturers to vary serving size declarations over time and manipulate label claims on the basis of per serving nutrient contents.

The significance of the chosen serving size is magnified by the fact that all nutrient values declared on the label are dependent upon this determination. For example, jelly and jam produced by the same manufacturer listing 1 or 2 teaspoons, respectively, as serving sizes illustrates the problem. Both labels offer the same information, and a careful comparison would reveal that the nutrient contents of the two products are virtually identical. Clearly, neither label is inaccurate. Yet, consumers who choose products mainly by examining the calorie content may think that one product has twice the calories of the other, when the calorie content of equal portions of the products is essentially the same.

The leeway given to manufacturers to set serving sizes offers them the opportunity to portray each food item in the most favorable light. In 1979, FDA expressed concern that "some manufacturers were using overly large serving sizes to inflate the nutritional value of their product in order to enhance its attractiveness (DHEW/USDA/FTC, 1979, p. 77)." The commercial rationale for doing so was the belief that consumers were seeking foods on the basis of increased nutritive value and, in particular, higher protein, vitamin, and mineral contents. FDA noted that the serving sizes recommended for many canned fruits and vegetables, as well as for some varieties of canned tuna, fruit juices, and frozen vegetables, had approximately doubled (in amount) since nutrition labeling was initiated.

Ten years later, the concern is that manufacturers have begun shrinking serving sizes in response to consumers' tendency to use label information for avoiding particular food constituents such as fat, sodium, and cholesterol (Heimbach, 1985, 1986, 1987). This tendency may be encouraged by current definitions of descriptors such as *low sodium,* which is based on a sodium content of less than 140 mg per serving. For example, an 8-oz food package that contains 360 mg of sodium does not qualify for a low-sodium descriptor if it is labeled as providing two 4-oz servings (with 180 mg of sodium per serving), but it may be labeled as *low sodium* if the package is declared to contain four 2-oz servings. Recent data from FDA's Food Label and Package Survey have shown that 19 of 44 product classes and both bread categories (white and nonwhite) moved toward smaller declared serving sizes in the period from 1977 to 1986 (Heimbach et al., 1990). The information contained in Table 7-2 dramatizes the considerable variability in serving size information on food labels, even for foods within the same product categories.

In some cases, food manufacturers keep the serving size unit constant and vary the volume of a serving or a container. For example, the serving size of ready-to-eat breakfast cereal is routinely listed as 1 oz, but the volume varies tremendously (from 2½ tablespoons to 1 cup of cereal) due to the wide variation in the densities of different products. Another example is juice, which is routinely listed as a 6-oz serving, but the number of servings varies from 1.4 to 8 per container. In other cases, the recommended serving size is varied in order to keep the number of servings per container constant, as is the case with single-serving canned soups, packets of instant oatmeal, or individual beverage boxes. Standardized serving sizes are needed so that information remains comparable within product categories, such as breakfast cereals, and across product categories.

Alternatives to Serving Size Specifications

If serving size is less than ideal as a reference standard, the alternatives need to be considered. One alternative would be to declare nutrient content per package or container and let consumers judge the proportion of that package that is being consumed at any eating occasion. Such a concept is useful for single-serving containers which are currently popular, but in the Committee's view could make it very difficult for the consumer to relate the nutrition data to the amount actually consumed, especially for packages containing large numbers of servings.

Another alternative would be to declare nutrient content per 100 g or other standard unit. This approach is used internationally where the metric system is in place, but it has not been widely used in the United States. Current law in Australia requires labeling per 100 g of product. However, it has recently been suggested that labeling on a per serving basis may be more appropriate for some foods (Farmakalidis, 1989). Canada required labeling per 100 g of product until recently, when research evaluating consumer understanding and usage of nutrition labels on ready-to-eat breakfast cereals revealed that consumers rely on and refer to information provided on a per serving basis rather than on a per 100-g basis. For example, 100 g is only about half the weight of a glass of milk but about seven times the weight of a pat of butter. The newest Canadian regulations, which were promulgated in 1988, express serving size "in the same units as the net quantity declaration, whether it be grams or milliliters, and as well in an equivalent household measure or common unit" (Gunner, 1989).

Farmakalidis (1989) provides further support for using the per serving rather than per 100 g designation:

> Consider, for example, very lightweight products such as desiccated coconut or a chocolate drink powder. Nutrition labelling on a per serving (in this case approximately 10 g) and a per 100 g serving (or ten ordinary servings) can only serve to seriously mislead consumers into thinking that the product, when consumed in an ordinary manner (i.e. a serving) will provide nutrients equivalent to that in a 100 g serving. Yet another example is puffed wheat cereal, one cup of which normally weighs only 15 grams. A 100 g serving would be equivalent to 6.6 cups, an amount which is highly unlikely even for the most dedicated puffed wheat eater. The extra nutrition information provided by the 100 g labelling merely clutters the label and confuses the consumer (p. 980).

Data from an FDA survey revealed that the per serving standard was preferred by majorities of consumers, food and nutrition professionals, and food industry representatives (Heimbach and Stokes, 1981). This preference was based on the belief that it would be less useful to consumers to have the nutrient content of all products calculated against a standard weight, which would often be larger or smaller than a usual serving.

Committee Recommendations

The main purpose of stating serving size on the food label is to provide a reference unit for the presentation of the nutrient composition about a product. If sizes are uniform and realistic, this manner of presentation provides consumers with comparable information about the nutritive value of products in the same category (e.g., breakfast cereals). Such label information should also enable consumers to compare the amounts of nutrients they consume with the amount of nutrients currently recommended. Without product-based information of this type, it may be more difficult for consumers to compare between alternative meals or meal components (e.g., between breakfast cereals and a bacon and eggs breakfast) or to plan daily diets. Despite the potential for misuses of the concept of serving, the Committee believes that it remains the best reference unit for expressing the nutrient composition of foods.

The Committee recommends that:

- Given the alternatives available (serving size, nutrient values per package or container, 100-g portions), *serving* should continue to be the reference unit for presenting nutrition information on foods.
- Serving sizes should be expressed in common household measures, followed by the weight in grams (in parentheses) to facilitate comparisons across product categories. Serving sizes should be standardized across food categories on the basis of volume or weight measures. For example, milk beverages should be listed in 1-cup servings, whereas breakfast cereals may be standardized by weight (e.g., 1 oz), as long as the corresponding volume measure is specified (e.g., 1 cup or 2 tablespoons, dry weight). All serving sizes should be rounded down to the nearest whole numbers; fractions or decimals should be avoided.
- The number of servings per package or container should be specified. For a single-serving container, 50 to 150 percent of the commonly consumed unit would be acceptable. The number of servings per container should be expressed rounded down to the nearest whole number.
- Consistent with the recommendation that serving sizes should be standardized, quantities specified by dietary guidance recommendations should serve as the main criteria for selecting the amount of food to be described as a serving. This preference for recommended, rather than as consumed, has the advantage that it can be more readily applied in educational programs and will ensure consistency between serving sizes as presented in dietary guidance materials and on the food label.
- FDA and USDA should jointly establish serving sizes for a limited number of different food categories (i.e., fruit juices, breads, cereals, fruits, vegetables, spreads, and salad dressings) since serving size-based information will be more valuable for consumers if it applies to broad categories of food. The Committee favors fewer, rather than more, categories so that nutrition information can readily be used by consumers for product comparisons and reference purposes.
- If a food manufacturer desires a serving size different from that set by the agencies, it should be permitted to petition the responsible agency to allow a deviation or to create a new subclass of foods with its own serving size.
- FDA and USDA should establish uniformity in serving size specifications within product categories and between agencies. As noted in the NRC report, *Designing Foods: Animal Product Options in the Marketplace*, "consistency [among serving sizes] would facilitate comparisons among products, labels, point-of-purchase information, and federal and private data bases" (NRC, 1988, p. 5). However, it will still be important for nutrition

education programs to provide the type of guidance and information to help consumers make appropriate types of food product comparisons.

- Research should be conducted to determine how consumers comprehend food label information and how they interpret serving sizes declared on the food package.

U.S. RECOMMENDED DIETARY ALLOWANCES

The first explicit, comprehensive effort to establish national dietary recommendations occurred in 1941. The poor nutritional status of military recruits and the prospect of some limitations on food availability were the immediate impetus, adding to existing concerns about health problems due to nutrient deficiency diseases. In response, the Food and Nutrition Board (FNB) issued guidelines in the form of Recommended Dietary Allowances (RDA). These recommendations included protein, six vitamins (A, C, D, and thiamin, riboflavin, and niacin), and two minerals (iron and calcium), expressed as the amounts needed (NRC, 1941). Revisions of this document issued in 1943, 1948, 1953, 1958, 1963, 1968, 1974, 1980, and 1989 showed an evolution in the science and the approaches used to arrive at the recommendations. The range of substances covered has increased, with the most recent 10th edition (NRC, 1989b) covering 11 vitamins and 7 minerals, and providing estimated safe and adequate daily dietary intakes (ESADDIs) for 2 vitamins and 5 minerals. Accumulating scientific data have also made the recommendations more precise. RDAs are defined as the levels of intake of essential nutrients that, on the basis of scientific knowledge, are judged by FNB to be adequate to meet the known nutrient needs of practically all healthy people.

Also in 1941, FDA established regulations for Minimum Daily Requirements (MDR) for use in the labeling of foods (41 Fed. Reg. 5921–5926, Nov. 22, 1941). The concept was designed to address the problem of labeling foods for special dietary uses and foods to which nutrients had been added. The nutrients of particular interest were vitamins A, C, and D, and thiamin, riboflavin, and niacin. Experience revealed, however, that many people misinterpreted the name MDR. Some believed that nutrients had to be consumed in at least the stated amounts daily, even though the goal had been to describe a desirable average to be consumed over time. People also misunderstood the term *minimum* to mean that there was a real health risk if at least those amounts were not consumed daily.

Current Provision of Desired Information

When FDA initiated nutrition labeling regulations in 1973, it was necessary to establish an appropriate way to convey the content of a certain nutrient contained in a food. The obvious choice might have been listing the amount of the vitamins and minerals in a food by weight. However, the agency chose to create a system whereby the nutrients for which there was an RDA (protein, vitamins, and minerals) would be listed as a percentage of a standard, so that consumers could determine the contribution a food would make to the daily intake of a given nutrient. Because the RDAs are set for numerous age and sex groups, FDA devised a scheme that generally took the highest RDA value for any of the nutrients involved and established it as the standard or U.S. RDA for that nutrient. Current U.S. RDA values are derived from the 1968 RDAs set for adults (NRC, 1968). U.S. RDAs were proposed for infants, children, and pregnant and lactating women, but were never finalized; instead, FDA guidelines exist for these three groups. Except for infant, baby, and junior-type foods for which special regulations apply, adult U.S. RDA values are used as the basis for the percentage reporting of protein, vitamins, and minerals listed on food labels. USDA's policy follows FDA's regulations for use of the U.S. RDA (USDA, 1989b).

Although the U.S. RDAs have not been revised as subsequent editions of the RDAs have been published, the 1968 figures are considered generous by most standards. The values are based on the RDAs for adult males or females, whichever value is higher, except for thiamin, niacin, iodine, and magnesium, which are based on the adolescent male RDAs; these values exceed those for adults. The U.S. RDAs for calcium and phosphorus are also higher than the adult RDAs, but lower than those for teenagers, and pregnant and lactating women. The 1989 RDA provided values for vitamins A, C, D, and E, thiamin, riboflavin, niacin, B_6, B_{12}, folate, calcium, phosphorus, magnesium, iron, zinc, and iodine (NRC, 1989b). The 1968 RDA did not include recommendations for zinc, copper, biotin, or pantothenic acid (NRC, 1968). Estimates were made to establish a value so that the percentage of the U.S. RDA for labels could include these essential nutrients if the manufacturer wished to provide them on the label. Table 7-3 provides a comparison of the current U.S. RDAs with the 1968 and 1989 RDAs. The regulations state that the U.S. RDA may be amended "from time to time as more information on human nutrition becomes available" (21 CFR § 101.9(c)(7)(b)(ii)).

On the food label, the percentage of U.S. RDA is "a statement of the amount per serving (portion) of the protein, vitamins, and minerals." According to FDA regulations, U.S. RDA percentages are expressed in 2 percent increments up to the 10 percent level, 5 percent increments from 11 to 50 percent levels, and 10 percent increments above the 50 percent level (21 CFR § 101.9(c)(7)(i)). Nutrients present in amounts less than 2 percent are indicated by a zero or an asterisk referring to another asterisk at the bottom of the table and followed by the statement "contains less than 2 percent of the U.S. RDA of this (these) nutrient (nutrients)." When a food product contains less than 2 percent of the U.S. RDA for each of five or more of the eight required nutrients (protein, vitamins

TABLE 7-3 Comparison of U.S. RDAs[a] with 1968 and 1989 RDAs[b,c]

Nutrient	1968 RDA Adult Male	1968 RDA Adult Female	U.S. RDA	1989 RDA Adult Male	1989 RDA Adult Female
Required nutrients on current nutrition information panel					
Protein (g)	65	55	65	63	50
Vitamin A (RE)	1,000	800	5,000 IU[d]	1,000	800
Vitamin C (mg)	60	55	60	60	60
Thiamin (mg)	1.4	1.0	1.5	1.5	1.1
Riboflavin (mg)	1.7	1.5	1.7	1.7	1.3
Niacin (mg)	18	13	20	19	15
Calcium (mg)	800	800	1,000	800	800
Iron (mg)	10	18	18	10	15
Optional nutrients on current nutrition information panel					
Vitamin D (IU)	—	—	400	5 μg[e]	5 μg[e]
Vitamin E (IU)	30	25	30	10 α-TE[f]	8 α-TE[f]
Vitamin B_6 (mg)	2	2	2	2	1.6
Folic acid (mg)	0.4	0.4	0.4	0.2	0.18
Vitamin B_{12} (μg)	6	6	6	2	2
Phosphorus (g)	0.8	0.8	1.0	0.8	0.8
Iodine (μg)	120	100	150	150	150
Magnesium (mg)	350	300	400	350	280
Zinc (mg)	—	—	15	15	12
Copper (mg)	—	—	2	1.5 –3.0[g]	
Biotin (mg)	—	—	0.3	0.03–0.1[g]	
Pantothenic acid (mg)	—	—	10	4 –7[g]	

[a] 21 CFR §101.9 (7).

[b] NRC (National Research Council). 1968. Recommended Dietary Allowances, 7th ed. Food and Nutrition Board, Assembly on Life Sciences. National Academy of Sciences, Washington, D.C. 101 pp.

[c] NRC (National Research Council). 1989. Recommended Dietary Allowances, 10th ed. Report of the Subcommittee on the Tenth Edition of the Recommended Dietary Allowances, Food and Nutrition Board, Commission on Life Sciences. National Academy Press, Washington, D.C. 284 pp.

[d] 1,000 RE.

[e] 5 μg as cholecalciferol = 200 IU of vitamin D.

[f] α-Tocopherol equivalents (1 α-TE = 1 mg of d-α-tocopherol).

[g] Estimated safe and adequate daily dietary intakes (ESADDI) for both males and females.

A and C, thiamin, riboflavin, niacin, calcium, and iron), the manufacturer may choose to declare no more than three of those eight required nutrients and none of the optional nutrients. In that case, it must be accompanied by the statement "contains less than 2 percent of the U.S. RDA of . . . ," listing whichever of the eight required nutrients are not declared, directly following the declared nutrient in the same type size. When vitamins and minerals are added to a food, or a claim is made about them, the percentage of the U.S. RDA contributed by the food must be declared. U.S. RDA percentages of other optional micronutrients may also be listed.

The percentage of the U.S. RDA for protein is currently required to be declared on the label (21 CFR § 101.9(c)(7)(ii)(a), (b)). There are two U.S. RDA adult values for protein because of the difference in protein quality. The U.S. RDA of the protein efficiency ratio (PER) in a food is 45 g if the product is equal to or greater than that of casein, and 65 g if the PER of the total protein in the product is less than that of casein. Total protein with a PER less than 20 percent of the PER of casein is not allowed on the label in terms of percentage of U.S. RDA, and the statement of protein in grams per serving is to be modified by a statement that the food is not a significant source of protein content regardless of the actual amount of protein present.

There are special labeling requirements for infant, baby, and junior-type food (21 CFR § 101.9(h)(1)). The U.S. RDA levels for infants from birth to 12 months of age and children under 4 years of age may be declared for foods intended for use by these two age groups. If such dual declaration is used on any label, it is to be included in all labeling, and with equal prominence given to both values in all promotional material. The U.S. RDA PER values for infants are 18 g and 25 g, and for children under age 4, 20 g and 28 g depending on protein quality. In cases in which the food does not contain 40 percent of the PER of casein, the U.S. RDA may not be declared on the label of infant foods, and the label must carry the statement, adjacent to the protein content statement, that the food is not a significant source of protein for infants, regardless of the actual amount of protein.

If the adult U.S. RDAs continue to be used as the basis for labeling vitamins and minerals, they need revision since several adult nutrient levels and/or their units of measurement are out of date. Nutrient levels most notably in need of revision are those for biotin, vitamins B_{12} and D, folate, pantothenic acid, iron, niacin, and protein (Table 7-3). The current recommendation for biotin is one-tenth of the current U.S. RDA; for vitamin B_{12}, one-third; and for vitamin D, folate, and pantothenic acid, one-half. The current U.S. RDA for protein is slightly above the 1989 RDA, with the 1989 reference protein allowance for adults now set at 0.75 g/kg/day. A moderate protein intake (no more than twice the RDA for all age groups) is now recommended (NRC, 1989a). The U.S. RDA does not use the official measurement unit, retinol equivalents (RE), for vitamin A activity, nor does it use the most appropriate measurement units for vitamins D or E, or niacin. Weights and heights for 1989 RDA reference adults are actual U.S. population mediums, but these figures do not imply that the height-to-weight ratios are ideal.

The technical nature of the U.S. RDA is not entirely overcome by using percentage comparisons on labels. Less emphasis on micronutrients on labels decreases the usefulness of comparisons with the U.S. RDA. Current regulations for the U.S. RDAs for protein, vitamins, and minerals include numerous exemptions and special requirements. The number of regulatory options further decreases consumer understanding, and hence, the value of the U.S. RDA in food labeling. U.S. RDAs are easily misconstrued as minimum requirements, especially because consumers often assume that more is better in their interpretation of the nutrient content of foods. The 1968-based U.S. RDA percentages on labels underestimate the relative amounts of several nutrients in foods.

The Committee believes that resolution of these problems and the emphasis on total diet, rather than daily consumption, should be the focus of reform. Ample assurance that all healthy individuals are covered should be the emphasis of any standard values used as the basis of nutrition labeling.

The current terms RDA and U.S. RDA have also been the source of confusion. FDA recently proposed new terms to replace the U.S. RDA: Recommended Dietary Intakes (RDIs) and Dietary Reference Values (DRVs) (56 Fed. Reg. 29,476–29,533, July 19, 1990). These two terms seem to compound the problem by continuing to use the letters R and D in some combination in the term. The Committee suggests that alternative terms such as Dietary Values, Reference Values, Reference Intake, or Standard Values be considered for the name of a dietary standard to describe nutrient content. Whether the RDAs or other dietary recommendations serve as the basis for reference values, the use of only one term both on the label and in the regulations will help to reduce the confusion, while still allowing the general concept to represent population-based, standard reference values.

"Source of" Listings of Micronutrients

The Committee was persuaded that the current manner of providing information about the levels of vitamins and minerals present in foods was dysfunctional. FDA's current regulations require the listing of protein and seven vitamins and minerals as a percentage of the U.S. RDA, which means that the user must understand both the concepts of the U.S. RDA and percentages. There is a good deal of evidence that many consumers do not (DHEW/USDA/FTC, 1979; Elizabeth Yetley, Center for Food Safety and Applied Nutrition, FDA, personal communication, July 1990). Furthermore, the use of percentages creates undesirable incentives for manufacturers to overfortify foods in order to achieve "100 percent of your [or the government's] requirements."

Accordingly, the Committee favors a system in which vitamins and minerals, when they are required or allowed to be listed, are described only qualitatively, using simple terms that convey usable information about a food as a source of micronutrients. The Committee recommends that the descriptors *very good source of, good source of,* or *contains* be used to characterize foods containing the required or optional micronutrients. These descriptors would be defined in terms of percent ranges of the U.S. RDA or any other system of recommended nutrient values that FDA and USDA might adopt.

Implementation of this scheme would require two types of decisions, and to an important degree, the choices the Committee made (or that FDA and USDA might make) are matters of judgment rather than of evidence. The first decision concerns the terminology to use. Current FDA regulations state that no claim may be made that a food is a *significant* source of a nutrient unless that nutrient is present in the food at a level equal to or in excess of 10 percent of the U.S. RDA in a serving (21 CFR 101.9(c)(7)(v)). FDA policies for shelf labeling allow a food to be characterized as an *excellent source of* a vitamin or mineral if a serving contains 40 percent or more of the U.S. RDA; the term *good source of* is assigned to foods containing 25 percent or more in a serving, and *source of* can be used by foods containing 10 percent or more of the U.S. RDA. The Committee recommends changing both the terms for and the content criteria to define these tiered source descriptors.

Two considerations led to this recommendation. First, the term *excellent source* appeared to provide its own incentive for unnecessary vitamin and mineral fortification. Second, on close review of the vitamin and mineral content of a variety of foods, including many fruits and vegetables, grains, meat, and poultry, it appeared clear that very few would be eligible for use of this accolade, even though many are recognized as important sources of nutrients. Furthermore, many vitamins and minerals do not occur naturally in high levels in any one food; a diet supplying nutritionally adequate levels of these nutrients must be assembled from a variety of different foods. This is the type of dietary pattern that labeling should encourage, not penalize. Applying FDA's own criteria, very few standard servings of unfortified foods could be characterized as an *excellent source* of any nutrient. Thus, the Committee opted for the more modest set of descriptive terms—*very good source of, good source of,* and *contains.*

The next choice the Committee faced was defining these terms. To aid in this exercise, the Committee examined micronutrient levels (per serving) in a selected sample of foods. The foods chosen for this exercise are listed in Table 7-4. The right-hand column indicates the percentage of the current RDA for the highest level of vitamin or mineral present, then the next highest, and so on. For the exercise, vitamins A, B_6, and C and folate, calcium, iron, sodium, and potassium are described. The purpose was to develop a preliminary understanding of how common foods which potentially comprise parts of a healthy diet might rate in the type of system the Committee was developing. It made little sense to define

TABLE 7-4 Nutrients Contained in a Standard Serving of Selected Foods[a] Ranked by Decreasing Percentage of the 1989 RDA[b]

Food	Nutrient	Percent RDA
Very good source of (greater than 20 percent of standard)		
Beef liver, pan-fried, medium (3 oz)	Vitamin A	1,000.0
Carrots, raw (100 g)	Vitamin A	310.0
Orange juice, canned (6 oz)	Vitamin C	100.0
Beef liver	Folate	95.0
Beef liver	Vitamin B	67.0
Milk, skim (1 c)	Calcium	35.0
Beef liver	Iron	35.0
Beef liver	Vitamin C	32.0
Tomatoes, raw (100 g)	Vitamin C	30.0
Chicken, white, no skin, fried (3 oz)	Vitamin B_6	29.0
Bread, whole wheat (1 slice)	Sodium	27.0
Kidney beans, canned (100 g)	Folate	26.0
Cheddar cheese (1 oz)	Calcium	25.0
Prunes, whole, dried, uncooked (100 g)	Vitamin A	22.0
Potatoes, baked, flesh and skin (100 g)	Vitamin C	22.0
Bread, white (1 slice)	Sodium	22.0
Good source of (from 11 to 20 percent of standard)		
Potatoes	Vitamin B_6	19.0
Bread, whole wheat	Iron	19.0
Cottage cheese, 4% fat, creamed ($1/2$ c)	Sodium	18.0
Prunes	Iron	17.0
Bread, white	Iron	17.0
Chicken, dark, no skin, fried (3 oz)	Vitamin B_6	17.0
Carrots	Vitamin C	16.0
Milk, skim	Vitamin A	16.0
Prunes	Potassium	15.0
Prunes	Vitamin B_6	14.0
Kidney beans	Sodium	14.0
Bread, whole wheat	Calcium	14.0
Tomatoes	Vitamin A	13.0
Hamburger, 19% fat, pan-fried, medium (3 oz)	Vitamin B_6	13.0
Tuna, canned, water-packed, light meat ($1/4$ c)	Iron	12.0
Tuna	Vitamin B_6	12.0
Hamburger	Iron	12.0
Flounder, fresh or frozen, raw (3 oz)	Vitamin B_6	10.0
Contains (between 2 and 10 percent of standard)		
Bread, white	Calcium	9.6
Cheddar cheese	Vitamin A	9.6
Apples, raw, with skin (100 g)	Vitamin C	9.5
Potatoes	Iron	9.3
Kidney Beans	Iron	8.7
Chicken, dark	Iron	8.7
Cottage cheese	Calcium	8.5

TABLE 7-4—Continued

Food	Nutrient	Percent RDA
Potatoes	Potassium	8.4
Orange juice	Vitamin B_6	8.3
Carrots	Vitamin B_6	8.3
Tuna	Sodium	8.0
Milk, skim	Potassium	7.6
Carrots	Folate	7.4
Cottage cheese	Folate	7.4
Cheddar cheese	Sodium	7.2
Bread, whole wheat	Potassium	6.6
Prunes	Calcium	6.4

[a] Based on data from Agriculture Handbook No. 8 (series), U.S. Department of Agriculture.

[b] Based on average values for adult men and women. NRC (National Research Council). 1989. Recommended Dietary Allowances, 10th ed. Report of the Subcommittee on the Tenth Edition of the Recommended Dietary Allowances, Food and Nutrition Board, Commission on Life Sciences. National Academy Press, Washington, D.C. 284 pp.

the third-tier descriptor, *very good source of*, in such a way that very few foods would be eligible to employ it.

Using the Committee's system, very few unfortified foods provide 100 percent of the RDA of any nutrient in a serving. Indeed, only five foods in the sample provide more than 40 percent. Only 16 foods in the sample provided more than 20 percent. With this array in mind, the Committee debated the appropriate range of a dietary standard (in this case, the 1989 RDA) to assign to the three tiers it had agreed on. It recommends that *very good source of* be used to describe any food that provides, in a serving, more than 20 percent of the dietary standard for a given vitamin or mineral. It recommends that *good source of* be used for any food that provides, in a serving, 11 to 20 percent of the dietary standard for a given nutrient. Any food that provides between 2 and 10 percent of the dietary standard for any nutrient would be permitted to say it *contains* that nutrient. A food that contained less than 2 percent of the dietary standard for any nutrient would not be required, or allowed, to list any vitamins or minerals on the nutrition information panel that were not present at a level above 2 percent of the dietary standard. These would appear on the nutrition information panel following the macronutrient listing as follows:

A very good source (over 20% [standard]) of: . . . .
A good source (11–20% [standard]) of: . . . .
Contains (2–10% [standard]) of: . . . .

This manner of listing would allow manufacturers to draw attention to the vitamin or mineral content of foods that are significant sources. It would assist consumers with recognizing, and choosing among, foods that are important sources of micronutrients. And it would discourage overfortification of processed foods by limiting those that contain substantially more than 20 percent of the dietary standard for any micronutrient to the term *very good source of.*

It should be repeated that the development of such a system of verbal rather than numeric description of vitamin and mineral content embodies decisions that are, if not arbitrary, ultimately matters of judgment. The Committee would not think it unwise for FDA and USDA to utilize a different set of terms to characterize macronutrient content, though it would consider any system unwise that retained terms such as *excellent,* which encourage needless fortification. Nor is the Committee absolutely convinced that the percent ranges of a dietary standard it has arrived at are the ideal ranges. Rather the recommendation put forward here is intended to reflect what is believed to be a sounder way of conveying label information about the vitamin and mineral content of foods.

Committee Recommendations

The Committee recommends that:

- The U.S. RDAs (or different reference term) should be updated, even if they are to play a smaller role in nutrition labeling in the future.
- FDA and USDA should require the use of the descriptors *very good source of, good source of,* or *contains* to characterize the content of required or optional micronutrients in foods.
- Use of the descriptive terms on the nutrition information panel would require that micronitrients meet the following or similar criteria: use of *very good source of* must provide, in a serving, more than 20 percent of the dietary standard for a given vitamin or mineral; use of *good source of* must provide, in a serving, 11 to 20 percent of the dietary standard for a given nutrient; use of *contains* must provide, in a serving, between 2 and 10 percent of the dietary standard for any nutrient; and a manufacturer would not be required or allowed to declare any nutrient present at less than 2 percent of the dietary standard.

INGREDIENT LABELING

One important source of information for consumers about the composition of packaged foods is the statement of ingredients that the Federal Food, Drug, and Cosmetic Act (FD&C Act), the Federal Meat Inspection Act (FMI Act), and the Poultry Products Inspection Act (PPI Act) require on most food labels. FDA and USDA require that ingredients be listed in order of predominance by their common, specific names. A complete, simple listing of ingredients can provide consumers with important information about the nutrient content of many foods (e.g., when an obvious source of protein or fat appears near the top of the list) or about its role in health-restricted diets (e.g., when eggs or salt appear as an ingredient). On foods that do not now have nutrition labeling, the ingredient statement may provide the only factual information about nutritional value. Furthermore, ingredient labeling can be a useful supplement to more elaborate nutrition labeling when the latter is provided.

FDA and USDA have similar requirements for ingredient labeling; however, they are subject to important exceptions. Some of these exceptions have nutritional implications and should, in the Committee's judgment, be eliminated by administrative action or, if necessary, by legislation. The Committee acknowledges that other criticisms have been lodged against the current rules governing ingredient labeling, such as the authority found in all three statutes, to declare spices, flavorings, and colors by function rather than by name. In declining to recommend modification of these provisions and other exceptions that have no direct relationship to the nutritional value of foods, the Committee does not mean either to dispute or to accept the criticisms; it is merely adhering to the boundaries of its charge.

The most important, and dubious, exception from the general requirement that the ingredients of a food be declared is the provision in the FD&C Act that allows, foods covered by a standard of identity, the omission of mandatory ingredients and the inclusion of only those optional ingredients that the standard requires to be declared (FD&C Act § 403(g)). This provision not only implies that mandatory ingredients need not generally be declared, but that FDA may not require their listing in specific instances. This is the agency's interpretation and it has been upheld by the courts (*LABEL, Inc. v. Edwards,* 1969–1974 F.D.L.I. Jud. Rev. 733 (D.C. Cir. 1973)). FDA responded to this ruling by announcing that it would require labeling of all optional ingredients in standardized foods and, furthermore, that it would take steps to amend existing standards of identity to recharacterize most heretofore mandatory ingredients as optional. By 1989, the agency had thus modified four-fifths of the existing food standards. USDA generally requires all ingredients to be listed on a food label, regardless of whether it is subject to a standard of identity.

In the Committee's view, FDA is to be commended for seeking to enlarge the share of foods that bear full ingredient labeling, but the statutory procedure that has made this slow and painstaking effort necessary is an anachronism that should be changed. The majority of packaged foods are not covered by standards of identity; accordingly, all of their ingredients must be declared on the food label. There is no longer any plausible basis, if there ever was one, for exempting standardized foods from this ingredient labeling requirement. There is also a troubling irony in FDA's announcement that an ingredient which for years has characterized a standardized food is now declared "optional" so that it can be required to appear on the label.

As this report notes, many important foods remain subject to FDA or

USDA standards of identity. Many of these foods, especially dairy products, contain nutrients in amounts that consumers should be attentive to and seek to modify in their diets. The Committee recommends that Congress amend the FD&C, FMI, and PPI Acts to make clear that the general requirement of full ingredient labeling applies to standardized as well as nonstandardized foods. In the meantime, it encourages FDA to continue the process of amending its standards to require ingredient labeling.

In addition, FDA and USDA should amend their regulations to require that the ingredients of standardized foods that are incorporated into other packaged foods are declared by name (and in order of predominance) on the label of the final product. The reasoning that supports full ingredient labeling of all packaged foods, including those covered by standards of identity, applies equally in this case.

FDA and USDA both require that ingredients be listed in order of predominance (by weight). Thus, the chief, often characterizing, ingredient is usually listed first, followed by ingredients used in smaller quantities. Each ingredient (other than spices, artificial flavorings, and colorings) must be named specifically. Thus, for example, corn syrup is identified by name and listed separately. This manner of listing, however, can obscure the total amount of sugars in the food. When different sugars are listed individually—e.g., dextrose, honey, and corn syrup—consumers may not always realize that all of these ingredients are sugars, and the quantities used may result in their dispersal throughout the listing of ingredients.

In such cases, listing of ingredients both by category and by name may be necessary. A revised regulation could require that all sugars be aggregated for purposes of the sequence of listing under the generic heading *sugars* and also be described by specific name. The label of a fruit pie might then bear the following listing: Cherries, Water, Flour, Sugars (Corn Syrup, Dextrose, etc.), Corn Starch, Salt, Artificial Flavoring. It would require only modest changes in FDA and USDA regulations to accomplish this change, and no change in existing legislation would be necessary. Although it could be argued that other ingredients, such as complex carbohydrates (starches), should also be grouped, current recommendations advise that it is the amount of simple carbohydrate consumed that should be reduced.

Neither FDA nor USDA generally requires that food labels disclose the proportions or relative quantities of individual ingredients, beyond the information that the consumer can infer from the sequence in which ingredients are listed. In some cases, FDA has adopted regulations requiring that the amount of characterizing ingredient in a food be declared as part of the product name (e.g., Peanut Spread Containing 45 Percent Peanuts), but in each instance, the FDA Commissioner has made a finding that the amount of this ingredient (but not others) has a material bearing on price or consumer acceptance (Hutt and Merrill, 1990). It is doubtful that FDA or USDA could now mandate a percentage declaration of ingredients for all foods. Some critics of current labels, however, argue that legislation should require, or at least allow the agencies to require, such labeling.

The Committee takes no position on these proposals, which may or may not be justified in terms of protecting consumer economic interests. The Committee has not been persuaded that, if the ingredients of all processed foods were listed and full nutrition information were required, the costs of percentage ingredient labeling would be worth its possible contribution to consumer assessment of the nutrient content of foods. However, this does not mean that the case for percentage labeling, at least of major ingredients, cannot be made on other grounds.

Finally, the current FDA and USDA format for declaring ingredients has been criticized. Although this format is not dictated by agency regulations, the typical mode of disclosure has a common and, in the view of critics, unfriendly appearance. Following the heading "ingredients," ingredients appear in a margin-to-margin, flattened column printed entirely in capital letters, separated only by commas, without other breaks or classifications, and occasionally parenthetical phrases describing ingredient functions. Moreover, only a minority of consumers appear to understand the rationale of the prescribed order of listing (Heimbach, 1982). The Committee has been impressed by proposals for making this portion of the food label more user friendly by, such changes as, using capital and lowercase letters, separating major from minor ingredients, and employing contrasting colors. The Committee recommends that when FDA and USDA test different basic formats for nutrition labeling, they should also seek information about consumer reactions to and use of different formats for depicting the ingredients in foods. If the ingredient panel is to contribute to consumer understanding of the nutritional characteristics of different foods, serious efforts should be made to improve its readability.

Committee Recommendations

The Committee recommends that:

- Congress should amend the FD&C, FMI, and PPI Acts to make clear that the general requirement of full ingredient labeling applies to standardized as well as nonstandardized foods.
- FDA and USDA should take steps to amend their requirements for ingredient labeling to require that the ingredients of standardized foods that are incorporated into other processed foods are declared by name on the label of the final product.
- When FDA and USDA test different formats for nutrition labeling, they should also seek information about consumer reactions to and use of different formats for depicting the ingredients in foods.

STANDARDS OF IDENTITY

This report focuses on the desired content and appropriate format for nutrition information on food labels, but the Committee was also urged to examine other regulatory practices that impinged on efforts to improve Americans' diets. One of the most controversial issues is the system of food standards of identity created and enforced by FDA. In broad terms, a *standard of identity* represents the official recipe for a food; it defines the composition of products entitled to use the name of a food. For example, the FDA standard of identity for ice cream specifies the ingredients that any product labeled ice cream must include, lists other optional ingredients that it may include, and prescribes the amount of milk fat—10 percent—that the final product must contain. In specifying the amount of this presumably valuable constituent, the ice cream standard is like numerous others that FDA has adopted under the authority of the FD&C Act. Many such standards cover dairy products, including cheeses, yogurt, and milk.

FDA's authority to establish definitions and standards of identity for foods is not unique (FD&C Act § 401). USDA exercises similar powers under both the FMI and the PPI Acts and has established standards for many meat and poultry products. Claims that food standards can impede consumer efforts to choose more nutritious foods have focused primarily on many of those issued by FDA several decades ago, when concerns about nutrition and the goals of regulation were quite different. USDA standards may not raise the same issues since they do not require a minimum fat content as some FDA standards do; most USDA standards establish maximum fat limits and minimum meat/poultry requirements.

With the time constraints it faced, the Committee was not able to study these claims thoroughly. It was persuaded, however, that certain aspects of FDA's current food standards system require reform. The criticisms of many FDA standards of identity fall into three categories: (1) Standards for such foods as ice cream and other dairy products require the presence of high levels of undesired constituents, chiefly fat; (2) FDA's enforcement of these food standards discourages the marketing of substitutes for the standardized products containing reduced levels of fat or other less desirable constituents; (3) current labeling requirements for standardized foods under the FD&C Act fail to require a full listing of ingredients, a criticism dealt with in the previous section.

A fourth criticism of the current FDA regimen concerns the procedure by which standards of identity must be adopted and, correspondingly, amended. This procedure, dictated by section 701(e) of the FD&C Act, is known as formal rulemaking. It entails, in addition to the conventional publication of a proposal followed by the submission of written comments and promulgation of a final regulation, the opportunity for a formal evidentiary hearing, the administrative equivalent of a judicial trial. This last requirement means that a proceeding to establish, amend, or repeal a standard of identity may take 2 or 3 years to complete. One notorious proceeding, to set a standard for peanut butter, took over a decade. This procedural feature of the food standards provision of the FD&C Act has implications for the substantive criticisms of the FDA system.

Two concerns motivated Congress in 1938 when it conferred this power on FDA. One was a concern for consumers, whom Congress (and FDA) believed often could not distinguish a debased product by sight or taste alone—for example, fruit preserves in which less expensive sugar was substituted for more costly fruit. The second concern was for producers, who claimed that manufacturers of cheapened products were competing unfairly. These concerns combined to yield the statutory authority under which FDA has defined and standardized nearly 300 foods, products that at one time accounted for almost half of consumers' food expenditures (Merrill and Hutt, 1980). In 1990, less skepticism exists about consumers' abilities, aided by informative labeling, to protect themselves against debased or diluted products. As *The Surgeon General's Report on Nutrition and Health* (DHHS, 1988) and the NRC *Diet and Health* report (NRC, 1989a) confirm, attention is now focused on the consumption of too much fat rather than the possibility that some products will be made using less of an ingredient that was historically considered a valuable constituent. Accordingly, it seems clear to the Committee that any system that significantly impedes the marketing of reduced-, low-, and non- or no-fat substitutes should be reexamined and, presumably, changed.

In theory, FDA food standards need not impede the marketing of such products, but there is reason to believe that they sometimes do (see Lorman, Appendix D). It is clear that the current standard of identity for ice cream prevents the marketing of a product called *ice cream* that contains less than 10 percent milk fat which would violate the food standards provision of section 403(g) of the FD&C Act. A possible response would be to amend the standard of identity and reduce the required level of fat, or eliminate any minimum fat requirement. However, the procedural impediments to such an action are formidable. Current manufacturers of ice cream would likely oppose any change in the standard that would make it easier for new and presumably more healthful products to compete with their formulations. Such opposition, even from only a few manufacturers, would ensure that FDA would have to follow the Act's full panoply of procedural requirements.

Amending the ice cream standard would not be the only way to facilitate the marketing of lower-fat alternatives. In theory, a frozen dessert product containing only 5 percent milk fat, or even less, should be marketable, and in fact it is. The problem comes in deciding the name for it. The law allows three possibilities but, as administered by FDA, forecloses the one possibility that manufacturers would most prefer (see Lorman, Appendix D). The lower-fat alternative could be standardized under an entirely new name, but this possibility confronts the same procedural hurdles as an effort to amend the ice cream standard does. It is unattractive for another reason because FDA is likely to be reluctant to allow the use of the name ice cream in any new standard. That name, in the agency's view, belongs to the original 10 percent milk fat formulation.

Another possibility would be to market the lower-fat alternative, without a standard of identity, under a name that distinguished it from standardized ice cream. Under FDA's view of the law, this descriptive name may not include the words *ice cream*. *No-fat ice cream* would not be allowed because the characterizing ingredient, cream, would not be part of the product, although a reduced-fat ice cream would be allowed. According to FDA, such a product would purport to be ice cream and, because it would not meet the standard, would be adulterated. (FDA would allow reduced-fat ice cream because it would contain at least some cream.) A name such as *frozen dairy dessert* would probably suffice, but many food marketers believe that this or any similar alternative name would make it more difficult for the product to attract the consumer's attention as a lower-fat substitute for the real thing. In short, they assert that fewer consumers would make the nutritionally sound choice to buy the substitute.

Based on case law, there is another alternative to which FDA would not object and which would permit the use of the name *ice cream*. The new product could be marketed as *imitation ice cream* (Merrill and Hutt, 1980). Many food marketers believe, however, that such a name would clearly mark the product as inferior to traditional ice cream and make it even harder to sell.

It is difficult to assess the merits of the arguments that FDA standards of identity, and the agency's refusal to permit the use of standardized names in the names of reformulated substitutes, are in fact discouraging the marketing of more healthful alternatives to traditional foods. Supermarket shelves are full of new products bearing novel names that have gained consumer acceptance. A firm prepared to spend large sums of money to promote a product as new, different, and more healthful can often compete effectively with a traditional formulation without using the standardized name. This strategy, however, selectively favors large producers. The criticisms of current FDA food standards policy seem plausible enough to warrant a recommendation that both the agency's current enforcement policy and the law itself should be reexamined.

Whether or not substantial reform is merited, the Committee believes that two changes need to be made in the FD&C Act: The current procedural requirements for adopting, amending, and repealing standards of identity cannot be justified, either in terms of efficient administration or of ensuring fair opportunities in FDA rulemaking. The majority of FDA regulations, which resolve issues of great moment and that govern commercial practices of profound significance to consumers and producers, are promulgated through informal rulemaking. Section 701(e) is an anachronism and should be repealed. At the very least, Congress should amend the FD&C Act to exempt standards of identity from its requirements.

This change in the law would accomplish two things: First, it would make it easier for FDA to amend old food standards that embody restrictions that no longer make sense, nutritionally or economically. Correspondingly, it would facilitate the adoption of standards for new substitutes for traditional foods when that seems appropriate. Second, FDA's 20-year effort to recharacterize mandatory ingredients of standardized foods as optional and require their complete listing on the label would be expedited if it were easier to amend food standards. However, the Committee believes this exercise will no longer be necessary if full ingredient labeling is required for foods with standards of identity.

The latter advantage would be significant only if Congress failed to make the second change that the Committee recommends. As noted elsewhere, the listing of ingredients on a food's label conveys information about the nutrition contents that can help attentive consumers make sounder nutrition choices. The FD&C Act effectively exempts standardized foods from this otherwise universal requirement. This exemption, in the Committee's judgment, should be repealed promptly.

Committee Recommendations

The Committee recommends that:

- FDA's food standards should be carefully examined for their effects on the marketing of low-, lower-, and no-fat substitutes for high-fat foods.
- Congress should amend the FD&C Act to eliminate the requirement that standards be adopted and amended through formal rulemaking.
- Congress should eliminate the exemption from full ingredient labeling for standardized foods.

PRINCIPAL DISPLAY PANEL DESCRIPTORS

Food labels have probably always been used to promote as well as to describe foods. In the current marketing environment, merchandisers of food think carefully about every facet of label design, from color to typography to size and location. Many choices are influenced by government requirements, but this does not mean that the entire contents are dictated by governmental directives. Manufacturers of foods, even those within USDA's jurisdiction, have a good deal of freedom to decide the information to include on a label and how to display it. Label and package size, of course, operate as important constraints on choice, but it is the rare food label that does not reflect the thoughtful efforts of the manufacturer to make the food appear attractive, tasty, or nutritious, and often all three. In recent years, the growing interest in nutrition in general, and such components as fiber, fat, and calcium in particular, has led manufacturers to try to characterize their products as being nutritionally beneficial. Examples are almost numberless, but the most common are familiar: *low calorie, fat free, no cholesterol, fiber rich,* and *light* (or *lite*). Current sales data reveal that about 32 percent of the packaged foods on the market bear some type of descriptor (FLAPS, 1988).

The verbal formulas used to describe nutrient contents take many forms, but they have been given the name *descriptors* or, sometimes, *adjectival descriptors.* The proliferation of terms and the growth in their usage have drawn a good deal of attention from regulatory bodies and health professionals, as well as from competitors. The reactions have been ambivalent, if not schizophrenic. On the one hand, the popularity of these terms probably signals a rising interest among consumers in the links between diet and long-term health. On the other hand, the potential for confusion, exaggeration, and outright deception has prompted some to argue that nutrient descriptors should be forbidden.

The problem stems in part from failures in the system for regulating food labels and has several facets. For many descriptors in common commercial use, neither FDA nor USDA has any official definition against which to measure individual product labels. This is not as serious a problem for USDA, which, by virtue of its power to approve labels, is able to resolve the issue through policy development. For FDA, however, the lack of standard definitions for many common descriptors is a serious problem, because the agency has no effective way to prevent manufacturers from using terms that are meaningless or potentially deceptive.

A distinction should be drawn between the lack of formal definitions embodied in regulations and the failure to have an agreed-upon definition. FDA has adopted regulations defining certain descriptors, such as terms describing sodium content, but in most cases it has relied on informal advice. For example, agency officials appear to have come to agreement on the meaning of *high fiber,* but the agency has not adopted any regulation to this effect, and thus, compliance is dependent both on knowing the informal position and being willing to adhere to it. With little risk of enforcement, a manufacturer who holds a different view has little reason to abide by the FDA rules.

The problem is amplified where USDA has formally defined a descriptive term but FDA has not. Examples include the terms *natural* and *lite,* and quantitative descriptors of fat content. Compliance with the USDA criteria is likely to be near universal, whereas manufacturers of FDA-regulated foods are as likely to be as concerned about their competitors' actions as about the suggestions or threats of agency officials. Finally, there are descriptors, such as reduced-calorie and reduced-fat, on whose meaning the two agencies differ. In such cases the same term may mean different things on two different foods displayed in different aisles of the supermarket.

Without formal definitions for common descriptors, some food manufacturers have been able to exploit consumer interest in foods that appear to be more healthful. For example, companies have been using the term *lite* in two very different ways. On some products it implies reduced calories, fat, or sodium; on others, the term is intended to convey lighter texture, flavor, or even color. For example, Frito Lights, San Giorgio Light 'n Fluffy Egg Noodles, Keebler Crispy Light Crackers, and Wesson Light and Natural Vegetable Oil do not provide fewer calories or less fat than their original counterparts do; only lighter taste. Yet, an FDA survey of 1,000 adults revealed that 70 percent who had seen foods labeled *lite* assumed that it meant lower in calories. The rest thought variously that it referred to sugar, salt, fat, cholesterol, or weight (Heimbach, 1982). The multiple-message problem is compounded in this case, because USDA has adopted a regulation that permits the term *lite* to be used to refer to breading and other components, as well as to the more familiar caloric, fat, or sodium content.

Some uses of nutrient descriptors border on the deceptive. It is a common practice to highlight a single desirable component in which the labeled food contains a significant amount of an undesirable component that the food lacks or contains in reduced amounts. Usually, there is no effort to provide a balanced statement on the nutritional characteristics of the food. This practice can be viewed merely as an example of aggressive merchandising, but some examples are arguably misbranding. Many observers, including members of the Committee, are troubled, for example, by foods with labels that state *no cholesterol* but that contain substantial amounts of saturated fat. Equally disconcerting, if not so serious, are such claims on products such as bananas and peanut butter, in which nature never put cholesterol.

The following pages describe the regulatory policies of FDA and USDA, and Table 7-5 details the agencies' key definitions for descriptors.

Current Regulation of Descriptors

Caloric Content and Body Weight

In 1978, FDA issued a final rule that regulates label statements relating to usefulness in reducing or maintaining caloric intake or body weight. The general requirement ensures that nutrition labeling must appear on any food that carries a caloric-related claim. If the product achieves its special dietary character because a nonnutritive ingredient is present in the food, then the ingredient and its percentage by weight must be specified on the label.

The regulation also establishes definitions for low-calorie and reduced-calorie foods and other comparative claims. A low-calorie food is defined by an absolute standard: the food must provide less than or equal to 40 calories per serving and less than or equal to 0.4 calorie per gram. The term *low calorie* or similar phrase must be displayed on the food's principal display panel. A reduced-calorie food must have at least one-third fewer calories, but otherwise be nutritionally equivalent to the food it replaces. Such claims must also be

TABLE 7-5 Status of Current Federal Policy for Selected Descriptors

Nutrient and Term	FDA Criteria	USDA Criteria
Calcium	No regulation; informal policy developed for trial shelf labeling programs[a]	No regulation
Source	At least 100 mg of calcium per serving	
Good source	At least 250 mg of calcium per serving	
Excellent source	At least 400 mg of calcium per serving	
Calories		
Low calorie	Less than or equal to 40 calories per serving and less than or equal to 0.4 calories/g (21 CFR §105.66(c))	Less than or equal to 40 calories per serving and less than or equal to 0.4 calories/g (USDA, 1982a)
Reduced calorie	At least one-third fewer calories, but otherwise nutritionally equivalent to the food it replaces; requires a statement of comparison (21 CFR § 105.66(d))	At least a 25 percent reduction is required along with an explanatory statement and quantitative information (USDA, 1982a)
Sugar free No sugar	Must be low calorie, reduced calorie, have a comparative claim, or descriptor must be followed by a phrase indicating it is not a low calorie food (21 CFR §105.66(f))	Negative claims are permitted if it is not clear from product name that the ingredient is not contained in the product (USDA, 1987a)

Cholesterol		
Cholesterol free No cholesterol	Tentative final rule; less than 2 mg of cholesterol per serving and 5 g or less of total fat per serving and 20 percent or less of total fat on a dry weight basis and 2 g or less of saturated fatty acids per serving and 6 percent or less of saturated fatty acids on a dry weight basis[b]	No such claims expected for meat products[c]
Cholesterol free food	Tentative final rule; must meet conditions for free of cholesterol, cholesterol free, or no cholesterol and inherently contain less than 2 mg of cholesterol per serving without the benefit of special processing or reformulation to alter cholesterol content; provided that such labeling clearly refers to all foods of that type and not merely to the particular brand to which the labeling attaches[b]	No regulation (see low cholesterol meal)
Low cholesterol Low in cholesterol	Tentative final rule; less than or equal to 20 mg of cholesterol per serving and 0.2 mg or less of cholesterol per g of food, and 5 g or less of total fat per serving and 20 percent or less of total fat on a dry weight basis and 6 percent or less of saturated fatty acids per serving and 6 percent or less of saturated fatty acids on a dry weight basis[b]	No regulation; tentatively using FDA's proposed definition[c]
Low cholesterol meal	No regulation	No regulation; working policy of no more than 20 mg/100 g of product[c]

TABLE 7-5—Continued

Nutrient and Term	FDA Criteria	USDA Criteria
Reduced cholesterol Cholesterol reduced	Tentative final rule; at least 75 percent reduction of cholesterol content compared with that in the food it resembles in organoleptic properties and for which it substitutes, provided that the label of such a food also bears clear and concise quantitative information comparing the product's per serving cholesterol content with that of the food it replaces[b]	No regulation; tentatively permitting comparative claims that are reduced at least 25 percent from the regular policy[c]
Fat		
Lean	No regulation	May contain no more than 10 percent fat (except for ground beef and hamburger, which may contain a 25 percent reduction from standard of 30 percent fat—i.e., no more than 22.5 percent fat); brand names must meet standard or lower-fat definition except dinners/entrees designed for weight loss or maintenance, which must include abbreviated nutrition label (USDA, 1987b)
Extra lean	No regulation	May contain no more than 5 percent fat (except for ground beef and hamburger—the exception described above will also qualify for extra lean) (USDA, 1987b)

237

Low fat	No regulation; policy guideline states that less than or equal to 2 g of fat per serving and less than or equal to 10 percent fat on a dry weight basis[d]	May contain no more than 10 percent fat (USDA, 1987b)
Reduced fat Lower fat	No regulation; policy guideline states that at least 50 percent reduction from the regular product accompanied by a statement of comparison[d]	Comparative claims must have achieved at least a 25 percent reduction (or difference) in fat (or lean) (USDA, 1987b)
Fiber	No regulation; informal policy developed for trial shelf labeling programs[a]	No regulation[c]
Source	At least 2 g of fiber per serving	No regulation[c]
Good source (FDA) Significant source (USDA)	At least 5 g of fiber per serving	No regulation; working policy of at least 3 g of fiber per serving[c]
Excellent source (FDA)	At least 8 g of fiber per serving	No regulation[c]
Fresh	May not be applied to foods that have been subjected to any form of heat or chemical processing (Compliance Policy Guide 7120.06)	May be used if not cured, canned, hermetically sealed, dried, or chemically preserved—not shelf stable; for poultry, cannot be used if frozen at or below 0°F; brand names exempt (USDA, 1989a)
Lite and Light	No regulation; working policy considers lite to mean reduced calorie, one-third fewer calories, unless defined elsewhere (i.e., a food standard, for example, light cream, or an obvious example, light versus heavy syrup)[e]	May refer to fat, salt, sodium, breading, and/or other components; a 25 percent reduction is required along with an explanatory statement and quantitative information; dinners/entrees designed for weight loss or maintenance must include abbreviated nutrition label (USDA, 1982a)

238

TABLE 7-5—Continued

Nutrient and Term	FDA Criteria	USDA Criteria
Natural	No regulation	May be used if product contains no artificial flavor, coloring, or chemical preservative and the product and its ingredients are not more than minimally processed, along with explanatory statement (USDA, 1982b)
Organic	No regulation	No regulation; not permitted
Sodium		
Sodium free	Less than 5 mg of sodium per serving (21 CFR §101.13(a)(1))	Less than 5 mg of sodium per serving (USDA, 1984)
Very low sodium	Less than or equal to 35 mg of sodium per serving (21 CFR §101.13(a)(2))	Less than or equal to 35 mg of sodium per serving (USDA, 1984)
Low sodium	Less than or equal to 140 mg of sodium per serving (21 CFR §101.13(a)(3))	Less than or equal to 140 mg of sodium per serving (USDA, 1984)
Reduced sodium	At least 75 percent reduction of sodium compared with that in the food it replaces; also requires a statement of comparison; additional comparative claims are permitted if at least 25 percent sodium reduction is achieved and is accompanied by explanatory statement (21 CFR §101.13(a)(4))	At least 75 percent reduction of sodium compared with that in the food it replaces; also requiresa statement of comparison; additional comparative claims are permitted if at least 25 percent sodium reduction is achieved and is accompanied by explanatory statement (USDA, 1984)

. . . source of	No regulation; informal policy developed for shelf labeling programs[f]	No regulation; FDA's definitions used as basis for working policy[c]
Fair Significant	At least 10 percent or more of U.S. RDA per serving	
Good	At least 25 percent or more of U.S. RDA per serving	
Excellent	At least 40 percent or more of U.S. RDA per serving	

[a] Letter to J.S. Kahan and B.L. Rubin, Hogan and Hartson, Washington, D.C., by R.J. Ronk, Center for Food Safety and Applied Nutrition, Food and Drug Administration, DHHS, August 26, 1988.

[b] 55 Fed. Reg. 29,456–29,473 (July 19, 1990).

[c] S. Jones, Standards and Labeling Division, Food Safety and Inspection Service, USDA, personal communication, 1990.

[d] Pennington, J.A.T., V.L. Wilkening, and J.E. Vanderveen. 1990. Descriptive terms for food labeling. J. Nutr. Ed. 22(1):51–54; and R.E. Newberry, Division of Regulatory Guidance, Center for Food Safety and Applied Nutrition, Food and Drug Administration, DHHS, personal communication, 1990.

[e] Letter to M.E. Thompson, Kraft, Inc., Glenview, Ill., by S.A. Miller, Center for Food Safety and Applied Nutrition, Food and Drug Administration, DHHS, July 9, 1987; and R.E. Newberry, Division of Regulatory Guidance, Center for Food Safety and Applied Nutrition, Food and Drug Administration, DHHS, personal communication, 1990.

[f] Letter to O. Mathews, Giant Food, Inc., Washington, D.C., by Sanford A. Miller, Center for Food Safety and Applied Nutrition, Food and Drug Administration, DHHS, July 16, 1986.

accompanied by a statement that clearly describes the comparison upon which the claim is based (21 CFR § 105.66(a), (c), (d)).

Terms such as *sugar free, sugarless,* and *no sugar* are also defined. FDA suggests that consumers would assume that products with these descriptors would be significantly reduced in calories. Therefore, the food must be labeled *low calorie* or *reduced calorie* or carry the comparative claim or the term, or every time the term is used it must be followed by a phrase indicating the product is not a low-calorie food (21 CFR § 105.66(f)).

USDA has guidelines for label claims related to the caloric content of a product in its usefulness for the reduction or maintenance of body weight. Such claims trigger a requirement for disclosing limited nutrition information including calories, and protein, carbohydrate, and fat content. Additional statements may be required if necessary for consumer understanding.

USDA's definition of *low calorie* is identical to the FDA definition: less than or equal to 40 calories per serving and less than or equal to 0.4 calorie per gram. Reduced calories or other comparative claims using the term *lite* must achieve at least a 25 percent reduction along with an explanatory statement and quantitative information (USDA, 1982a). Negative claims, such as *no sugar,* are permitted (USDA, 1986).

Cholesterol

In July 1990, FDA issued a tentative final rule defining cholesterol descriptors. The definition for *cholesterol free* would be allowed on foods that contain less than 2 mg of cholesterol per serving; 5 g or less of total fat and 20 percent or less of total fat on a dry-weight basis; and 2 g or less of saturated fatty acids and 6 percent or less of saturated fatty acids on a dry-weight basis. *Low cholesterol* would be allowed for foods containing 20 mg or less of cholesterol per serving and 0.2 mg or less of cholesterol per gram of food; 5 grams or less of total fat per serving and 20 percent or less of total fat on a dry-weight basis; and 2 g or less of saturated fatty acids per serving and 6 percent of saturated fatty acids on a dry-weight basis. *Reduced cholesterol* would be allowed on foods that contained at least 75 percent less cholesterol compared with the level in the food it replaces accompanied by an explanatory statement of comparison (e.g., cholesterol content has been reduced from 100 mg to 25 mg per serving). The notice also provided guidelines for use of the terms *cholesterol free* food and *low cholesterol* food, which would not permit the use of defined terms for foods that normally contain low cholesterol, such as applesauce, unless such labels refer to all foods of that type (e.g., applesauce, a cholesterol-free food) (55 Fed. Reg. 29,455–29,473, July 19, 1990).

The proposal also would delete the requirement that any reference to the cholesterol content of a food be accompanied by a statement that the information is provided for individuals who are modifying their diets on the advice of a physician, although this statement is little used in recent practice. Also to be deleted is the present requirement that the percentage of calories from fat must accompany fatty acid labeling. A declaration of either fatty acid composition or cholesterol content would require that quantitative information about both be provided, except for low-fat foods. Additionally, if a food with a cholesterol descriptor is represented as a substitute for a traditional food, it must be its nutritional equivalent.

USDA has no formal policy on cholesterol descriptors. The agency is waiting for FDA to issue its final rule on cholesterol claims before proposing its own. At present, USDA is using FDA's 1986 proposed definition of *low cholesterol,* which is less than or equal to 20 mg of cholesterol per serving. *No cholesterol* claims are not expected to be used for meat products. USDA permits comparative cholesterol claims if the cholesterol content per serving has been reduced by at least 25 percent from a similar product, as described in Agriculture Handbook No. 8 or similar source. USDA rejected FDA's proposed definition of a *low cholesterol meal* because it allowed for too high a cholesterol level. USDA's working policy limits a *low cholesterol meal* to no more than 20 mg of cholesterol per 100 g of product (Sally Jones, Standards and Labeling Division, FSIS, USDA, personal communication, 1990).

Fat

FDA has no regulations on fat descriptors which is currently under review at FDA. The agency expects to propose a rule on fat descriptors (including *fat free, low fat, reduced fat and low in saturated fat*) by October 31, 1990 (R.E. Newberry, Division of Regulatory Guidelines, FDA, personal communication, 1990). However, FDA has announced policy guidelines for *low fat* and *reduced fat* claims. The present working definition of *low fat* is a food that provides less than or equal to 2 g of fat per serving and less than or equal to 10 percent fat on a dry-weight basis. The policy guideline for *reduced fat* suggests that it may be used for foods that have achieved at least a 50 percent reduction in fat from the regular product as well as display a statement of comparison (Pennington et al., 1990; R.E. Newberry, Division of Regulatory Guidelines, FDA, personal communication, 1990). FDA has no regulation for *lean* claims. Rules defining saturated and polyunsaturated fatty acids have existed for some time; the July 1990 tentative final rule defined monounsaturated fatty acids.

USDA has issued guidelines for labeling claims concerning the fat and lean contents of meat and poultry products. Emphatic expressions, such as *lean,* as well as comparative claims, such as *leaner,* may be used. *Low fat* products may contain no more than 10 percent fat. *Lean* products may contain no more than 10 percent fat (except for ground beef and hamburger). *Extra lean* products are limited to those with no more than 5 percent fat (except for ground beef and hamburger). In all cases, total fat must be disclosed on the label, for example, contains 4 percent fat (USDA, 1987b).

If ground beef or hamburger is labeled *lean* or *extra lean*, the fat content must be reduced by 25 percent from the regulatory standard of 30 percent fat. Thus, they may contain no more than 22.5 percent fat. The actual fat and lean percentages must be included prominently on the label. USDA illustrates this as follows: ground beef with 20 percent fat could be labeled as "Lean Ground Beef, contains 80 percent lean and 20 percent fat." Fat percentages, with no fat descriptors, may be provided on labels (USDA, 1982b, 1987b).

Comparative claims regarding lean or fat content must be based on at least a 25 percent reduction or difference in fat or lean. If a market-basket survey shows comparable products have a different amount of fat than that in the standard, then the survey must form the basis for comparison. The amount of fat in a similar product as described in applicable references such as Agriculture Handbook No. 8 may be used. An explanatory statement must accompany a comparative claim. For example, leaner italian sausage could be labeled as, "This product contains 24 percent fat, which is 30 percent less fat than allowed by the USDA standard for Italian sausage" (USDA, 1987b, p.2).

USDA permits a loophole in these guidelines for fanciful names, brand names, and trademarks that include the term *lean*. Products, such as lean entrees or dinners, need only provide USDA's abbreviated labeling requirements. USDA assumes that for such foods, the term is used to suggest usefulness in weight reduction or maintenance (USDA, 1987b).

To protect consumers from literally watered down a products, lean claims are supposed to be limited to products composed solely of fat and lean material with no added substances such as water or extenders. Comparisons with leading brands, or the company's regular product, are no longer permitted. USDA viewed these comparisons as limited in value, because sometimes the comparison product was unavailable at the same supermarket or was not typical of marketplace products.

Lite *and* Light

FDA has no regulations covering the use of *lite* or similar terms. FDA's working policy considers lite to mean reduced calorie under 21 CFR § 105.66, which requires one-third fewer calories, unless the term is defined elsewhere (such as a standardized food, or light cream) or is obvious (light syrup as opposed to heavy syrup) (letter to J. Edward Thompson, Kraft, Inc., by Sanford A. Miller, July 7, 1987; R.E. Newberry, Division of Regulatory Guidance, FDA, personal communication, 1990).

The USDA policy memorandum on *lite* allows food manufacturers leeway to creatively use such terms as *lite, light,* and *lightly* (USDA, 1986). The memo notes that such terms generally imply that a product has significantly fewer calories than expected in the product it replaces. However, the agency condones the use of *lite* to refer to fat, salt, sodium, breading, and/or other components. The reference component must be reduced by at least 25 percent.

USDA requires the term *lite* to be explained either adjacent to its use or by an asterisk with an accompanying explanation on the principal display panel or information panel. Quantitative information must be provided about the component along with a qualitative comparison to (1) the amount permitted by an applicable standard if it is representative of the majority of products in the marketplace, (2) the amount found in similar products in a market-basket survey, or (3) the amount in similar products as described by an applicable reference source such as Agriculture Handbook No. 8.

Products that meet an absolute *low* standard as defined by USDA may provide only disclosure of the actual amount of the substance without a comparative statement. For this purpose, calories can be no more than 40 per serving and no more than 0.4 calorie per gram of product. For fat and breading, the limit for *low* is no more than 10 percent of the product. For salt and sodium, the product can contain no more than 35 mg of sodium per 100 g of the product to qualify for a *low* descriptor.

Products that use the term *lite* in the brand name need only meet USDA's abbreviated nutrition labeling requirements. The agency suggests that when *lite* is used in this manner it is assumed to represent usefulness in weight reduction or maintenance (USDA, 1982a).

The Bureau of Alcohol, Tobacco, and Firearms (BATF) has jurisdiction over alcohol labeling (45 Fed. Reg. 83,530–83-545, Dec. 19, 1980). In 1988, BATF proposed a rule to regulate the use of the words *lite* and *light* in the labeling (and advertising) of wine, distilled spirits and malt beverages. BATF proposed two alternative ways a beverage could qualify for a *lite* claim: (1) if it contains 20 percent fewer calories than the producer's regular product or, if the producer does not make a regular product, 20 percent fewer calories than a competitor's same or similar regular product; or (2) if the product is labeled with both the number of calories in the producer's lite and regular products or, if the producer makes no regular product, the number of calories in a competitor's specifically named regular product (53 Fed. Reg. 22,678, June 17, 1988). This proposal has not been finalized.

Organic, Natural, *and* Fresh

FDA has taken no formal position on the use of the descriptors *organic* and *natural.* According to a 1978 article, the agency "has not tried to arrive at a legal definition of these terms because enforcement would be difficult or impossible, and costly. Organically grown foods, once they are removed from the field, cannot be told from commercially fertilized plants" (Stephenson, 1978). In a December 16, 1988, letter to the National Association of State Departments of Agriculture on organic food standards, FDA stated, "We believe it would serve no useful purpose to create standards for foods which are virtually the same, regardless of methods of production" (Food Chemical News, 1988, pp. 16–17).

The agency also has not defined the term *natural*. Informal agency policy considers *natural* to mean that there is nothing artificial or synthetic in the product, and that includes any color (e.g., beet juice in lemonade to make it pink would not be natural) (R.E. Newberry, Division of Regulatory Compliance, FDA, personal communication, 1990).

FDA has a policy guideline that defines the term *fresh*, which states that the term should not be applied to foods that have been subjected to any form of heat or chemical processing" (Compliance Policy Guide 7120.06). Additionally, to avoid misrepresentation and provide information needed to ensure proper storage, food labels are supposed to include in the name or statement of identity appropriate descriptive terms such as *pasteurized* or *frozen*. Recently, certain food labels using the descriptor *fresh* for foods from cooked tomatoes have been challenged by consumer organizations and competing manufacturers; however, the issue has not been resolved (Food Chemical News, 1990).

USDA has no formal policy on *organic* claims, and it has never approved the use of the term *organic* on any label (Sally Jones, Standards and Labeling Division, FSIS, USDA, personal communication, 1990).

Though FDA suggests that *natural* is too difficult to define, USDA has had a policy memorandum defining the term *natural* since 1982 (USDA, 1982b). Under its policy, *natural* claims may be made if the product meets two criteria: (1) no artificial flavor, coloring ingredient, or chemical preservative or any other synthetic ingredient is contained in the product; and (2) the product and its ingredients are not more than *minimally processed*. USDA considers minimal processing to mean any traditional process used to make food edible, such as freezing or drying. Additionally, the agency requires an explanatory statement on the packaging, such as "the product is natural because it contains no artificial ingredients and is only minimally processed." USDA's policy memorandum on use of the term *fresh* permits its use on any product that is not cured, canned, hermetically sealed, dried, or chemically preserved, that is, not shelf-stable (USDA, 1989a). For poultry, *fresh* cannot be used on poultry frozen at or below 0°F. The agency makes exceptions if *fresh* is used as part of a brand name.

(Note: There are about 20 states that encourage producers and marketers of organic food through labeling laws and/or programs that certify growers'/producers' claims for food buyers [TDA, 1989]. In addition, there was legislation pending in the 101st Congress which contained provisions defining the term *organic*.)

Sodium

In June 1982, FDA issued a proposed rule to amend the food labeling regulations concerning sodium labeling. That proposed rule established definitions for four claims: *sodium free, low sodium, moderately low sodium,* and *reduced sodium.* It provided for the proper use of these terms in food labeling. The appropriate uses of the terms *without added salt, unsalted,* and *no salt added* were also included. Additionally, FDA specified that sodium content of foods be included in nutrition labeling information whenever it was used on food labels. FDA explained that its goals for this program were to increase the availability of, and make more effective, sodium content labeling, as well as to reduce the amount of sodium added to processed foods, when it was safe and technically possible (47 Fed. Reg. 26,580–26,595, June 18, 1982).

Two years later, FDA issued a final rule on sodium content labeling, defining the number and terms as well as the numeric basis for the above descriptors (49 Fed. Reg. 15,510–15,535, Apr. 18, 1984). Four sodium-related descriptors were established by the final rule. *Sodium free* may be used to describe foods that contain less than 5 mg of sodium per serving (21 CFR § 101.13(a)(1)). *Very low sodium* may be used for foods that contain 35 mg or less of sodium per serving (21 CFR § 101.13(a)(2)). *Low sodium* may be used for foods that contain 140 mg or less of sodium per serving (21 CFR § 101.13(a)(3)). *Reduced sodium* may be used in labeling if the product contains 75 percent less sodium than the regular product and is represented as a direct substitute for that food. Additionally, if reduced sodium is claimed on a food, its label must also provide a sodium comparison per serving with the original product (21 CFR § 101.13(a)(4)).

If any of these four terms is used in labeling, or any other truthful statement about sodium content is used in labeling, the product label must provide quantitative sodium information. This information must be provided as part of full nutrition labeling (21 CFR § 101.9). If the food is represented for special dietary use for low salt or low sodium intake, then either full nutrition labeling or only the number of milligrams of sodium per portion needs to be provided (21 CFR §§ 105.69, 101.13(b)(5)).

The final rule also permits references on labeling to salt content, such as *unsalted, no salt added,* or *without added salt.* Such terms, or their equivalents, are permitted only if (1) no salt is added during processing, (2) the food it resembles normally is processed with salt, and (3) either nutrition labeling or sodium content labeling is provided (21 CFR § 101.13(b)).

In its final rule on sodium labeling, FDA discusses several important aspects of descriptors. The agency noted that the 1982 survey documents that consumers object to the use of too many descriptor terms as too confusing (49 Fed. Reg. 15,510–15,535, April 18, 1984. Yet, truthful and nonmisleading descriptors were described as "useful and desirable for highlighting products, particularly when quantitative information does not appear on the display panel.

A total of 93 percent of respondents to the 1982 FDA consumer survey who reported concern about sodium intake wanted descriptor labeling in addition to quantitative content. FDA concluded that its sodium definitions were "simple terms that are easily understood and that will not mislead the consumer."

In situations in which manufacturers use descriptors that are not defined in its final rule, the agency has, basically, punted. For example, one comment on the proposed rule asked FDA to prohibit the use of undefined claims such as "naturally low in sodium." It strongly urged manufacturers to use only those descriptors defined in section 101.13(b) to minimize consumer confusion. It did not limit manufacturers in any other way, however. FDA mentioned its case-by-case review for false and misleading claims as a means to protect consumers from labeling pandemonium.

USDA policy on sodium labeling differs from the FDA approach. USDA requires quantitative information on the sodium content per serving only if a claim is made about sodium and/or salt content of a meat or poultry product (USDA, 1984). Otherwise, sodium content information is provided on a voluntary basis. Like FDA, USDA permits manufacturers to provide sodium content information without other nutrition information on foods for special dietary use.

The USDA definitions of *very low sodium, low sodium, sodium free,* and *unsalted, no salt added,* or *without added salt,* or equivalent terms, are identical with the FDA definitions. USDA also allows reduced-sodium claims to be used if the product has achieved a 75 percent reduction in sodium content and the label provides quantitative information comparing it to the original product.

Like FDA's sodium labeling regulations, USDA's policy memorandum on sodium specifically describes how a comparative sodium claim may be used, such as: "This bologna has 25 percent less sodium per serving than our regular bologna" (USDA, 1984). Comparative claims may not be made unless (1) a product's sodium content is at least 25 percent less than the product to which it is compared and (2) the comparative claim is accompanied by (in immediate conjunction with the claim or referenced by an asterisk) an identification of the product(s) with which the comparison is being made and a quantitative statement of the difference in sodium content per serving (using equivalent serving sizes) of the products being compared. USDA encourages companies to reduce the sodium contents of their products to even lesser amounts, though such foods would not qualify for sodium comparative claim labeling.

USDA's earlier sodium labeling policy contained provisions for the qualitative sodium claims before FDA had such regulations. Some of them were adopted by FDA, such as *unsalted, no salt added,* and *without added salt* (Wolf et al., 1983).

No *or Negative*

FDA has no written policy on negative descriptors and no plans to develop such a policy (R.E. Newberry, Division of Regulatory Guidance, FDA, personal communication, 1990).

In 1987, USDA modified its policy on negative ingredient labeling, because the agency believed that negative descriptors can be useful and meaningful to consumers as an aid in understanding product contents. Also, such claims offer a simple and direct means of alerting consumers to the absence of ingredients they might not want to consume for health, ethnic, or personal reasons (USDA, 1987a). The phrase *no preservatives* exemplifies negative descriptors.

USDA guidelines permit negative labeling if it is not clear from the product name that the ingredient is not contained in the product. The agency uses as an example the term *no beef* on the label of turkey pastrami as an example. Negative labeling is also allowed if the food processor can show that the statement would be beneficial for health, religious preference, or similar reasons. Other statements are also allowed to describe product packaging, such as *no refrigeration needed*. Negative labeling may also be used to highlight the absence of ingredients that are prohibited by regulation, as long as the label prominently indicates this absence. USDA gives the following example for ground beef: "USDA federal regulations prohibit the use of preservatives in this product" (USDA, 1987a).

FDA Descriptors for Shelf Labeling in Grocery Stores

Some retail grocery stores have wanted to provide consumers with point-of-purchase shelf labeling nutrition information. At the request of Giant Food, Inc. (Washington, D.C.), and other stores, FDA has, on a case-by-case basis, developed policies that exempted stores from certain nutrition labeling requirements on a temporary basis to permit in-store food labeling experiments. The terms used by Giant Food, Inc., are listed in Table 7-6.

International Use of Descriptors

Descriptors are used in many countries through the world. Canada and the United States have defined a larger number of descriptors than other countries or international entities through efforts to achieve consistency and address significant health matters. The Council of the European Community and the Codex Alimentarius Commission have proposed or defined terms for reduction or absence of nutrients, calories, sodium, natural, organic, fresh, wholesome, healthful, and sound. An overview of the terms Canada has defined appear in Table 7-7. Further discussion of the international use of nutrition labeling is provided in Appendix C.

TABLE 7-6   Descriptive Terms Used in a Supermarket Shelf Labeling Program[a]

Term	Criteria Per Serving
Micronutrients	
Fair source	10 percent or more of U.S. RDA
Good source	25 percent or more of U.S. RDA
Excellent source	40 percent or more of U.S. RDA
Fiber	
Source	2 g
Good source	5 g
Excellent source	8 g
Calcium	
Source	100 mg
Good source	250 mg
Excellent source	400 mg
Low calorie	40 calories or less and 0.4 calories/g or less
Low fat	2 g or less of fat and less than 10 percent fat on a dry weight basis

[a] Adapted from letter to O. Mathews, Giant Food, Inc., Washington, D.C., by S.A. Miller, Center for Food Safety and Applied Nutrition, FDA, DHHS, July 16, 1986, and letter to J.S. Kahan and B.L. Rubin, Hogan and Hartson, Washington, D.C., by R.J. Ronk, Center for Food Safety and Applied Nutrition, FDA, DHHS, August 26, 1988.

Summary of the Current Use of Descriptors

It is not easy to summarize the problems associated with the current widespread use of nutrient descriptors on food labels. The variety of terms used makes generalization difficult, and efforts to group the terms into smaller, similar categories is challenging. No doubt this explains, in part, the two agencies' failure to establish official definitions for more of them, much less to agree upon a framework for establishing definitions for terms that may be used in the future. The central concern, in the Committee's view, is that the unregulated use of a growing variety of nutrient descriptors will nullify the efforts of consumers to make intelligent use of the factual information required on the nutrition label. There is a second concern as well, however. The absence of authoritative definitions for many descriptors works to the disadvantage of manufacturers that are reluctant to use terms that distort or exaggerate nutritionally unimportant differences. If calling a product high fiber produces a 0.5 percent increase in market share, the temptation to exploit this consumer interest will be difficult to resist.

Accordingly, the Committee believes that FDA and USDA could contribute to consumer understanding of nutrition labeling by adopting and enforcing

TABLE 7-7 Criteria for Descriptive Terms Used in Canada[a]

Term	Criteria
Low calorie	Less than 1 calorie/100 g
Low calorie food	Greater than 50 percent reduction, less than 15 calories per serving, and less than 30 calories per reasonable daily intake
Calorie reduced	Greater than 50 percent reduction
Low fat	No more than 3 g of fat per serving and not more than 15 percent fat in the dry matter (about 30 percent calories from fat)
Fat free	Less than 3 g per serving
Low saturates	No more than 2 g of saturated fatty acids per serving and not more than 15 percent calories from saturated fatty acids
Low cholesterol	No more than 20 mg of cholesterol per serving and per 100 g and low in saturated fatty acids
Cholesterol free	No more than 3 mg of cholesterol per 100 g and low in saturated fatty acids
Sodium free	Less than 5 mg/100 g
Low sodium food	Greater than 50 percent reduction and less than 40 mg/100 g with some exceptions
Fiber	
Source or moderate source	At least 2 g/serving
High source	At least 4 g/serving
Very high source	At least 6 g/serving
Descriptive terms	
Contains or source	At least 5 percent of RDI[b]
High or good source	At least 15 percent of RDI (30 percent for vitamin C)
Very high or excellent source	At least 25 percent of RDI (50 percent for vitamin C)

[a] Steele, P.J., and M.C. Cheney. 1989. Canada's system of nutrition labeling. Rapport 4(2):1-2.
[b] Recommended Daily Intake.

official and uniform definitions for a much larger number of nutrient descriptors. For many descriptors it will not be possible to say with confidence which of several possible definitions is the best. It seems improbable that consumers possess clear notions about the meaning of different descriptors. The choice of definitions, in some cases, will be arbitrary; the key is to be sure a definition is chosen.

The Committee does not believe that the exercise must always be arbitrary. There is a category of descriptors, comprising many of those now in wide use, for which it would appear to be possible to establish generic definitions. These are terms used to characterize the relative amount of a component in a serving of food, such as low-fat and high-fiber. As these examples suggest, there appear to be two subcategories for which different criteria probably apply. One category includes quantitative descriptors of nutrients whose consumption should be encouraged, such as vitamins, minerals, and carbohydrates, and the second would include descriptors of nutrients whose consumption should be controlled or curtailed, such as fat, cholesterol, and sodium.

This section incorporates this distinction in suggesting a uniform set of criteria for quantitative descriptors of such components as fat, cholesterol, fiber, and complex carbohydrates. However, in those instances in which FDA or USDA has already adopted official definitions (and there is no conflict between the agencies), the Committee recommends that no change be made. Stability in meaning is more important than theoretical consistency across nutritional components. It is the Committee's hope that such criteria might provide a general framework for establishing official definitions for quantitative descriptors (sometimes termed nutrient content claims) in the future.

Suggested Framework for Defining Descriptors

If present practices offer any lessons, innumerable descriptors and derivatives thereof may be proposed in the future. To control future proliferation and possible misunderstanding of these descriptors, the Committee suggests that all such descriptors could be assigned to one of three classes: (1) those that allege or imply a health benefit, (2) those that describe various other features and that require specific definitions and criteria, and (3) those that describe relative amounts of nutrients and other constituents.

The first group of descriptors—those that imply a health claim (e.g., *heart healthy* or *safe for diabetics*)—presumably would be regulated under the current proposed FDA regulations for public health messages (55 Fed. Reg. 5176–5912, Feb. 13, 1990). The second group of descriptors represents a more diverse and creative list of terms that characterize other features (e.g., *fresh, natural,* or *organic*). This group ought to be defined on the basis of reasonable and reliable scientific evidence. Indeed, there is legislation currently pending before Congress to establish a legal definition for the term *organic*.

The third group consists of descriptors that relate to the quantity of nutrients and other constituents. The following proposal is intended to cover all food constituents—nutrients and nonnutrients—for which there may be future interest in this quantitative category. Therefore, the term *nutrient* will be used generically to reflect all possible food components, regardless of whether there are current published RDAs or other dietary standards for their consumption.

The message conveyed by quantitative descriptors should be consistent, clear, and reliable. Consistency can be obtained by including under the umbrella of the following criteria all nutrients contained in all food products. This is a reasonable assumption because *low sodium*, for example, should have the same meaning, whether it is applied to soup, frozen peas, or meat.

Clarity of message may be achieved by using simple rules. Thus, the Committee suggests that descriptors be limited to two categories of nutrient contents that deviate from the norm, that is, low and very low, or high and very high. The first category, demarcated by words such as *low* or *high* or their equivalents, should represent a relative nutrient content that can be expected to have significantly different biological effects, whereas the second category, *very low* or *very high*, is demarcated by a level one-half (or twice) this amount. A third category is obvious but pejorative and irrelevant in the marketplace. Although it might be useful to consumers if they had some way of knowing that a food contained a low level of a desirable nutrient or a high level of an undesirable nutrient, manufacturers would have no interest in describing a food as containing an *average* or *low* level of a desirable nutrient or an *average* or *high* level of an undesirable nutrient.

Descriptors that depict nutrient amounts should be indexed against authoritative dietary recommendations for upper and lower benchmarks. This notion suggests that nutrient intake recommendations should be expressed as ranges, not as single numbers, because they reflect the fact that every nutrient or other dietary constituent is toxic when consumed at high enough levels. Ranges are essential if regulation of these quantitative descriptors is to be consistent rather than ad hoc. Beneficially low levels of nutrients should be indexed against recommended upper limits, whereas beneficially high levels should be indexed against recommended lower limits. Accordingly, a consistent and reasoned scheme applicable to all nutrients requires the development of consistent and rationally developed ranges of optimal intakes for all nutrients.

Unfortunately, except for two vitamins and five minerals with ESADDIs (NRC, 1989b), dietary intake recommendations are not given as optimal intake ranges for most nutrients. For most nutrients (protein, 11 vitamins, and 7 minerals), only single numbers (i.e., RDAs) are published, which are designed for the maintenance of good nutrition of practically all healthy people in the United States. These single numbers are not minimum requirements for individuals. In the absence of alternative reference limits, however, for purposes of illustration, these RDAs may be considered as comparable lower benchmarks for the various nutrients to which they apply. For a few nutrients (total fat, cholesterol, sodium, and dietary fiber), recommended upper benchmarks have been published, although traditional RDAs do not exist.

This suggested scheme, as it applies to a few nutrients, is illustrated in Table 7-8. It is important to emphasize the tentative nature of the suggested descriptor reference points; they have been selected only from varied and somewhat fragmentary information to illustrate the scheme and to give approximate estimates of descriptor benchmarks. If the logic of this scheme is appealing, it would be necessary to produce appropriate benchmarks for all nutrients. The scheme illustrates the need for a broader definition of nutrients. If minimal intakes of constituents such as dietary fiber, carotenoids, total fat, and any other naturally occurring food constituents are essential for optimal health, it would be reasonable to establish RDAs or some equivalent standard for them, especially when current dietary recommendations provide clear indications on such values as the percentage of calories from fat and desirable fiber intake. Also, it will be necessary to develop rational benchmarks for each of the four categories of descriptors (*high* and *very high, low* and *very low*). The Committee suggests that these benchmark limits be kept conceptually consistent for all nutrients in order to simplify the message.

This scheme could also lend itself to establishing the terms of reference and criteria for nutrition information panel descriptors. For macronutrients, the benchmark criteria could be based on the existing FDA criteria of *excellent/very good source* (greater than 40 percent), *good/high source* (greater than 20 percent), *low source* (less than 2 percent), and *very low source* (less than 1 percent) of the standard for a nutrient. Thus, macronutrient content claims on the principal display panel would be supported by the quantitative values listed on the nutrition information panel. Similarly, the criteria proposed by the Committee for the listing of micronutrients on the nutrition information panel—*very good source of* (greater than 20 percent), *good source of* (11 to 20 percent), and contains (2 to 10 percent)—could serve as the same criteria and descriptors for the micronutrients on the principal display panel. The micronutrients would not be supported by quantitative values on the nutrition panel, but the reference range (e.g., 11 to 20 percent of standard) would be provided based on the rationale provided in the section on U.S. RDAs in this chapter. Use of the terms *no* or *free* could be based on the criteria that macronutrients so classified on the label are present at a level that is less than 1 percent of the maximum benchmark.

Comparative Descriptors

Descriptors also have been used to compare similar products, although the product being compared is not always identified. The Committee recommends that use of comparative descriptors be strictly regulated to ensure that the products being compared are clearly identified and that the extent of nutrient

TABLE 7-8 Descriptors Indexed Against Upper and Lower Intake Benchmarks[a]

Nutrient Intake (per day)	Good/High Source (>20% min.)	Excellent/Very High Source (>40% min.)	Lower Benchmark	Low Source (<2% max.)	Very Low Source (<1% max.)	Upper Benchmark
Fat (kcal)	—	—	None	12	6	600[b]
Sodium (mg)	—	—	500[c]	66	33	3,300[d]
Energy (kcal, males)	—	—	—	58[e]	29[e]	2,900[f]
Energy (kcal, females)	—	—	—	44[e]	22[e]	2,200[f]
Energy (kcal, average and rounded off for both sexes)	—	—	—	50[e]	25[e]	2,550[f]
Cholesterol (mg)	—	—	None	6	3	300[g]
Protein (g, males)	11.2	22.4	63[h]	—	—	—
Protein (g, females)	9.6	19.2	50[i]	—	—	—
Protein (g, average and rounded off for both sexes)	10	20	20[j]	—	—	—
Fiber (g)	4	8	20[j]	—	—	—

[a] In previous FDA correspondence, criteria have been established both according to richness of source (fiber, calcium) and comparative adjectives.
[b] Based on recommendation to reduce total fat intake to 30 percent of calories or less and 2000 kcal daily intake.
[c] "Minimum requirement of healthy persons" (adults, >18 years) from 1989 RDA.
[d] "Safe and adequate intake" from 1989 RDA; no estimate was published in the 1989 report.
[e] Compares with "low calorie" limit of "40 calories per serving or less" proposed by FDA.
[f] Based on reference body weights which are actual medians rather than arbitrary ideals; therefore, there are no minimum or maximum allowances.
[g] Based on recommendation to reduce total cholesterol intake to 300 mg/day or less.
[h] Based on recommendation of 0.8 g/kg and 70 kg of body weight.
[i] Based on recommendation of 0.8 g/kg and 60 kg of body weight.
[j] Based on recommendation of ideal intake of 20 to 35 g/day.

modification is specified. The Committee suggests that for the use of comparative descriptors (e.g., *reduced* and *lower than*), modifications of at least 20 percent be required. Descriptors should not be allowed for nutrients unless they are normally present in physiologically significant amounts. A suggested benchmark for a physiologically significant amount might be the same 1 percent of the maximum allowance used to define the limits for *very low* in Table 7-8. On the basis of this reasoning, a *no cholesterol* descriptor would not be allowed on foods that do not normally contain cholesterol, because they normally would contain less than 1 percent of the maximum daily allowance in a serving.

Such a scheme would provide a logical and consistent system for regulation of quantitative descriptors of food constituents which may be proposed or discovered in the future. Without some such a scheme, regulation will, of necessity, remain ad hoc and invite continued confusion.

LABEL FORMAT OPTIONS

This section examines the history of the current label format, sets forth the Committee's criteria for label redesign, and proposes specific examples of improved labels. Recommendations are made for a mechanism for testing label revisions prior to implementation in the next section.

Selection of Current Label Format

In 1972, when the nutrition labeling program was in preparation, FDA investigated the various options that might be appropriate for the nutrition panel of the food label. A study conducted for FDA sought to determine the best way to convey the nutritional value of a food to consumers (CRI, 1972). In that study, three methods were tested: (1) a numeric system, (2) a verbal system, and (3) a pictorial system. In the numeric system, the amount of the RDA provided by the product for each of seven key nutrients was presented as a numeric percentage. In the verbal system, adjectives were used to rate the product as a source of a nutrient. In the pictorial system, symbols such as stars or smiling faces were used to indicate the quantity of nutrient present in the product. The study measured consumer reaction to all three systems on (1) how well the information could be understood and used in making food purchase decisions, (2) how each method affected the actual purchasing behaviors of consumers, and (3) how well each of the three alternative formats was liked.

A majority of those surveyed, including consumers representing underprivileged minority groups, seemed to understand the nutrition information regardless of the method used. Consumer responses to all three systems were reported as encouragingly high, but the verbal system was consistently less well received by consumers than the other two format systems were. There were no major differences among the formats in terms of influencing product choice, although consumers indicated that, under certain conditions, they would switch to products that were nutritionally superior. Consumers reported that they preferred nutrient information presented in terms of numeric percentages rather than in terms of words or pictures, which were considered too vague to communicate precise nutrition information. Consumers stated that they expected the nutrition information to be precise (even though it cannot be; see Chapters 4 and 5) and felt that words were too vague for this purpose. In addition, because they considered nutrition to be a serious subject, consumers felt that use of symbols such as faces was childish and condescending. On the basis, at least in part, of these results, FDA decided to use numbers and percentages, which were determined to be the best of the three alternatives under consideration.

The usefulness of listing nutrient information for all key nutrients, regardless of their presence in the product, was tested. Consumers seemed to find it easier to determine the best nutritional value when the label listed only nutrients that were actually present rather than all key nutrients, even when some were not present.

Consumers provided with information on the percent composition of fat, carbohydrate, and protein in a product showed a tendency to switch to products with lower fat contents compared with consumers who did not receive such information.

The results of this study influenced FDA's decision to select the current label format using the numeric system that presently appears on the current nutrition panel. As part of the interagency review of all aspects of food labeling in the late 1970s, FDA commissioned a study to explore nutrition label format alternatives. That study developed five alternative labels for consumer testing which included the present label and four others described as simplified numeric/numeric, simplified numeric/verbal, simplified numeric/graphic, and simplified graphic/graphic (or unitary nutrient density) (USDA/DHHS, 1982). Unfortunately, further consumer testing of these label alternatives was never funded.

Experience with Other Label Formats

Some research has assessed how well the current label format and various alternatives convey nutrition information to consumers. Studies conducted before nutrition labeling was instituted were primarily focused on ascertaining consumers' reactions to the novel concept. The early research did not evaluate certain alternative formats, such as various graphic presentations. However, later studies did test such formats, including nutrient density, but none of the studies on nutrition labels tested various elements of a nutrition label in graphic format against themselves or against other elements. A review of these format studies is included in the section "Consumer Understanding of Nutrition and Use of Food Labels" in Chapter 4 (see Asam and Bucklin, 1973; Babcock and Murphy,

1972; Betteman, 1979; CNCFL, 1990; Geiger et al., 1990; Hammonds, 1978; Lenahan et al., 1972; McCullough and Best, 1980; Mohr et al., 1980; Muller, 1985; ORC, 1990; Rudd, 1986, 1989; Vankatesan, 1977, 1986; Yankelovich, Inc., 1971)

Revised Nutrition Label Information

The studies cited above have established that consumers want more relevant nutrition information on the products they purchase, even though they display less than a complete technical understanding of current label information. Further improvements in consumer ability to make dietary choices will be seriously hampered if deficiencies in the current labeling requirements are not corrected. Daly (1976) concluded that unless product information is easily accessible at the point of purchase, can be easily understood by the consumer, and is presented in a format allowing direct comparisons of alternatives, it is unlikely to be used in making food choices.

In evaluating various label format alternatives, the Committee used the following criteria: health relevance of content, clarity to consumers, consistency, space requirements, and compatibility with existing labeling practices.

Relevant Content Information

Declaration of nutrient content information on the label should reflect the goals of the current dietary recommendations as summarized in the Surgeon General's report (DHHS, 1988) and the NRC *Diet and Health* report (NRC, 1989a). Although knowledge of the relationship between nutrition and long-term health will continue to evolve, these two reports set forth a reasonable consensus for action. The objective of label revisions suggested in this report is to provide consumers with the food label information necessary to apply these dietary recommendations to their food purchase and consumption decisions.

The Committee's recommendations for information on nutrient content are based on the discussion in Chapter 6. Included are recommendations on the disclosure and presentation of total calories, fats, cholesterol, carbohydrates, protein, fiber, sodium, potassium, calcium, iron, and other micronutrients. Contained earlier in this chapter are discussions of and recommendations for serving size and qualitative disclosure of micronutrients.

Clarity of Information

In addition to standardizing and limiting the number of categories of serving size and providing for the organized grouping of fats and carbohydrates, several other issues are of concern that have an impact on label formats.

Units of Measurement The appropriate measure for most macronutrients is grams. However, for macronutrients such as cholesterol, sodium, and potassium, the measure should be milligrams, to avoid the need to use decimal declarations. The Committee recommends that components listed in milligrams be grouped together following the macronutrients declared in grams.

Nutrient Groupings For clarity of information and to facilitate the education process, consumers should expect that nutrients will be presented in logical groupings. Consumers should also expect that the quantities declared for nutrient subgroupings added together will equal the amount appearing on the line for the group as a whole (e.g., required fat components [except cholesterol] and, if provided, carbohydrate components [except fiber]).

Presentation Issues Consumer understanding of label information is undoubtedly influenced by the manner of presentation. Many of the formats that have been suggested are modifications of the current format, which either expand on the existing components (breakdown of fats) or add new items not previously required (fiber, cholesterol) to the list. Several visual representations (graphics) of nutritional value have been suggested, but their usefulness to consumers has yet to be successfully demonstrated. Graphics include such options as bar graphs, pie charts, and symbols.

Use of graphics for a combination of several nutrients makes it difficult to convey the information that consumption of some nutrients, such as complex carbohydrates, is to be encouraged whereas others, such as saturated fatty acids, are to be discouraged. Graphics based on a calorie reference require selection of a single calorie consumption standard, even though individuals vary widely in their requirements. A decision must also be made as to whether graphic information is to be expressed with or without water. For example, on a weight basis, milk, including the water, makes the product appear to be very low in protein, whereas excluding the water makes it appear to be very high in fat and carbohydrates.

Space is another serious constraint for any graphic format. A graphic representation would result in a significant expansion of the size of the nutrition information panel, since graphic presentations must be supported by numeric information. As a result, the type size for the numeric section would be reduced on many products, and the number of products of a size too small to support the revised label would increase the number of products that would be exempt from mandatory labeling. Another problem with graphics is that manipulations of the scale used, i.e., ratio of height to width, can produce serious visual distractions and consequent potential for abuse. For these reasons, the Committee recommends that the use of any graphic representations be optimal.

An additional presentation issue concerns the provision of dietary recommendation standards against which consumers can compare the nutritional value of a food to their dietary patterns. The current consensus on dietary recommendations provides a set of standards for the provision of such information to make such a comparison. However, the listing of such information will take up precious space on the label, requiring another column of comparative values.

Consistency

Consistency has three dimensions: internal consistency, consistency of format across products, and consistency over time. Internal consistency means that the same measurement should be used for all similar groups of nutrients. All fats, for example, should be expressed both in grams and as calories from fat. Consistency of format across products means that all nutrition labels should list the same nutrients in the same order. A zero declaration, in other words, is preferable to omission. As a result, consumers would be presented with a familiar format each time, thus simplifying education programs. Consistency over time means that the format selected should not include information about constituents that do not yet have a well-established diet-health relationship and, therefore, require frequent revision.

Consistency of format becomes more critical with the age of the user. Younger individuals tend to be better able to separate relevant information from a cluttered presentation. Older individuals are more field dependent; that is, they rely more on consistency of placement and presentation to aid their information gathering. Cross-sectional studies indicate that after people reach their late 30s, the rate of change toward greater field dependence accelerates (Cole and Gaeth, 1990; Eisner, 1972).

Space Requirements

Although space limitations should not be decisive when there is a compelling health reason for including information, space is an important consideration in designing any label. Currently, over half of the food packages that bear nutrition labeling confine this information to an area no larger than 2 square inches, which is the average space allotted to the nutrition panel on food packages (FLAPS, 1988). A significant expansion of space requirements would necessitate major redesign of many labels, delaying compliance and increasing food costs.

Space requirements are a major problem with graphic displays. Although these should be allowed on a voluntary basis, as mentioned above, the Committee does not recommend that they be required. There may be a perception that manufacturers could enlarge the size of the package to accommodate any new labeling requirements, but this perception is distorted. Government limits on slack fill of packages place an upper limit on the size of the container. Even when this is not a factor, consumer perception of deception due to slack fill limits the freedom of the manufacturer to expand the size of the package at will.

Compatibility with Existing Labeling Practices

To the extent that recommendations for label reform can be made compatible with existing practices, the costs of compliance will be minimized, the speed of compliance will be enhanced, existing private-sector educational materials will remain useful, and consumers will not need to relearn a different protocol. It is important to recognize that consumers have a 17-year investment in the current label format. Consumers have become accustomed to the current format over a long period of time, and a wide variety of information and educational programs have been developed to support the understanding and use of current label information. In addition, manufacturers also have experience in using the current label format. Although familiarity should not prevent beneficial change, neither should this 17-year investment be abandoned lightly.

Committee Recommendations

A number of recommendations were made in the previous sections and chapters concerning the content and manner by which to better convey nutrition information to consumers on food labels. To summarize those issues that apply to format changes, the Committee recommends that:

- Serving size should be prominently displayed on the nutrition information panel and should appear in household units.
- The amount of the serving should appear in grams or milliliters in parentheses following household units.
- Nutrient information should appear for the food as it is packaged, with the option of providing information relevant to the manner in which the food is prepared.
- Macronutrients should be listed in grams or milligrams.
- Macronutrients should be listed first, and then other food components, electrolytes, and micronutrients, and similar food components should be grouped together, except dietary fiber and cholesterol should not appear in groupings.
- Various issues related to placement and prominence of food components on the nutrition label (e.g., increased prominence of fat components, decreased prominence of protein, and ordering of macro- and micronutrients) should be subjected to consumer testing.
- Comparison with dietary recommendations should be optional.

Sample Formats

The sample formats in Figure 7-1 illustrate the Committee's recommendations for nutrient content disclosure on and format of the nutrition information panel. The Committee is not endorsing any one of these samples; they serve only to illustrate ways in which the various recommended components could appear on a nutrition panel. Given the Committee's recommendation for the need to test label formats, graphic options were not included.

TESTING OF LABEL FORMATS

Although there is considerable information about the beneficial changes that might be made in the content and formats of nutrition labels, consumer understanding and acceptance of any new design will determine the success or failure of this effort. This information cannot be determined without direct tests of the proposed revisions.

The Committee believes that alternative label formats should be subjected to both qualitative and quantitative consumer testing prior to issuance of any final nutrition labeling requirements. However, this testing must be carefully structured to produce measurable results and, given the level of expectation for this process, must be carried out within a reasonable period of time. It is also assumed that before any testing procedures begin, the agencies will have determined through the comment and rulemaking process the nutrient content information to be conveyed on the label, as this will affect the required nutrition information to be presented in any format tested.

As to the experimental design, it would be a mistake to structure format comparisons amounting to little more than popularity poll choices among alternatives. First, the revisions must be based on sound science. That is, the objective must be to provide the kind of label information to the public that will allow consumers to apply current dietary recommendations to their everyday food purchase and consumption decisions. Therefore, all formats to be tested should be consistent with this objective. For this reason, it is unnecessary and unwise simply to test all label revisions that have been proposed. A screening process must first be carried out to eliminate formats that do not pass the tests of sound science and at least an initial screen of reasonableness.

Second, the level of detail provided should be consistent with the type of information needed to make informed dietary choices and a reasonable size requirement for labeling. Consumers have a strong tendency, in purely attitudinal surveys, to favor greater levels of detail, even when that detail is of questionable relevance (ORC, 1990). That is, consumers tend to say they want more information, regardless of whether they are likely to use it. However, unnecessary detail would expand the size of the nutrition information panel and would therefore exempt a higher percentage of foods in packages too small to accommodate the new labeling requirements.

Third, the popularity of a format alone is not enough to recommend its use. Consumers must be able to use the new format to make improved dietary choices. After an initial screening of label formats for preference, it is therefore essential that actual formats be tested in an environment closely approximating marketplace conditions. For this to take place, some minimal level of education will need to be given to the test subjects. Since new label formats will be used, test subjects will need some instruction as to their use. If this is not done, clearly inferior formats might surface as the labels of choice simply because they are similar to a preexisting frame of reference.

The Committee recommends that:

- A brief test panel education program reviewing the current dietary recommendations and explaining the basics of the new label formats should precede label format testing.
- A format testing procedure should be initiated that ensures adequate consumer input and evaluation of whichever label format is chosen as the standard and should include the following elements:
    1. An advisory panel, consisting of individuals familiar with dietary guidance and an understanding of how consumers use label information to make decisions, should be assembled to work with the relevant agencies. This group should be charged with assisting the agencies to select the label formats to be tested and with overseeing the nature of the testing process.
    2. The first stage in any testing process would be the mock-up of several label formats in order to submit them to comprehensive qualitative review by consumers. Such a review would probably be performed by using a number of focus groups of consumers with varying interest and ability levels to determine their preference for the amount of information presented and the label format of choice.
    3. In-depth consumer evaluation of the most preferred choices would be necessary to assess consumers' ability to apply the food label information in making food choices. Individual protocols to determine how they process the label information can be used. Such protocols to determine cognitive responses to nutrition information have previously been developed and tested (Sims and Shepherd, 1987). By such techniques, it is possible to determine before-and-after label use.
    4. On the basis of results from the cognitive response protocol testing, revisions to the label format should be made. Large-scale surveys can then ascertain overall consumer acceptance and compre-

A

```
┌──────────────────────────────────────────────────┐
│                  2% LOWFAT MILK                    │
│            Nutrition Information Per Serving        │
│  SERVING SIZE ........................    ONE CUP  │
│  SERVINGS PER CONTAINER ..    8                    │
│  CALORIES ...............................  120     │
│  PROTEIN ................................    8  GRAMS │
│  CARBOHYDRATE.....................   11  GRAMS     │
│  FAT .........................................    5  GRAMS │
│  SODIUM ...................................  130  mg │
│                                                    │
│                 Percentage of U.S.                 │
│       Recommended Daily Allowances (U.S. RDA)      │
│  PROTEIN ..........   20   RIBOFLAVIN .....   25   │
│  VITAMIN A ........   10   NIACIN .............    *  │
│  VITAMIN C ........    4   CALCIUM.........   30   │
│  THIAMINE .........    6   IRON ................    *  │
│  *CONTAINS LESS THAN 2% OF THE U.S. RDA FOR THESE NUTRIENTS │
└──────────────────────────────────────────────────┘
```

B

```
┌──────────────────────────────────────────────────┐
│                  2% LOWFAT MILK                    │
│  Serving size................................ 1 cup (8 fl oz) │
│  Servings per container.................................  8 │
│                                                    │
│           Nutrition Information Per Serving         │
│                                                    │
│  Calories .......................................... 120 │
│  Total Fat ...............................   5   g  (45 kcal) │
│     Saturated Fat ....................   3   g  (27 kcal) │
│     Unsaturated Fat .................   2   g  (18 kcal) │
│  Carbohydrate .......................   11  g      │
│  Protein...................................    9  g      │
│  Total Dietary Fiber ...............    0  g      │
│  Cholesterol ...........................   20  mg     │
│  Sodium ................................. 120  mg     │
│                                                    │
│  A very good source (over 20% [standard]) of:      │
│  Calcium.                                          │
└──────────────────────────────────────────────────┘
```

FIGURE 7-1 Current nutrition label and samples of revised nutrition labels based on the Committee's recommendations. The U.S. RDA was used as the standard for *source of* listings. (A) Sample nutrition information panel for 2% lowfat milk (½ gallon) under current FDA regulations (minimum requirements). (B) Sample nutrition information panel for 2% lowfat milk (½ gallon) incorporating the Committee's mandatory content recommendations. *Total dietary fiber* is included on the nutrition information panel, but could be exempted for milk products (see Chapter 6). Iron is not declared in the *source of* listings because its value is less than 2 percent. (C) Sample nutrition information panel for 2% lowfat milk (½ gallon) incorporating the Committee's mandatory and voluntary recommendations. Note that *carbohydrate* changes to *total carbohydrate* when its components are listed. Listing of complex carbohydrate and sugar content are optional. Declaration of calories from total carbohydrate, complex carbohydrate, sugars, and protein are optional. Aside from calcium and iron (not listed; less than 2% standard), all *source of* listings of micronutrient content are optional. (D) Sample nutrition information panel for macaroni and cheese dinner incorporating the Committee's mandatory and voluntary content recommendations contained in Sample C, and the optional *as prepared* format.

C

2% LOWFAT MILK

Serving size .... 1 cup (8 fl oz)
Servings per container 8

Nutrition Information Per Serving

Calories			120
Total Fat	5	g	(45 kcal)
Saturated Fat	3	g	(27 kcal)
Unsaturated Fat	2	g	(18 kcal)
Total Carbohydrate	11	g	(44 kcal)
Complex Carbohydrate	0	g	(0 kcal)
Sugars	11	g	(44 kcal)
Protein	9	g	(36 kcal)
Total Dietary Fiber	0	g	
Cholesterol	20	mg	
Sodium	120	mg	
Potassium	430	mg	

A very good source (over 20% [standard]) of:
Vitamin D, Calcium, Riboflavin, Phosphorus.
A good source (11-20% [standard]) of:
Vitamin A, Vitamin B12.
Contains (2-10% [standard]): Vitamin B6,
Vitamin C, Magnesium, Pantothenic Acid,
Thiamin, Zinc.

D

MACARONI & CHEESE DINNER

Serving size (as prepared) .... 3/4 cup (50 g)
Servings per container 4

Nutrition Information Per Serving

	As Packaged		As Prepared	
Calories	190		290	
Total Fat	2 g	(18 kcal)	13 g	(117 kcal)
Saturated Fat	1 g	(9 kcal)	9 g	(81 kcal)
Unsaturated Fat	1 g	(9 kcal)	4 g	(36 kcal)
Total Carbohydrate	36 g	(144 kcal)	34 g	(136 kcal)
Complex Carbohydrate ...	30 g	(120 kcal)	28 g	(112 kcal)
Sugars	6 g	(24 kcal)	6 g	(24 kcal)
Protein	9 g	(36 kcal)	9 g	(36 kcal)
Total Dietary Fiber	1 g		1 g	
Cholesterol	5 mg		5 mg	
Sodium	425 mg		525 mg	
Potassium	850 mg		900 mg	

As Packaged
A very good source (over 20% [standard]) of: Niacin, Riboflavin,
Thiamin.
Contains (2-10% [standard]): Calcium, Iron.

As Prepared
A good source (11-20% [standard]) of:
Riboflavin, Thiamin.
Contains (2-10% [standard]): Vitamin A, Calcium, Iron, Niacin.

hension of the label information. In addition, testing of the label with consumers under conditions approximating marketing environments should be carried out. This latter testing would involve determination of consumer ability to describe the nutritional contents of individual food products, compare nutritional contents across product categories, and choose among relevant food alternatives.

Given the normal time requirements for research of this type, and given the extensive material already available in this report and elsewhere on suggested label revisions, it is reasonable to set a minimum timetable of 1 year for this testing to be completed. Following that period, the agencies will then be ready to propose the new format.

EDUCATING CONSUMERS TO USE NUTRITION INFORMATION ON FOOD LABELS

Given the current wave of authoritative reports linking diet and chronic disease, coupled with an era of public responsiveness to dietary recommendations, a unique opportunity exists to positively influence the future health of the U.S. population. Rising consumer awareness of the relationship between nutrition and long-term health has stimulated the food industry to develop a variety of new, more healthful products, has encouraged increased use of experimentation with health claims on food labels, and in some cases, has promoted the development of innovative consumer information programs. Whether raising public awareness of the dietary risk factors for disease can lead to the desired fundamental changes in dietary behavior in the United States depends on many factors, such as the availability of foods with high nutritional quality in the food supply and consumer ability to make more healthful food choices.

The proposed *Year 2000 Objectives for the Nation* provide a number of nutrition objectives that relate to consumer knowledge of foods, nutrition labeling, and availability of improved food products. The nutrition objectives are designed to enable consumers to adopt sound dietary practices (reduce dietary fats and sodium; increase calcium and dietary fiber), and identity the dietary factors associated with chronic disease. Objectives specific to labeling are to:

- increase to at least 80 percent the proportion of people age 21 and older who use food labels to make food selections;
- increase nutrition labeling that provides information to facilitate choosing foods consistent with the *Dietary Guidelines for Americans* to at least 80 percent of processed foods and 40 percent of fresh meat, poultry, fruits, vegetables, baked goods, and ready-to-eat foods;
- increase to at least 5,000 brand items the availability of processed food products that are reduced in fat, saturated fat, and cholesterol; and

- increase to at least 5,000 brand items the availability of processed foods with lowered sodium (DHHS, 1989).

Strategies for Promoting Dietary Changes

Two general approaches have been suggested to promote dietary changes: (1) environmental or structural intervention, and (2) personal or direct-influence strategies (Glanz and Mullis, 1988; Sims and Smiciklas-Wright, 1978). *Environmental* or *structural interventions* are strategies that encourage positive behaviors by creating opportunities for action and removing barriers to follow health-promoting practices. Such strategies focus on modifying the environment first, without requiring the individual to make conscious (often unwanted or unpopular) choices or to participate voluntarily in educational activities.

In terms of promoting dietary change, such strategies take the form of modifying some aspect of the food supply or improving consumer access to food. Examples of such strategies would be to directly provide or distribute food, improve consumer's ability to purchase food, directly alter the nutritional quality of food products (e.g., by enrichment or fortification), or limit the food selections available to population groups in certain locations, such as institutions, work site cafeterias, or vending machines. In economic terms, environmental strategies can be said to affect the supply side, whereas direct or personal strategies are used in an attempt to alter the demand side of the supply-and-demand equation.

Personal or *direct-influence* strategies are based on providing information or applying educational, persuasion, and behavior modification techniques directly to individuals or small groups. Over the past two decades, educational techniques have evolved from simple information transmission (based on the premise, "If they know the facts, they will change their behavior") to a variety of direct behavior modification techniques that are designed to lead directly to the development of health-promoting skills and practices. Although such strategies have grown increasingly sophisticated and behaviorally oriented, they appear to be inefficient and ineffective means of reaching large population groups (Glanz and Mullis, 1988).

The provision of nutrition information on food labels is an interesting amalgam of the environmental and personal strategies. On the one hand, it is unquestioningly a personal informational strategy. One stated goal of nutrition labeling is that the nutrient composition information provided on the food label should enable the public to make informed food choices. To the extent that nutrition labeling leads to improvements in the nutritional qualities and varieties of foods that are consumed, labeling can be expected to have positive health benefits.

Yet, government has been encouraged to adopt this information provision strategy in order to facilitate and enhance the application of nutritional considerations to food consumption behavior (Quelch, 1977). Rather than prohibit all information on food labels that would promote the importance of the relationship between diet and long-term health, FDA adopted the current policy strategy in the early 1970s that the manufacturer could present factual information on the nutrient composition of foods and then proceeded to promulgate regulations governing the content, format, and placement of nutrition labeling (Hutt, 1986). With such action, a personal strategy was transformed into an environmental strategy, those described as being more efficient and practical than one-to-one programs (Syme, 1986) and having the potential for reaching wider audiences and yielding a greater health-promoting impact (Glanz and Mullis, 1988).

Promoting Health Through Informational Campaigns

Various public information campaigns aimed at promoting healthy behavior (including those for coronary heart disease, high blood pressure, and cancer) have focused on enhancing knowledge, changing attitudes, and improving skills. Two beliefs characterize many of the health promotion campaigns conducted in the United States over the past two decades. The first belief is that if people are just given the facts, they will proceed to change their behavior in accordance with this guidance. The second belief is that if people can be induced to hold favorable or unfavorable attitudes about a particular practice, they will change their behaviors to correspond with the appropriate attitude. Unfortunately, the research evidence does not fully support the efficacy of presenting just information or improving attitudes to cause individuals to follow health-promoting practices (Bettinghaus, 1986).

Consumers must have an information base in order to make long-lasting dietary changes. Yet, information alone cannot possibly be expected to produce behavioral changes unless adequate quantities of appropriate foods are available from which consumers can make choices. Educational approaches make sense only as far as there are environmental resources available to enable the consumer to implement the advice. The challenge is to combine effectively both types of strategies in nutrition labeling programs in order to capitalize on the relative strengths of each approach, with the ultimate goal being to achieve long-lasting positive behavioral changes among consumers.

Communication diffusion research (Rogers, 1983), in particular, has demonstrated that mass media—whether print or audiovisual as in radio or television—are best used to create awareness or expand knowledge about a particular new concept or program. In order to effect longer-lasting attitudinal and behavioral changes, however, information is best delivered by interpersonal communication channels, such as instructional sessions or friendly advice.

Mass media can be effectively used to introduce a new concept or piece of information to target populations and thus create a better knowledge base about the meaning of that new concept or idea. In order to effect behavior change, however, it is essential to employ interpersonal communication channels, such as small group discussions, individual counseling sessions, or personal demonstrations (Sims, 1979).

Obstacles To Effecting Dietary Changes

There are a myriad of factors that affect dietary habits, from environmental and cultural to personal and idiosyncratic. It is little wonder that dietary change, no matter how sought after or desired, is difficult to achieve. Many foods, and often those most laden with saturated fatty acids, sodium, or cholesterol—offer psychological comfort. Yet, others are imbued with symbolism of a cultural heritage, such as foods eaten on spacial occasions.

Most diet-related health problems develop gradually, and often they do not present immediate or dramatic symptoms. In turn, risk-factor reduction and disease prevention through dietary means require individuals to make long-term and often arduous changes in their habitual food intakes. Furthermore, some dietary changes (e.g., weight loss) provide obvious physical feedback, but others (e.g., increased fiber intake and cholesterol reduction) do not. Dietary recommendations, such as those contained in the Surgeon General's (DHHS, 1988) or the NRC (NRC, 1989a) reports, advise the public to forego immediate satisfaction in order to experience health benefits in the distant future. Most Americans consider themselves reasonably healthy and question whether such major alterations in their life-styles will really provide long-term benefits.

Some believe (Glanz and Mullis, 1988) that in order to achieve health improvement by promoting healthy diets, nutrition interventions must reach large segments of the population and effectively influence the diverse factors that determine eating patterns. Most one-on-one nutrition education efforts are directed toward individuals identified as being at risk for disease or as having conditions requiring therapeutic dietary intervention. Nutrition information on food labels has the unique function of being able to offer something for all: consumers trying to avoid or reduce the percentage of certain elements in their diet (e.g., fat, cholesterol or sodium) or to maximize other elements (e.g. fiber, vitamins, or minerals); patients with congestive heart failure assiduously monitoring their sodium and/or potassium intake; consumers who want to see if the *no cholesterol* claim on the front of the label is, in fact, correct in terms of the nutrient composition of the product; or consumers who wish to compare two comparable products (e.g., breakfast cereals) for their nutrient composition. It was the responsibility of this Committee to make recommendations to ensure that the information-seeking consumer is able to make informed dietary decisions with the facts presented on the food label in the most understandable and usable format.

Using Food Label Information To Make Food Choices

Consumers define the quality of a diet in terms of types of foods, not nutrients (Liefeld, 1983). In order to facilitate dietary changes, consumers must understand the contributions that specific foods and food types make to the overall diet. From this perspective, science-derived diet and disease messages must be supplemented by information about the nutritional characteristics of specific foods and food types, and how to buy and prepare appropriate foods and meet appropriate quantitative goals. Without such understanding, attempts to modify dietary intake may not meet with success.

From the perspective of helping consumers make intelligent food selections, one difficulty with diet and disease messages is that these messages usually are based on food components whose scientific role is not well understood by consumers. For most consumers, cholesterol, fatty acids, fiber, and sodium are relatively new terms when they are applied to making food choices. As a consequence, consumers may need to acquire knowledge about specific nutrients, food components, or food and nutrition processes in order to implement the generic dietary advice implied by such messages. To apply the general recommendations to reduce the intake of saturated fatty acids or sodium or to consume more dietary fiber, for example, an individual must understand the major food sources of these components, the contribution of different foods to the total diet, and how one's present diet may be excessive or deficient in these food components. Appropriate dietary behavior depends on consumer's ability to recognize foods with desirable properties, to understand relevant terminology and apply it to food choices, to critically evaluate claims, and to assess the relative benefits of possible dietary changes in their own diets.

Committee Recommendations

The very concept of a comprehensive national nutrition policy suggests that not only should adequate supplies of safe, nutritious foods be available but that consumers should be given the educational means for making informed food choices (Helsing, 1989; Quelch, 1977). The Committee understands that a nutrition labeling program is only one component of a comprehensive education program, but believes that a well-designed nutrition label can help consumers to make informed food choices. However, nutrition information on food labels is just that, an information provision strategy, not an education program. The provision of information is only the first stage in the behavioral change process. Nutrition labeling can provide information about food and nutrition to the public, but it cannot be a substitute for comprehensive nutrition education programs. It is imperative that nutrition education programs be designed to complement nutrition labeling in order to give consumers the information and skills to make healthful food choices.

A comprehensive, coordinated program of nutrition education will enable consumers to make individual food choices within the context of their own comprehensive program for health maintenance and disease prevention. The Committee urges the establishment of a public- and private-sector initiative to better help consumers understand and apply the information on the revised nutrition label. However, the Committee refrains from providing a discussion of or recommendations about the specific aspects of nutrition education programs in deference to the pending Institute of Medicine/FNB report by the Committee on Dietary Guidelines Implementation which will address this subject in depth (IOM, in press).

The Committee recommends that comprehensive nutrition education programs be developed in order to assist consumers to understand the information on food labels to plan diets and make appropriate food choices. It is the responsibility of those designing such public information programs to ensure that consumers can process the information easily and accurately. This means that more attention must be given to thorough message testing research to determine the most effective format for delivering nutrition information on food labels.

The Committee recommends that:

- Public- and private-sector initiatives should be established to help consumers understand and apply the information on the nutrition label.
- Comprehensive nutrition education programs should be developed in order to help consumers to understand the information on food labels to enable them to plan diets and make appropriate food choices.

COSTS OF NUTRITION LABELING REFORM

Any reform of food labeling to provide more complete nutrition information and any expansion of the coverage of current nutrition labeling requirements will impose costs on producers, manufacturers, retailers, and, ultimately, consumers. It is not only the Committee's recommendations that would result in such costs; FDA's recent nutrition labeling proposal and the nutrition labeling legislation currently before Congress would impose similar costs.

The Committee was not charged with assessing the costs of its or any other set of proposals for reform. But it would be irresponsible not to acknowledge that expanded and improved nutrition labeling will have costs and that the magnitude of these costs ought to be taken into account by FDA and USDA in their formulation of the details of and, even more important, the timing of a revised nutrition labeling system.

In 1990, FDA commissioned a study on the costs of implementing the type of changes in nutrition labeling that it was planning to propose (55 Fed. Reg. 29,476–29,533; July 19, 1990). The agency's notice of proposed rulemaking contains a preliminary analysis of the private-sector and consumer costs in the first four areas of implementing revised nutrition labeling regulations: (1) extending mandatory nutrition labeling to all packaged foods, (2) standardizing serving sizes, (3) revising the U.S. RDAs, and (4) listing all optional ingredients in standardized foods. FDA estimated that 21,000 firms would be affected and that the cost per U.S. household will be $3.15 in the first year of implementation of its proposal, and $0.60 per U.S. household each year afterward. This estimate, if accurate, may provide some guide as to the costs of the Committee's more ambitious set of recommendations.

The added costs of expanded nutrition labeling must be compared to the savings through improved health that consumers are expected to realize by having and using improved, more comprehensive nutrition information. The Committee believes that potential long-term savings in health care costs and gains in longevity would outweigh the cost of its recommendations.

Overview of Costs To Manufacturers and Retailers

The costs incurred by food producers will include those for administrative activities, nutrient analysis of foods, changes in label design, printing new labels, and in some instances, reduced ingredient flexibility. Within the first category are the costs of discovering and interpreting new requirements, assessing their impact on products, and developing a product compliance system. In addition, retail food stores, which under the Committee's proposal would be required to post nutrition information about produce, meat, poultry, and seafood, would incur costs in preparing and maintaining this information. Some costs, however, notably the costs of assembling the information about nutrient content, will be borne by the suppliers of fresh foods. Ultimately, most additional costs will be passed on to consumers.

FDA noted in its proposal that a firm's costs for nutrient analysis would depend to a great extent on which and how many of its products currently carry nutrition labeling or have nutrient analysis data available (55 Fed. Reg. 29,476–29,533; July 19, 1990). For foods that have not previously provided nutrition labeling, the start-up costs of obtaining the required information may be substantial. Costs for relabeling would include label design, printing, and inventory costs. The latter could be minimized by scheduling the effective date of new regulations to conform with the already-scheduled "uniform compliance dates" for incorporating other mandated label changes and by allowing existing label stocks to be exhausted.

For some foods there could conceivably be costs associated with reduced flexibility in the choice of ingredients. The Committee recommends that man-ufacturers be allowed to continue to use "and/or" labeling for fats and oils, on the condition that the food label state the highest level of saturated fatty acids achievable by any combination of listed fats and oils. This approach should not constrict choice of fats and oils unless manufacturers, worried about disclosing high levels of saturated fatty acids, decide to curtail their use of some highly saturated fats or oils. But the associated product costs of such changes would be offset by direct nutritional benefits for consumers. FDA's proposal is designed to require more detailed listing of fatty acid content, which could curtail flexibility in formulation. By limiting the breakdown of fat components to saturated and unsaturated fatty acids, however, the agency expects that most manufacturers will be able to maintain sufficient flexibility in their selection of ingredients to minimize any increase in the cost of the final product.

Costs for Different Food Categories

Four major sectors of foods will be affected by the adoption of new requirements for nutrition labeling: (1) foods that currently carry nutrition labeling; (2) food that do not currently carry nutrition labeling but have been analyzed; (3) produce and fresh seafood under FDA jurisdiction, and fresh meat and poultry under USDA jurisdiction, and (4) restaurant foods. Under the Committee's recommendation (as well as FDA's proposal and proposed legislation), virtually all packaged foods would be required to bear nutrition labeling. In addition, foods now bearing nutrition labeling would be required to provide different information.

Cost for Foods That Currently Carry Nutrition Labeling

It is the Committee's judgment that its recommendations for the content of nutrition labels would require very little information that producers do not already possess. Possibly, the requirements that sodium and dietary fiber be listed will require reanalysis of some products. However, the requirements for listing the content of fat, fatty acids, protein, carbohydrates, vitamins, and minerals do not appear likely to demand new testing. For foods in this sector (now 60 percent of all packaged foods), the Committee's recommendations would mainly require changes in the presentation of information that manufacturers already have.

The timing of the imposition of such requirements could affect the cost of compliance. If new labels had to be prepared and applied on a schedule that took no account of the normal, commercially driven evolution of food labels, or other government-mandated label changes, the extra cost could be substantial. But labels undergo relatively frequent changes, and FDA customarily establishes a "uniform compliance date" for all required label changes far in advance of the effective date. The Committee believes that recommended changes in nutrition labeling should be implemented on the same schedule already fixed for other mandated changes, which should allow utilization of old label stocks. USDA should also follow this same approach for implementing changes in nutrition labeling for meat and poultry products.

Cost for Foods That Do Not Currently Carry Nutrition Labeling

For foods that do not now bear nutrition labeling of any sort, additional costs will be incurred. It is likely that manufacturers do not currently have complete information about the nutrient content of some products. The cost of analysis of these foods may not be trivial, though adequate methods and laboratory resources are available to analyze, at a reasonable cost, virtually all packaged foods for all of the nutrition components that the Committee recommends. It is reported that many packaged foods that do not currently bear nutrition labeling have nonetheless been analyzed by their manufacturers (Daniel Padberg, Texas A&M University, personal communication, 1990). The growth in voluntary nutrition labeling over the past decade and the willingness of most sectors of the packaged-food industry to accept, and in many instances support, mandatory nutrition labeling suggests that these costs will not be significant. The costs of relabeling can be controlled in the same fashion as for foods that already bear nutrition labeling, by allowing reasonable lead time and schedules, coupled with the mandated label changes.

Costs for Labeling Fresh Foods

Produce and Seafood   The Committee is recommending nutrition labeling, broadly defined, for selected produce and fresh seafood. Retailers will incur modest costs in displaying and maintaining the required information, but the major costs are likely to occur in assembling the data base to support the required nutrient declarations. The Committee acknowledges that FDA may have to adjust the timing of its requirement for such information in light of the costs, and time required, to comply.

The Committee recognizes, as does FDA, that providing point-of-purchase nutrition information for produce and fresh seafood will impose significant new costs on retailers and on consumers. Some 235,000 food stores were estimated to be in operation in 1987. FDA's proposal does not provide any estimate of total compliance costs. It does estimate that 50 percent of stores could supply the required information at an annual cost of $200 per store, but it acknowledges that this figure does not include the cost of generating the data bases to support such displays, and a portion of this cost is likely to be borne by food stores and, ultimately, consumers.

Meat and Poultry   Unlike either the FDA proposal or pending legislation, which do not mention meat and poultry products, the Committee is recommending nutrition labeling of all packaged meat and poultry products and point-of-purchase information for fresh meat and poultry products. A share of USDA-regulated packaged foods now bear nutrition information, and the abbreviated

USDA format demands less information than FDA, only requiring information about calories, protein, carbohydrate, and fat. Fresh meat and poultry do not provide significant amounts of dietary fiber. Analysis for sodium, calcium, and iron would be an expense only if they were not included in the original analysis. Costs for labeling fresh meat and poultry products would be from printing and maintaining point-of-purchase information in retail food stores, since the data would be taken from existing nutrient data bases. Broadly speaking, however, it would appear that the cost of implementing the Committee's recommendations for meat and poultry should not differ substantially, on a per product basis, from those incurred by FDA-regulated packaged foods and for produce and fresh seafood.

A caveat should be added here, however. It is possible that USDA's rigorous criteria for approving nutrient statements on the labels of meat and poultry products would impose higher per product costs than those of FDA. The department's prior approval system, like other premarket approval systems, appears to invite the type of skepticism that drives up the cost of product testing. The Committee believes that it is important for FDA and USDA to agree on uniform criteria for assessing the accuracy of label statements of nutrition content as well as on consistent standards for approving data bases as the source of nutrient composition data for fresh foods (see Chapter 5).

Costs for Labeling Restaurant Foods

In one respect, the costs of the Committee's recommendations will differ sharply from those of FDA's proposal or the pending legislation. The Committee is recommending that limited-menu restaurants be required to display point-of-purchase nutrient content (and ingredient) information on their foods and that all other restaurants be required to have such information available to consumers on request. The first half of this recommendation is not likely to entail substantial additional costs, either for the limited-menu restaurant or for consumers. The products sold by these operations are standardized, carefully controlled for content and quality, and generally uniform throughout the country, and the world. Major limited-menu restaurant franchise chains have previously reported that they have already analyzed their products for nutrient content. The only significant new cost involved is likely to be that of preparing and maintaining the posted nutrient information. The recent willingness of several major chains to display information of the type recommended by the Committee suggests that this expense is, on a per restaurant basis, modest.

The costs of the Committee's recommendation to require all other restaurants to have their menus evaluated and to offer nutrient information on request to consumers are considerably less certain and more speculative. The Committee believes that computer programs for evaluation of the nutrition profile of menus is widely available and inexpensive, but even modest expense may prove high for small operators (see Chapter 5). Printing the statement "nutrition information is available on request" on menus would be essentially costless. If requests were frequent, however, the cost of preparing, duplicating, and maintaining menu information could prove more than trivial, particularly for operators that changed menus frequently. This is an area in which close study of potential costs is warranted.

REFERENCES

Asam, E.H., and L.P. Bucklin. 1973. Nutrition labeling for canned goods: A study of consumer response. J. Market. 37:32–37.

Babcock, M.J., and M.M. Murphy. 1973. Two nutrition labeling systems. J. Am. Diet. Assoc. 62:155–161.

Betteman, J.R. 1979. An Information Processing Theory of Consumer Choice. Addison-Wesley, Reading, Mass. 402 pp.

Bettinghaus, E.P. 1986. Health promotion and the knowledge-attitude-behavior continuum. Preventive Med. 15:475–491.

CNCFL (Committee on the Nutrition Components of Food Labeling). 1990. Workshop on Label Formats, CNCFL, Food and Nutrition Board, Institute of Medicine, April 25, 1990. Unpublished.

Cole, C.A., and G.J. Gaeth. 1990. Cognitive and age-related differences in the ability to use nutritional information in a complex environment. J. Market. Res. May:175–184.

CRI (Consumer Research Institute). 1972. Interim Report of the First Two Phases of the CRI/FDA Nutrition Labeling Research Program. CRI, Washington, D.C. 223 pp.

Cronin, F.J., A.M. Shaw, S.M. Krebs-Smith, P.M. Marsland, and L. Light. 1987. Developing a food guidance system to implement the Dietary Guidelines. J. Nutr. Ed. 19(6):281–302.

Daly, P.A. 1976. The response of consumers to nutrition labeling. J. Consumer Affairs 10(Winter):170–178.

DHEW/USDA/FTC (U.S. Department of Health, Education, and Welfare, U.S. Department of Agriculture, and Federal Trade Commission). 1979. Food Labeling Background Papers. Government Printing Office, Washington, D.C. 124 pp.

DHHS (U.S. Department of Health and Human Services). 1988. The Surgeon General's Report on Nutrition and Health. Government Printing Office, Washington, D.C. 727 pp.

DHHS (U.S. Department of Health and Human Services). 1989. Promoting Health/Preventing Disease: Year 2000 Objectives for the Nation. Draft for public review and comment. Public Health Service, Washington, D.C.

Eisner, D. 1972. Developmental relationships between field independence and fixity-mobility. Perceptual Motor Skills 34(June):767–770.

Farmakalidis, E. 1989. Nutrition labelling—an industry perspective. Food Aust. 41(10): 979–981.

FLAPS (Food Labeling and Package Survey). 1988. Status of Nutrition and Sodium

Labeling of Processed Foods. Division of Consumer Surveys, Center for Food Safety and Applied Nutrition, FDA, Washington, D.C. 19 pp.

Food Chemical News. 1988. FDA declines to establish "organic" food labeling standards. 26(December):16–17.

Food Chemical News. 1990. FDA action against Ragu "Fresh Italian" sauce asked by Public Voice 12(March):20.

Geiger, C.J., B.W. Wyse, C.R.M. Parent, and R.G. Hansen. 1990. The use of adaptive conjoint analysis (ACA) to determine the most useful nutrition label for purchase decisions. Abstract No. 4587. Presented at Federation of American Societies for Experimental Biology, Washington, D.C.

Gersovitz, M., J.P. Madden, and H. Smiciklas-Wright. 1978. Validity of the 24-hour dietary recall and seven-day records for group comparisons. J. Am. Diet. Assoc. 73:48–55.

Glanz, K., and R. Mullis. 1988. Environmental interventions to promote healthy eating: A review of models, programs, and evidence. Health Ed. Q. 15(4):395–415.

Gunner, S.W. 1989. Nutrition labelling—the Canadian experience. Food Aust. 41(10): 984–987.

Guthrie, H.A. 1984. Selection and quantification of typical food portions by young adults. J. Am. Diet. Assoc. 84:1440–1444.

Hammonds, T.M. 1978. Testimony before the Subcommittee on Nutrition, Committee on Agriculture, Nutrition, and Forestry, U.S. Senate. August 9–10, 1978.

Heimbach, J.T. 1982. Public Understanding of Food Label Information. Food and Drug Administration, Washington, D.C. 24 pp.

Heimbach, J.T. 1985. Cardiovascular disease and diet: The public view. Public Health Rep. 100:5.

Heimbach, J.T. 1986. The growing impact of sodium labeling of foods. Food Technol. 40(12):102.

Heimbach, J.T. 1987. Risk avoidance in consumer approaches to diet and health. Clin. Nutr. 6:159.

Heimbach, J.T., and R.C. Stokes. 1981. Nutrition Labeling for Today's Needs: Opinions of Nutritionists, the Food Industry and Consumers. Food and Drug Administration, Washington, D.C. 52 pp.

Heimbach, J.T., A.S. Levy, and R.E. Schucker. 1990. Declared serving sizes of packaged foods, 1977–86. Food Technol. 44:82–90.

Helsing, E. 1989. Nutrition policies in Europe—the state of the art. Eur. J. Clin. Nutr. 43(Suppl.):57–66.

Hunter, D.M., L. Sampson, M.H. Stampfer, G.A. Colditz, B. Rosner, and W.C. Willett. 1988. Variability in portion sizes of commonly consumed foods among a population of women in the United States. Am. J. Epidemiol. 127:1240.

Hutt, P.B. 1986. National nutrition policy and the role of the Food and Drug Administration. Currents 2(2):2–11.

Hutt, P.B., and R.A. Merrill. 1990. Food and Drug Law: Cases and Materials. Foundation Press, Inc., Mineola, N.Y. In press.

IOM (Institute of Medicine). In press. Improving America's Diet and Health: From Recommendaions to Action. Committee on Dietary Guidelines Implementation, Food and Nutrition Board. National Academy Press, Washington, D.C.

Krebs-Smith, S.M., and H. Smiciklas-Wright. 1985. Typical serving sizes: Implications for food guidance. J. Am. Diet. Assoc. 85:1139–1141.

Lansky, D., and K.D. Brownell. 1982. Estimates of food quantity and calories: Errors in self-report among obese patients. Am. J. Clin. Nutr. 35:727–732.

Lenahan, R.J., J.A. Thomas, D.A. Taylor, D.L. Call, and P.I. Padberg. 1972. Consumer reaction to nutrition information on food product labels. Search Agric. 2(15):1–26.

Lewis, C.J., A.M. Beloian, and E.A. Yetley. 1988. Serving size issues in estimating dietary exposure to food substances. J. Am. Diet. Assoc. 88:1545–1552.

Liefield, J.P. 1983. Nutrition Labeling and Consumer Behavior: A Review of the Evidence. Prepared for the Bureau of Nutritional Sciences, Health & Welfare Canada, Ottawa, Ontario, Canada.

Madden, J.P., S.J. Goodman, and H.A. Guthrie. 1976. Validity of the 24-hour recall. J. Am. Diet. Assoc. 68:143–147.

McCullough, J., and R. Best. 1980. Consumer preference for food label information: A basis for segmentation. J. Consumer Affairs 14(1):180–192.

Merrill, R.A., and P.B. Hutt. 1980. Food and Drug Law: Cases and Materials. Foundation Press, Inc., Mineola, N.Y. 959 pp.

Mohr, K.G., B.W. Wyse, and R.G. Hansen. 1980. Aiding consumer nutrition decisions: Comparison of a graphical nutrient density labeling format with the current food label system. Home Econ. Res. J. 8(3):162–172.

Muller, T.E. 1985. Structural information factors which stimulate the use of nutrition information: A field experiment. J. Market. Res. May:143–157.

NRC (National Research Council). 1941. Recommended Dietary Allowances. Committee on Food and Nutrition. National Research Council, Washington, D.C. 13 pp.

NRC (National Research Council). 1968. Recommended Dietary Allowances, 7th ed. Report of the Committee on the Seventh Edition of the Recommended Dietary Allowances, Food and Nutrition Board. National Academy of Sciences, Washington, D.C. 101 pp.

NRC (National Research Council). 1988. Designing Foods: Animal Product Options in the Marketplace. Committee on Technological Options to Improve the Nutritional Attributes of Animal Products, Board on Agriculture. National Academy Press, Washington, D.C. 367 pp.

NRC (National Research Council). 1989a. Diet and Health: Implications for Reducing Chronic Disease Risk. Report of the Committee on Diet and Health, Food and Nutrition Board, Commission on Life Sciences. National Academy Press, Washington, D.C. 749 pp.

NRC (National Research Council). 1989b. Recommended Dietary Allowances, 10th ed. Report of the Subcommittee on the Tenth Edition of the Recommended Dietary Allowances, Food and Nutrition Board, Commission on Life Sciences. National Academy Press, Washington, D.C. 285 pp.

ORC (Opinion Research Corporation). 1990. Food Labeling and Nutrition: What Americans Want. Survey conducted for the National Food Processors Association, Washington, D.C. 178 pp.

Pao, E.M., K.H. Fleming, P.H. Guenther, and S.J. Mickle. 1982. Foods Commonly Eaten by Individuals: Amount Per Day and Per Eating Occasion. Home Economics

Research Report No. 44. Human Nutrition Information Service, U.S. Department of Agriculture, Washington, D.C. 431 pp.

Pennington, J.A.T., V.L. Wilkening, and J.E. Vanderveen. 1990. Descriptive terms for food labeling. J. Nutr. Ed. 22(1):51–54.

Quelch, J.A. 1977. The role of nutrition information in national nutrition policy. Nutr. Rev. 35(11):289–293.

Rogers, E.M. 1983. Diffusion of Innovations, 3rd ed. The Free Press, New York. 367 pp.

Rudd, J. 1986. Aiding consumer nutrition decisions with the simple graphic label format. Home Econ. Res. J. 14(3):342–346.

Rudd, J. 1989. Consumer response to calorie base variations on the graphical nutrient density food label. J. Nutr. Ed. 21:259–264.

Sims, L.S. 1979. The community nutritionist as change agent. Fam. Community Health 1(4):83–92.

Sims, L.S., and S.K. Shepherd. 1987. An Information Processing Approach to the Evaluation of Nutrition Education Materials. Final Report submitted to the Human Nutrition Information Service. USDA, Washington, D.C.

Sims, L.S., and H. Smiciklas-Wright. 1978. An ecological systems perspective: Its application to nutrition policy, program design and evaluation. Ecol. Food Nutr. 7(3):173–180.

Stephenson, M. 1978. The confusing world of health foods. FDA Consumer 12(6):19–20.

Syme, S.L. 1986. Strategies for health promotion. Preventive Med. 15:492–507.

TDA (Texas Department of Agriculture). 1989. Statement of the Texas Department of Agriculture before the U.S. Food and Drug Administration hearing on food labeling. San Antonio, Tex., Nov. 1, 1989.

USDA (U.S. Department of Agriculture). 1958. Food for Fitness: A Daily Food Guide. Leaflet No. 424. Institute of Home Economics, Agricultural Research Service. Government Printing Office, Washington, D.C.

USDA (U.S. Department of Agriculture). 1975. Nutritive Value of American Foods in Common Units. Agriculture Handbook No. 456. Government Printing Office, Washington, D.C. 291 pp.

USDA (U.S. Department of Agriculture). 1976. Composition of Foods. Agriculture Handbook No. 8 series. Government Printing Office, Washington, D.C. Revised continuously.

USDA (U.S. Department of Agriculture). 1981. Nutritive Value of Foods. Home and Garden Bulletin No. 72, revised. Government Printing Office, Washington, D.C. 72 pp.

USDA (U.S. Department of Agriculture). 1982a. FSIS Policy Memorandum 039. Food Safety and Inspection Service, Washington, D.C.

USDA (U.S. Department of Agriculture). 1982b. FSIS Policy Memorandum 055. Food Safety and Inspection Service, Washington, D.C.

USDA (U.S. Department of Agriculture). 1984. FSIS Policy Memorandum 049C. Food Safety and Inspection Service, Washington, D.C.

USDA (U.S. Department of Agriculture). 1986. FSIS Policy Memorandum 071A. Food Safety and Inspection Service, Washington, D.C.

USDA (U.S. Department of Agriculture). 1987a. FSIS Policy Memorandum 019A. Food Safety and Inspection Service, Washington, D.C.

USDA (U.S. Department of Agriculture). 1987b. FSIS Policy Memorandum 070B. Food Safety and Inspection Service, Washington, D.C.

USDA (U.S. Department of Agriculture). 1989a. FSIS Policy Memorandum 022C. Food Safety and Inspection Service, Washington, D.C.

USDA (U.S. Department of Agriculture). 1989b. FSIS Standards and Labeling Policy Book. Standards and Labeling Division, Food Safety and Inspection Service, Washington, D.C.

USDA (U.S. Department of Agriculture). 1990. Report of the Dietary Guidelines Advisory Committee on the Dietary Guidelines for Americans, 1990. Report to the Secretary of Agriculture and the Secretary of Health and Human Services. Government Printing Office, Washington, D.C. 48 pp.

USDA/DHHS (U.S. Department of Agriculture and U.S. Department of Health and Human Services). 1980. Nutrition and Your Health: Dietary Guidelines for Americans. Government Printing Office, Washington, D.C. 20 pp.

USDA/DHHS (U.S. Department of Agriculture and U.S. Department of Health and Human Services). 1982. Design and Evaluation of Nutrition Label Formats: Information Kit. Government Printing Office, Washington, D.C. 20 pp.

USDA/DHHS (U.S. Department of Agriculture and U.S. Department of Health and Human Services). 1985. Nutrition and Your Health: Dietary Guidelines for Americans, 2nd ed. Government Printing Office, Washington, D.C. 24 pp.

Vankatesan, M. 1977. Providing Nutritional Information to Consumers. Paper presented at a Special NSF/MIT Conference on Consumer Research for Consumer Policy, Cambridge, Mass., July.

Vankatesan, M., W. Lancaster, and K.W. Kendall. 1986. An empirical study of alternative formats for nutritional information disclosure in advertising. J. Public Policy Marketing 5:29–43.

Webb, C.A., and J.A. Yuhas. 1988. Ability of WIC clientele to estimate food quantities. J. Am. Diet. Assoc. 88:601–602.

Wolf, I.D., N.R. Raper, and J.C. Rosenthal. 1983. USDA activities in relation to the sodium issue: 1981–1983. Food Technol. 37:59.

Yankelovich, Inc. 1971. Nutrition labeling: A consumer experiment to determine the effects of nutrition labeling on food purchases. Chain Store Age January:55–77.

Yuhas, J.A., J.E. Bolland, and T.W. Bolland. 1989. The impact of training, food type, gender, and container size on the estimation of food portion sizes. J. Am. Diet. Assoc. 89:1473–1477.

8

Legislation and Regulation

The Committee was specifically asked to consider the implications of its food labeling proposals for existing legislation governing nutrition and ingredient labeling and to propose policy options for modifying current statutory and regulatory directives. This language was interpreted by the Committee as a request to consider whether the laws under which the Food and Drug Administration (FDA) and the U.S. Department of Agriculture (USDA) now regulate food labels or the regulations they have issued should be changed to implement the recommendations set forth in earlier chapters. Chapters 5, 6, and 7 addressed the adequacy of current FDA and USDA regulations, and endorsed some changes and pointed out deficiencies in others. The changes in regulations required to implement the Committee's recommendations should be obvious from that discussion, and thus, they are not itemized here.

This chapter deals with the other facet of the Committee's charge, that is, to assess the adequacy of existing statutes to support the changes in food labeling requirements that the Committee endorses. It examines the current statutory authorities of FDA and USDA and discusses the arguments for and against efforts to elicit new legislation. The Committee concludes that such legislation is desirable to foreclose disputes about existing authority and to ensure that FDA and USDA proceed in tandem to implement the needed changes in food labels. The enactment of appropriate legislation cannot be assumed, however, so the chapter concludes with a discussion of the desirability of administrative initiatives to improve nutrition labeling.

The three statutes chiefly involved in nutrition labeling are the Federal Food, Drug and Cosmetic Act (FD&C Act), the Federal Meat Inspection Act (FMI

Act), and the Poultry Products Inspection Act (PPI Act). The Committee recommends that the U.S. Congress amend all three of these laws to eliminate doubt about the agencies' authority to expand the coverage and revise the content of current nutrition and ingredient labeling requirements. (The types of amendments that would be desirable are discussed below.) This key recommendation does not reflect the judgment that FDA or USDA would be held to lack the authority to adopt the reforms endorsed in this report. Rather, it is a recognition that doubt about the existence of such authority may impede agency action and result in court challenges that could delay the implementation of needed reforms. Furthermore, the Committee recognizes that existing arrangements for internal executive branch review of agency rulemaking initiatives, whatever their general merit, will also cause delay. The enactment of legislation that directed both FDA and USDA to broaden the coverage and reform the content of nutrition labeling and set a timetable for the adoption of implementing regulations would accelerate the administrative process and discourage court challenges.

CURRENT LEGAL AUTHORITY
TO EXPAND NUTRITION LABELING

The difficult questions concerning the authority of FDA and USDA under existing laws to implement the Committee's recommendations relate to recommendations to extend nutrition labeling to all packaged foods; foods sold in restaurants; and produce and fresh and frozen meats, poultry, and fish. Although the matter is not entirely free from controversy, discussions between the Committee and legal experts did not reveal serious doubt about either agency's authority to prescribe the content and format of nutrition information when such labeling can otherwise be required.

With respect to the issue of coverage, it is not clear that FDA and USDA are in the same situation. The FD&C Act is perhaps less generous than either the FMI Act or the PPI Act, which give USDA the power to approve in advance all labels used on meat and poultry products. Therefore, this discussion begins with the question of whether FDA could, under current law, require that all packaged foods within its jurisdiction (subject to administratively determined exceptions) bear nutrition labeling. It then turns to the questions of FDA's authority to require nutrition labeling for foods sold in restaurants and its authority to require some point-of-sale nutrition information, that is, some form of nutrition *labeling*, for produce and seafood.

An additional reason to begin this discussion with an examination of FDA's authority to broaden the coverage of mandatory nutrition labeling is that the products that fall within its jurisdiction comprise well over half of all foods purchased by Americans. In the Committee's view, a conclusion that FDA lacks, or might be held by a court to lack, such authority would alone be sufficient to justify a recommendation that Congress should act, regardless of the conclusions that might be reached regarding USDA's current legal authority.

FDA's Legal Authority To Mandate
Nutrition Labeling on All Packaged Foods

The term *legal authority,* rather than *statutory authority,* is used to draw a distinction between what might be termed the literal interpretation of statutory provisions and an assessment of the maximum scope of authority over food labels that courts would approve if FDA chose to exert that authority. (Lawyers would use the terms *express* and *implicit* legal authority to capture the same distinction.) This distinction may puzzle some readers, who might assume that such issues of agency power are clear-cut. They would be surprised by the vagueness of many laws, particularly older laws, as they apply to contemporary problems that very likely were not contemplated by the Congress that enacted them. In fact, important questions of administrative power are often not answered by the language or the history of statutes that support major regulatory programs. For a lawyer, however, such a concession does not end the analysis. Modern U.S. regulatory law has a dynamic character, both by legislative design and through judicial interpretation. In addition to conveying specific powers to an agency, Congress will often include a general grant of authority to an agency to adopt the regulations needed to implement a statute's general objectives. The Supreme Court has held that when Congress does so, an agency's exercise of this residual authority should be sustained unless it exceeds clear limits on its power (*Chevron, U.S.A. v. Natural Resources Defense Council,* 467 U.S. 837 (1984)).

The point of this abstract discussion is that FDA has the authority to do more than the specific language of the FD&C Act might at first appear to allow. Many of its current requirements for food labels represent the assertion of a general authority to adopt the regulations needed to implement the goals of the Act. For example, no provision of the FD&C Act states, in so many words, that FDA may prescribe the content of nutrition information provided voluntarily or require nutrition labeling on foods for which nutrition claims are made or to which one or more nutrients have been added. Yet, this is precisely the requirements of FDA's current regulations, and their validity has never been challenged (nor, in truth, has it been upheld) in any court. Experienced legal experts believe that FDA's current regulations would be almost certainly sustained if they were now challenged. Accordingly, it is appropriate to begin this analysis with the legal theory on which FDA relied when it promulgated its original regulations in 1973.

Section 403(a) of the FD&C Act provides that a food is misbranded (and subject to seizure or other enforcement proceedings) if "its labeling is false or misleading in any particular." The courts have read this language expansively to prohibit not only false or clearly deceptive statements but also statements that, although literally true, are misleading in context. This treatment of the language of section 403(a) is reinforced by another key provision, section 201(n), which reads as follows:

> If an article is alleged to be misbranded because the labeling . . . is misleading, then in determining whether the labeling . . . is misleading there shall be taken into account (among other things) not only representations made or suggested . . . but also the extent to which the labeling . . . fails to reveal facts material in the light of such representations or material with respect to consequences which may result from the use of the article to which the labeling . . . relates under the conditions of use prescribed in the labeling . . . or under such conditions as are customary or usual.

When it issued the regulations in 1973, FDA made essentially two arguments. First, it argued that a standardized format for nutrition labeling was required to prevent deception of consumers who would otherwise confront a bewildering array of statements about nutrient content on food labels. Second, relying on section 201(n), it argued that the making of a nutrition claim for a food or the addition of any nutrient (which would be disclosed on the label) would be misleading unless consumers were provided with more complete information about the nutritional value of the food:

> Only by having available this full nutrition labeling for a food to which a nutrient is added or for which such claim or information is provided can such claim or information be evaluated and understood, and the food properly used in the diet. Without full nutrition labeling such claims or information would be confusing and misleading for lack of completeness, and could deceive consumers about the nutritional value of the food, its overall nutritional contribution to the daily diet, and its nutritional weaknesses as well as strengths (38 Fed. Reg. 2125, Jan. 19, 1973).

Some believe that this same theory could be extended to support the adoption of regulations mandating nutrition information on all packaged foods (or all except those that FDA chose to exempt) and perhaps others as well. In testimony made before the Committee in December 1989, a spokesman for the Grocery Manufacturers of America (GMA) articulated the argument FDA might make:

> The vast majority of the public is deeply interested in the nutritional composition of marketed food products. The nutritional composition of a food has come to be a material fact that is of inherent interest to the consumer . . . . Thus, the marketing of any food that makes a significant nutritional contribution to the daily diet is sufficient to trigger nutritional labeling under section 201(n) of the FD&C Act. GMA does not believe that new legislation is needed in order to require nutrition labeling for all food that makes a significant contribution to the daily diet, and

would support the promulgation of regulations by FDA to achieve this purpose (GMA, 1989).

Others would add to this argument the fact that the growth of voluntary nutrition labeling, which now appears on over half of all packaged foods, has itself contributed to consumer expectations that food labels will provide information about nutrient composition. This theory arguably represents the broadest interpretation of FDA's current authority to mandate nutrition labeling on all packaged foods. Some lawyers might consider it untenable. Although most would acknowledge that the theory might be upheld on judicial review, few would guarantee that it would be upheld.

A variant of the foregoing application of the half-truth principle of section 201(n) would proceed in two steps. Step one would focus on the precise language of section 201(n), which treats as misbranding the failure to disclose facts "material with respect to the consequences which may result from the use of the article to which the labeling relates." As documented in the reports of the National Research Council (NRC, 1989) and the Surgeon General (DHHS, 1988), excessive consumption of certain food components (including saturated fatty acids, sodium, and cholesterol) is associated with heightened chronic disease risk. It would not be farfetched to argue, therefore, that the failure of manufacturers of foods that contain significant amounts of these components to disclose their presence on the labels renders the foods misbranded under section 403(a). Step two of the analysis, tracking of FDA's original theory for standardizing nutrition labeling, would assert that consumers could be misled if all food labels did not declare these components. It would be a short step to conclude that FDA could also require label disclosure of other nutrients, including underconsumed complex carbohydrates, calcium, and fiber.

Although such legal arguments might puzzle laypeople and offend some lawyers, the Committee does not dismiss the possibility that, without any change in the current law, FDA could successfully mandate nutrition labeling on all packaged foods. Courts have upheld other assertions by the agency of its power to prescribe the contents of food labels. Perhaps the most notable example is a case that was decided in 1975, which upheld FDA regulations defining the common or usual names of several foods (*American Frozen Food Institute v. Mathews*, 413 F. Supp. 548 (1976), *aff'd*, 555 F.2d 1059 (D.C. Cir. 1977)).

Until recently, FDA had not publicly confronted the question of whether it has the authority to require nutrition labeling on all packaged foods. The agency made its 1973 requirements mandatory only for foods that contained added nutrients or that made nutrition claims, but it claimed then that this reflected a pragmatic judgment rather than doubt about its legal authority. The FDA 1979 background papers prepared in connection with the review of food labeling by FDA, USDA, and the Federal Trade Commission (FTC) did not discuss whether the agency's nutrition labeling requirements could be extended beyond these foods (DHEW/USDA/FTC, 1979). However, in congressional testimony in August 1989, then FDA Commissioner Frank Young suggested that agency officials believed that nutrition labeling could be required on all packaged foods under existing law (Young, 1989).

As this report was being completed, FDA proposed revisions of its nutrition labeling regulations that would, if adopted, apply to virtually all packaged foods within the agency's jurisdiction. This proposal asserts that the agency declined to mandate nutrition labeling of all foods in 1973 because knowledge of nutrient content was still incomplete and the methods of chemical analysis were inadequate in many cases. FDA now argues that these obstacles have since been removed. Furthermore, it stresses the growth in knowledge of the relationship between nutrition and long-term health, knowledge that makes choices among foods more important and justifies action to ensure that consumers can assess the consequences of the food selections they make. "[G]iven the history and use of nutrition labeling, the advances in nutrition science, and the public interest in healthful diets," the proposal concludes, "the nutritional content of a food is a material fact, and . . . a food label is misleading if it fails to bear the nutrition information that would be required . . ." (55 Fed. Reg. 29,476–29,533, July 19, 1990).

FDA's Authority To Prescribe the Content and Format of Nutrition Labeling

The adoption of mandatory nutrition labeling for all packaged foods would probably present the most serious test of FDA's current legal authority. The Committee's recommendations, however, go further. They call for changes in the content and format of current nutrition labels and for the extension of nutrition labeling to classes of food that do not now bear labeling that meets FDA requirements: produce, seafood, and foods sold in most restaurants. They also call for labeling of fresh meat and poultry, but the power to accomplish this lies, if it exists at all, with USDA (see discussion of USDA legal authority, below).

FDA's authority to prescribe the content and format of nutrition information in food labels, for whatever foods on which it may lawfully require such information, appears to be well established. The experts whom the Committee consulted generally concurred that the agency's authority to prevent misleading labeling and to force disclosure of the whole truth under section 201(n) would support any reasonable requirements for content and format, and the Committee agrees. Reasonable requirements are those requirements that are supported, on the one hand, by scientific evidence and, on the other, by studies of or reasoned judgments about consumer understanding and expectations, with appropriate consideration for simplicity, consistency, legibility, cost, and enforceability.

Similarly, FDA's decisions to exempt certain categories of packaged food from some or all nutrition information requirements, if supported by evidence and reasoning, would very likely be upheld. Thus, the agency could, under current law, properly decide to exempt foods sold in packages that are too small to bear full nutrition information or foods that make no significant nutritional contribution, such as condiments, chewing gum, and coffee and tea. By mentioning these examples, the Committee does not mean to imply that they should be exempted either by FDA or by Congress. The Committee does agree, however, that the authority to exempt foods from some or all nutrition labeling requirements is essential; furthermore, it believes that decisions about which foods to exempt should be made by FDA or USDA and not specified by statute. Requests for exemption from, or modification of, the standard requirements are likely to be numerous. The merit of such a request for any food, or any category of foods, should require an examination of nutrient content (to assess the need for nutrition information) and the feasibility of alternative means of conveying desired information. These types of issues are better resolved at the agency level than by Congress.

FDA's Authority To Require Nutrition Labeling of Produce, Seafood, and Foods Sold in Restaurants

The Committee's recommendations that some form of nutrition labeling should be required for fruits and vegetables, seafood, and foods sold in limited-menu restaurants raises other serious issues. However, the experts whom the Committee consulted were in general agreement that if FDA could establish its authority to mandate nutrition labeling on all packaged foods, its extension of these requirements to produce, seafood, and foods sold in restaurants would likely be upheld. Nothing in the FD&C Act purports to exempt any of these categories of foods from its basic labeling requirements, although FDA, for practical reasons, has by tradition effectively, although never expressly, exempted all three areas.

Significant practical problems would accompany efforts to require nutrition information for any of these categories of food, whether authorized by new legislation or undertaken under existing law. In the case of produce and most seafood, FDA would have to devise, or require sellers to devise, a substitute for the conventional package label, presumably some form of above-bin sign or placard perhaps supplemented by information on the display carton, and would have to take account of such problems as seasonal changes, relocations of displays, and damage by customers. In the case of foods sold in restaurants, FDA would have to be able to demonstrate that the foods it required to be labeled were sufficiently well standardized in the restaurants covered that nutrition statements were reliable and were sold in a setting where labeling was practicable. It is worth reiterating that labeling need not be affixed to the product; any information displayed in conjunction with the foods described would qualify and would, in principle, be subject to regulation by FDA.

The general law governing U.S. administrative bodies requires that their requirements, even when authorized by legislation, be supported by facts and reasoning. The usual formulation of this principle is that agency regulations must not be arbitrary or capricious, and although this test accords agencies considerable deference, courts apply it seriously. Moreover, courts have been willing to overturn agency regulations that appear to require substantial expenditures in return for modest benefits (*National Tire Dealers and Retreaders Association v. Brinegar*, 491 F.2d 31 (1974)). Thus, FDA's efforts to extend nutrition labeling to produce, seafood, and some foods sold in restaurants would probably face the sternest test if they were challenged as impractical rather than as unauthorized.

FDA's few statements on the issue of its authority to regulate the labeling of produce, seafood, and foods sold in restaurants have betrayed some ambivalence. The problems of enforcement in these contexts, coupled with the judgment that food labeling violations generally rank low in priority, have made FDA reluctant to exert jurisdiction over such foods. Yet, when squarely confronted, FDA has generally claimed that it has the authority to regulate the labeling of produce (and, by implication, seafood) and foods sold in restaurants (Hutt and Merrill, 1990).

When it adopted the current nutrition labeling regulations, FDA at first decided that they should apply to fresh fruits and vegetables. The agency ultimately retreated from this position, but the reasons it offered had nothing to do with legal authority. In the mid-1970s the agency was urged to require ingredient labeling for foods sold in limited-menu restaurants. Again, its decision not to proceed chiefly reflected concern for the practical obstacles to federal enforcement, which overrode any doubts about statutory authority.

FDA revisited these issues in 1979 during the joint DHEW/USDA/FTC review of federal regulation of food labeling and advertising. For restaurants, the immediate issue was again the labeling of ingredients, which some parties had urged the agencies to require. The agency's entire discussion of the legal aspects of this possibility reads as follows:

> [P]resent legal authority would be adequate to extend ingredient labeling to those restaurant foods that come in "containers" or that have "wrappers," but it is questionable whether this authority could be applied to other kinds of restaurant foods. A change in the law may be needed in order to require ingredient listings of food served in traditional restaurants (DHEW/USDA/FTC, 1979, p. 14).

The July 1990 FDA proposal would extend nutrition labeling to produce, but the preamble does not address the specific issue of authority. The agency explicitly does not propose to require nutrition labeling for foods sold in restaurants, but it implies that this decision represents a pragmatic judgment, not a concession that it lacks legal authority.

FDA's authority under current law to require nutrition information, in some form, for produce, fresh and frozen seafood, and foods sold in restaurants therefore remains unresolved. No court decision squarely addresses the issue, but neither does any court decision cast doubt on FDA's power. The FD&C Act's labeling requirements extend to foods "held for sale after shipment in interstate commerce" (21 USC § 301(k)). The agency's failure historically to attempt to control the information that restaurants provide about the foods they serve and its extremely modest efforts to influence the information that sellers of produce and seafood provide to consumers could undermine any effort now to exert long-dormant and, perhaps, debatable statutory authority. It remains the judgment of many experienced lawyers, however, that if FDA could devise nutrition labeling requirements for these foods that could be implemented economically and enforced without huge expenditures, courts probably would uphold its regulations against the outright claim that the FD&C Act does not provide the authority for their adoption.

USDA's Authority To Expand Nutrition Labeling of Meat and Poultry Products

The issues surrounding USDA's existing authority to expand the coverage of nutrition labeling parallel those discussed in connection with FDA, although the analysis does not. Unprocessed meat and poultry are usually sold fresh and frozen in wrappers that bear very simple labels. Processed meat and poultry products appear in a wide variety of forms in supermarkets, and many of the dishes featured by restaurants include meat or poultry. Perhaps the chief significant difference between the FDA and USDA sectors of the retail food business is that meat and poultry products, unlike produce, are almost never sold without any packaging whatsoever.

With respect to the authority to extend nutrition labeling to all packaged meat and poultry products, USDA appears to stand on firmer ground than does FDA, although as noted above, FDA's claim is quite plausible. Under the FMI Act, a label must be affixed, under the supervision of a USDA inspector, to any meat product that is placed or packed "in any can, pot, tin, canvas, or other receptacle or covering." In addition to confirming that the contents have passed inspection, the label must include, at a minimum, the name of the food, a statement of the quantity of the contents (typically net weight), a list of ingredients (unless it is subject to a standard of identity), and the name and place of business of the producer. Furthermore, the label may not be "false or misleading in any particular" (FMI Act § 607). The FMI Act does not, however, contain an explicit general grant of authority to require affirmative disclosures of information. Nor is its prohibition of misleading labeling accompanied by an equivalent to section 201(n) of the FD&C Act, which directs consideration of what is omitted from a food's label in deciding whether it is misleading.

To this point one might conclude that the FMI Act provides weaker support for any attempt by USDA to mandate nutrition labeling on all processed meat products. Nonetheless, the Committee is persuaded that USDA could successfully assert such authority under the current law. Section 607(c) of the FMI Act empowers USDA, "whenever [the Secretary of USDA] determines such action is necessary for the protection of the public, [to] prescribe . . . the styles and sizes of type to be used with respect to material required to be incorporated in labeling to avoid false or misleading labeling." This language does not indicate that USDA may determine the material required to avoid deception but, together with the prohibition against misleading labeling, it may also empower the agency to mandate additional disclosures, and not merely to prescribe the style and type size in which the statutorily specified information must appear on labels. The primary source of USDA authority, however, stems from its power to require prior approval of every meat product label affixed at an inspected establishment. This power, in the agency's view, derives from its power to inspect and certify products shipped from such establishments, and it appears to be USDA's view that it can require nutrition information on meat product labels whenever the agency concludes that it is necessary to prevent the label from being misleading. Essentially the same analysis supports the conclusion that USDA could, under the PPI Act, require all processed poultry products to bear nutrition labeling.

An assertion by USDA of its authority to require nutrition labeling for unprocessed fresh and frozen cuts of meat and poultry and foods sold in limited-menu restaurants containing significant amounts of meat or poultry would raise more difficult issues of authority. These questions are analyzed separately.

USDA has largely ceded the authority to regulate the labeling of retail cuts of fresh and frozen meat, and to a lesser extent of poultry, to local public health agencies. So far as the Committee is aware, USDA has never sought to prescribe nutrition labeling for such products, and the same labels that appear on cuts of meat and of poultry prepared on site in supermarkets are not individually approved by USDA. However, retail cuts of meat do bear the USDA inspection stamp, as well as its grade rating. Furthermore, the FMI Act empowers USDA to "regulate marketing, labeling, or packaging of meat . . . to prevent the use of any false, or misleading mark, label, or container" (Kushner et al., 1990). In addition, the Act (like the FD&C Act) extends USDA jurisdiction to products "held for sale after shipment in interstate commerce . . . ." It appears to be USDA's position that the FMI Act (or the PPI Act) would allow it to prescribe the content of labels on unprocessed meat (or poultry) sold at the retail level but that local regulations have rendered the exercise of such authority unnecessary. The Committee, accordingly, believes that USDA would be held to have authority to mandate nutrition information on labeling of fresh and frozen unprocessed meats and poultry if it chose to assert it.

Whether USDA could assert the same authority over off-package labeling is less clear. The agency has previously said it has jurisdiction over point-of-purchase printed materials as "labeling," but it has never attempted to require prior approval of such materials (Kushner et al., 1990). On at least one occasion it took the position that placards posted beside meat product displays in supermarkets were not "labeling" (*American Meat Institute v. Pridgeon*, 74 F.2d 45 (1984)).

The Committee is less confident that USDA would be successful if, without change in the existing law, it attempted to prescribe labeling, including nutrition information, for meat- and poultry-containing foods sold by restaurants. The Committee found no evidence that USDA has ever sought to claim such jurisdiction over foods sold by restaurants.

For the purposes of this report, however, it suffices to state that USDA's authority to prescribe nutrition labeling for foods sold by limited-menu restaurants is by no means clear. This is of concern to the Committee, which recommends that nutrition information be required for foods provided in limited-menu establishments. Putting aside the practical problems of implementation, the Committee's recommendation requires that some federal agency have clear legal authority to act in this area. FDA's claim to such power may be stronger than USDA's but it may lack jurisdiction over those restaurant foods that contain substantial amounts of meat and poultry. A labeling scheme that omitted these products would be inadequate. Meat or poultry dishes provide most of the protein offered by limited-menu restaurants; the principal share of vitamins and minerals; and most significantly, most of the calories, fat, cholesterol, and sodium. It is their exclusion from current labeling requirements that prompts the Committee's recommendation that nutrition labeling be required for such foods.

DESIRABILITY OF SEEKING NEW LEGISLATIVE AUTHORITY FOR NUTRITION LABELING

The foregoing discussion of FDA and USDA legal authority to mandate nutrition labeling for all packaged foods and extend the requirement, or some variant, to produce, seafood, fresh and frozen meats and poultry, and foods sold in restaurants at least suggests the desirability of new legislation that would lay continuing doubts to rest. And for this reason the Committee, in principle, recommends that Congress amend the FD&C, FMI, and PPI Acts to enlarge and clarify the authority of the two agencies. However, the pursuit of new legislation could have disadvantages that should be acknowledged.

Disadvantages of Seeking New Legislation

One disadvantage of seeking new legislation lies in the possibility that the effort may not succeed. The negative implications of Congress's failure to act, although not necessarily final to any later assertion of present authority (see *Petroleum Refiners Ass'n v. FTC*, 482 F.2d 672 (D.C. Cir. 1973), *cert. denied*, 415 U.S. 951 (1974)), might give pause to supporters of expanded nutrition labeling.

A second disadvantage, from the Committee's perspective, stems from the propensity of Congress to enact statutory requirements of such detail that they restrict administrative flexibility and hamper responses to new circumstances. An example of the Committee's concern is labeling of fiber content. Current speculations about the role of dietary fiber in reducing the risk of cancer, its clear contribution to digestion, and obvious consumer interest have led the Committee to recommend that fiber content be a required component of nutrition labeling. Members of Congress might well agree. In the Committee's judgment, however, mandating of fiber content labeling by statute would be a mistake. Further study of the role of dietary fiber might undermine the scientific case for including fiber in nutrition labeling and diminish consumer interest in the fiber content of food. A statutory directive that this information appear, however, would leave FDA no choice but to require it.

The Committee's concern about statutory rigidity is obviously a function of the kind of legislation that might be enacted. Congress could, in theory, enact legislation that states little more than (1) all food shall bear nutrition labeling, and (2) FDA and USDA shall determine its content, taking into account recent scientific findings, official dietary recommendations, consumer desires, and the practicalities of effective implementation. It seems unlikely in the current climate, however, that Congress would refrain from specifying the content and coverage of nutrition labeling in considerable detail.

The Committee is more concerned that new legislation might restrict the coverage of nutrition labeling by excluding, either expressly or by implication, important categories of foods such as produce, seafood, fresh and frozen meats and poultry, or foods sold in restaurants. The Committee is confident about both the desirability and the practicability of its recommendation that all packaged foods, except those exempted by FDA or USDA, should bear nutrition labeling. The Committee is also convinced of the desirability of providing point-of-sale nutrition information for fruits and vegetables, fresh and frozen meats, poultry, and seafood, and some foods sold in restaurants, though it recognizes the need to adapt conventional labeling requirements to fit the market realities of these categories of foods. Accordingly, the Committee would consider legislation that omitted these foods from any new grant of authority to require nutrition labeling to be inadequate.

A final concern is that new legislation might encumber FDA or USDA with rulemaking procedures that would delay the adoption or impede the later amendment of regulations mandating more informative nutrition labeling. The Committee is not aware of any current proposals that would prevent either agency from utilizing informal rulemaking procedures to adopt regulations, but the risk of an unfriendly amendment is always present.

Advantages of Seeking New Legislation

The foregoing considerations may well have played a role in discussions within FDA, and perhaps within USDA, about whether to urge new legislation, and contributed to FDA's decision to rely on its existing statutory authority to expand the coverage of nutrition labeling. On balance, however, the Committee is convinced that carefully drafted legislation could advance the goals of public health by facilitating the expansion and modernization of nutrition labeling. This section outlines the desired features of such legislation and in the process explains why the Committee favors the legislative route for reform.

The chief advantage of new legislation is that it could lay to rest doubts about FDA's and USDA's legal authority to mandate nutrition labeling for all packaged foods (subject to administrative exceptions) and clarify the agencies' authority to require nutrition information to accompany foods that currently escape most federal labeling requirements. Such legislation would not only give the agencies' assertion of authority immediate legitimacy, it would also reduce the incentives that third parties might have to challenge regulations the agencies adopt and thereby delay the implementation of the Committee's recommendations.

A second advantage is that new legislation could expedite the administrative process of developing regulations for implementing new nutrition labeling requirements. Although the Committee has expressed concern that new legislation might place burdensome rulemaking requirements on FDA and USDA, it could as easily have confirmed that the agencies were empowered to proceed by informal rulemaking. More significantly, legislation could speed the process of internal executive branch review by setting deadlines for the promulgation of implementing regulations.

In the Committee's judgment, reform of food labels is overdue. Both the Surgeon General (DHHS, 1988) and NRC (1989) have documented the clear links between nutrition and long-term health and have urged improved nutrition information for consumers. It would be distressing indeed if the Committee's recommendations—to the extent that they earn endorsement from health professionals and consumers—were impeded by prolonged debate within the federal executive branch. Legislation that requires the adoption of expanded nutrition labeling requirements by a certain date would avert this possibility.

New legislation could also overcome other impediments to comprehensive reform of nutrition labeling. Currently, two federal agencies—FDA and USDA—share responsibility for regulating food labels. They have generally worked in a cooperative fashion, but never with complete unity on issues of food labeling. FDA took the initiative in adopting the first nutrition labeling requirements. Although both agencies sponsored the Committee's study, only FDA (with the support of the U.S. Department of Health and Human Services [DHHS]) has taken the first steps to implement reforms. Some USDA officials, by contrast, have publicly expressed skepticism about the need to change nutrition information requirements. The Committee believes that successful reform of nutrition labeling requires FDA and USDA to work in tandem. For consumers to be able to use nutrition labeling in choosing food and thereby translate the advice of the Surgeon General and NRC into practice, nutrition labeling should be comprehensive and uniform. Legislation that mandates consistency and places both agencies on the same schedule for implementing nutrition labeling reform could obviate many of the problems that often beset administrative efforts to achieve agreement between departments in the executive branch.

There is one other justification for legislation authorizing the food labeling reforms that the Committee recommends. The seriousness of the issues implicated by contemporary understanding of the relationships between diet and chronic disease, the significant role of food in social and community patterns, and the importance of the commercial interests involved in the production, distribution, and sale of food in the United States make seemingly small disputes over labels important issues of national policy. In the U.S. political system, Congress is the appropriate arena for the resolution of such issues and the adjustment of such interests.

Accordingly, the Committee broadly supports the current efforts within Congress to fashion and enact sound nutrition labeling legislation promptly. This judgment, however, is accompanied by clear views about what such legislation should and should not include. These subjects are discussed in the following section.

DESIGN OF FOOD LABELING LEGISLATION

This section recommends approaches to the major issues implicit in the Committee's recommendation that Congress should enact new legislation that addresses nutrition labeling of foods.

Goals of New Legislation

New food labeling legislation could serve many goals. From the perspective of the Committee, whose members believe that improvements in current labels are necessary and that many more foods should be accompanied by nutrition labeling, the central objectives are (1) to establish, beyond question, the legal authority of FDA and USDA to require nutrition labeling on all packaged foods within their jurisdiction and (2) to confirm that the agencies may require point-of-purchase nutrition information for produce, seafood, meats, poultry, and foods sold in restaurants.

New legislation should also effect reforms in food labeling that are compatible with modern science and promote improved eating habits as quickly as practicable. Thus, statutory provisions that facilitate the prompt adoption of regulations for the implementation of nutrition labeling are desirable. Any new legislation should afford FDA and USDA flexibility in prescribing the content and format of nutrition labeling. Scientific understanding of the relationship between nutrition and long-term health will not remain static during the next decade, and research may reveal new connections that should be reflected in nutrition labeling.

Central Issues To Be Resolved

Clarification of FDA and USDA Authority To Mandate Nutrition Labeling

It is essential that new legislation lay to rest all doubt that FDA and USDA have the authority to require that labels on all packaged foods within their jurisdiction bear nutrition information.

Coverage of Fresh Fruits and Vegetables

The Committee favors legislation that clearly empowers FDA to require point-of-sale nutrition information for produce, with the understanding that implementation may be postponed until analytical methods or data bases are better developed and may require modifications of the requirements for labels on conventional packages. Almost any form of point-of-sale nutrition information, whether in the form of placards, brochures, or tear-off notices, would fall within the current FD&C Act's definition of *labeling*, and that is the general term used here.

The Committee believes that the precise timing, the authorized method(s) for nutrition labeling of produce, and the role, if any, of data bases rather than analytical results should be worked out by FDA and should not be fixed by statute. The Committee supports the issuance of implementing regulations for nutrition labeling by a certain date, however, to make clear that the benefits of providing nutrition information have already been judged to outweigh the costs.

Coverage of Fresh and Frozen Meats and Poultry

Fresh and frozen meats and poultry should also be subject to mandatory nutrition labeling as soon as nutrient data bases have been established for use on these foods. The Committee recognizes that some modification of the requirements applicable to processed meat and poultry products may be necessary. Again, the Committee favors legislation that mandates the adoption of some form of point-of-sale nutrition information program by a certain date but leaves its design to USDA.

Coverage of Fresh and Frozen Seafood

The Committee urges that the same approach be followed in mandating nutrition labeling for fresh and frozen seafood as recommended above for fresh and frozen meats and poultry, and produce.

Coverage of Foods Sold in Restaurants

The Committee believes that the general authority of FDA and USDA to require nutrition information for foods sold in restaurants should be confirmed by legislation. The Committee's primary recommendation is that nutrition labeling should be mandated for foods offered by limited-menu restaurants, which are generally required to conform to system-wide composition and quality standards. It also recommends that other restaurants be required, on request, to provide their customers with nutrition information. Legislation that confirms the general authority of FDA and USDA should suffice for both purposes. Congress should not, however, purport to decide precisely how such information is to be provided. Because FDA and USDA potentially share jurisdiction over food sold in restaurants, their cooperation will be necessary for any nutrition information program to work, and Congress may wish to consider mandating a schedule for implementation, periodic progress reports, or other measures to ensure timely accomplishment of the goal of providing restaurant customers with point-of-sale information about this increasingly important segment of Americans' diets.

Issues of Label Content

Required Components

A threshold issue is whether new legislation should specify any of the dietary components that are to be required or allowed in nutrition labeling. The Committee believes that it would, in principle, be desirable to leave decisions about content to FDA and USDA, allowing the two agencies to respond to changes in scientific knowledge about nutrition and the relationships between diet and chronic disease. It may be unrealistic, however, to believe that Congress would confer such unchanneled authority, particularly when recommendations of agency scientists and nutrition experts will confront departmental and Office of Management and Budget review. However, if new legislation is to specify components that must be described in nutrition labeling, the Committee urges a restrained approach.

The factors to consider in deciding which components should always be included in nutrition labeling are a matter of debate, but the Committee suggests two. Components whose aggregate consumption should be restricted should be included. Based on current knowledge, this category includes fat, saturated fatty acids, cholesterol, and sodium. On the same basis, the Committee believes that legislation should require that labeling include the number of calories per serving. Components whose consumption should be increased should also be included. This category includes complex carbohydrates. The Committee does not believe that declaration of protein should be mandated by statute, even though inclusion of protein in nutrition labeling is currently required by FDA regulations and is among the mandatory components of the Committee's recommended label. There is evidence that many Americans now consume too much protein, and whether it should continue to be mandated (rather than simply permitted) in nutrition labeling ought to remain a matter of administrative judgment.

Inclusion of fiber in nutrition labeling should also be left to administrative judgment. There is evidence that consumption of dietary fiber may affect the risk of certain cancers, but this evidence is by no means conclusive. The recommended consumption of complex carbohydrates and more fruits and vegetables generally ensures adequate fiber intake. The Committee believes that the current evidence is sufficient to warrant an administrative requirement that fiber content be required in nutrition labeling, but concedes that the evidence could look very different a decade from now. Accordingly, this information should not be mandated by statute.

The Committee believes that decisions about all other components be left to FDA and USDA, with confidence that they would generally agree with the Committee that calcium, iron, and sodium should also be mandated by regulation.

As the foregoing discussion makes clear, the Committee draws a distinction between components that should be required by agency regulations and components that should be mandated by statute. The enactment of legislation is a slow process. That the food labeling provisions of the FD&C Act have remained essentially unchanged for over 50 years demonstrates that legislation in this field is not likely to be updated frequently. The Committee favors new legislation only on the assumption that it will be drafted to allow the administering agencies freedom to update and revise their labeling requirements as the discoveries of science and the realities of the marketplace dictate.

Serving Size

The Committee is persuaded that "serving" is the best, although by no means the ideal, reference for conveying information about the nutrient content of foods to U.S. consumers. Accordingly, FDA and USDA should continue to require that nutrition information be stated per serving. They should also prescribe uniform serving sizes for major food categories.

It does not appear to be feasible, nor would it be wise, for Congress to attempt to specify serving sizes for different food categories. Indeed, the Committee is not persuaded that Congress should mandate that serving be the standard reference for nutrition information. Experience may demonstrate that some other reference standard is more readily understood by consumers or, even if not superior, better serves other objectives (such as unencumbered international commerce in packaged foods). Changes in the ways that foods are marketed and, perhaps, even in the ways or frequency with which they are consumed may render the concept of serving obsolete. The possibility that per serving references will not always prove to be the best standard for providing nutrition information argues against including such a requirement in legislation.

Two features of the current regimen do, however, require legislative attention. The first is the proliferation of serving sizes described on food labels. To reduce confusion in the marketplace, FDA and USDA should be directed to adopt regulations that establish one or more uniform standards for providing nutrition information.

A second troublesome feature of the current regimen is the reported disparity between serving sizes sanctioned by FDA and those formally approved by USDA. There may be instances in which such disparities can be justified, but they should have to be justified. Thus, if new legislation were to address the serving size (i.e., reference standard) issue, it should direct the two agencies to adopt uniform serving sizes (or other reference standards) for purposes of food labeling.

Descriptors

The Committee studied the current law and regulations governing nutrient content descriptors (or content claims), such as *low calorie, no fat,* and *high in fiber.* FDA and USDA should adopt uniform definitions of the most commonly used descriptors, though it is not likely to be feasible to standardize all of the phrases that manufacturers might wish to use to characterize their products. The question to be addressed is whether new food labeling legislation should expressly confer on the agencies authority to adopt uniform definitions. The Committee believes that current law provides the two agencies adequate legal authority to implement its recommendations on descriptors. Both agencies have already defined a number of descriptors (e.g., *low sodium*), and their legal authority to do so has not been challenged. However, the Committee agrees that if new legislation is to be enacted to resolve other questions of FDA and USDA authority, it should include explicit language confirming their power to define, through informal rulemaking, commonly used food descriptors. FDA and USDA should also have the authority to prohibit the use of any defined descriptor on a food that does not conform to the definition. Legislation should not attempt to specify the descriptors appropriate for definition or the components for which descriptors should be defined.

Prohibition of Descriptors

The Committee was troubled by labels that focus attention on the low level or absence of a constituent, such as cholesterol, on foods that contain high levels of other constituents whose consumption should be curtailed, such as saturated fatty acids or sodium. Another troubling practice is the use of a descriptor such as *no cholesterol* on a food, such as a banana, that has never contained cholesterol and would not ordinarily be thought of as a source of cholesterol. Both declarations are misleading, not because they are incomplete but because they exploit consumer misperceptions.

One response to such practices would be to forbid the use of descriptors under such circumstances. FDA and USDA should have the authority to forbid the use of descriptors when no full-disclosure alternative seems satisfactory. (An illustration of such an alternative would be something like *no cholesterol; high in saturated fat*.) Although both agencies probably already have such authority, either through product-specific enforcement actions or by general regulation, confirmation in new legislation would not be unwelcome. Prohibition of factually accurate, but misleadingly incomplete, content claims should, however, be a last resort. In most cases it should suffice to require the labels of foods to tell the whole truth about their nutritional composition. This could mean requiring a food whose label features a desired trait—for example, *cholesterol free*—to accord equivalent prominence to undesired traits such as *high in fat*.

The Committee accordingly recommends that new legislation confirm FDA's and USDA's legal authority to require, by regulation, such affirmative disclosures as are needed to ensure that labels are not misleading and to prohibit misleading, although factually accurate, statements when affirmative disclosures are not likely to prevent consumer deception.

Prohibition of Labeling of Constituents

The nutrition label that the Committee recommends (see Chapter 7) does not include all of the components that are currently required by FDA's nutrition labeling regulations, much less all of the components for which Recommended

Dietary Allowances have been established by the Food and Nutrition Board of the National Research Council or that sellers of food may desire to list. A label that included all of the mandated components and dozens of others added to or present in a food would often be difficult to read or understand. The question arises, therefore, whether FDA and USDA should be empowered to prohibit the listing of any components on the grounds that (1) they are not useful in human nutrition or are inevitably consumed in adequate quantities or (2) that their appearance crowds the label and risks confusion.

Although sympathetic with the concerns reflected in this reasoning, the Committee is reluctant to endorse any categorical ban on the truthful listing of nutrition components, absent a convincing showing that this is the only means of preventing consumer confusion. The Committee does, however, believe that FDA and USDA should be able to restrict the nutrition panel to specific components and to require that any other components that the seller chooses to include appear elsewhere on the label. Current law appears to provide FDA and USDA with this authority.

Exceptions from Mandatory Labeling

FDA and USDA already possess, and sometimes exercise, the authority to modify their general labeling requirements for specific foods. This authority to modify or, in appropriate cases, even to waive requirements is essential to the practicability of any comprehensive system of nutrition labeling. Explicit confirmation of this authority would be desirable, but it should be general rather than itemized. It would be appropriate for new legislation to describe, in general terms, the kinds of justifications that might support modifications of or exemptions from standard labeling requirements (e.g., small size of the package, lack of nutritional contribution, and perhaps even the modest resources of the manufacturer), but it should not codify exemptions. Final decisions about which foods or firms should be exempted from requirements or eligible for reduced requirements should remain with FDA and USDA.

Label Format Issues

Basic Label Design

Chapter 7 discussed the factors that should be weighed in prescribing a standard format for nutrition labeling. The Committee does not endorse a single format, and legislation should not do so either. Legislation should direct FDA and USDA to develop and then test different formats and ultimately specify, by regulation, a uniform format that must be followed by all sellers of food. (The issue of FDA-USDA uniformity is addressed in more detail below.)

Modifications of Standard Format

The two agencies should be empowered to approve modifications of the standard format in appropriate cases. For example, it may be appropriate to allow foods that contain very few of the mandatory components of nutrition labeling to use an abbreviated version of the standard format, although the Committee does not endorse such modifications for foods that are lacking in desirable components. It also appears clear that some changes, modifications, or alternative modes of presentation will be required for foods in very small packages.

There is an obvious tension between the goal of label uniformity, which will facilitate consumer use of nutrition labeling, and the possible need for modification for specific foods or markets. The Committee believes that uniformity should be a very high priority and that the burden of justifying adjustments of the uniform nutrition labeling format should rest on those who seek them. Legislation should not attempt, however, to determine whether that burden has been met; FDA and USDA are better equipped to resolve such claims on a case-by-case basis.

Process for Adopting a Standard Format

A single format should apply to all packaged foods, and for the purposes of this discussion, it is assumed that a uniform format will be agreed to by FDA and USDA.

The Committee is not convinced that there is one best procedure for deciding on the appropriate format for nutrition labeling. FDA and USDA should participate jointly in the effort, and their implementing regulations should be issued contemporaneously. The importance of interagency consistency is such that the Committee favors a statutory requirement that obliges either agency to justify publicly why it declines to subscribe to a common resolution of any format issue.

In the Committee's judgment, the process for selecting the standard label format should allow comment from members of the public, and it should accord substantial weight to the views of individuals in three sectors in particular: (1) the professional nutrition community, (2) experts in consumer understanding and behavior, and (3) state and local health and regulatory authorities. A statutory advisory committee might be a useful vehicle for ensuring that the views of individuals in these sectors are adequately considered.

It seems likely that the standard label format will require periodic revision as understanding of nutrition and health is improved by science, as food consumption patterns change, and as merchandising practices evolve. Accordingly, the Committee believes that a mechanism should be put in place for considering and recommending desired changes, including revisions in the content of the standard label.

Legislation should not describe in detail the process for establishing the standard label format. It should merely (1) direct that the job be done, (2) prescribe a deadline for its completion, and (3) mandate consideration of the views of the public and those in the three sectors mentioned above.

Institutional Issues

The Committee considered a cluster of issues surrounding allocation of responsibility for regulating food labeling, including the wisdom of the current bifurcation of federal authority between FDA and USDA, the occasions and justifications for discrepancies between FDA and USDA labeling requirements, the impact of the distinction between USDA's system of advance label approval and FDA's system of post hoc enforcement, and the sensitive issue of the power of the states to regulate the labels of foods sold within their borders. Although some of these topics were not directly relevant to the Committee's charge, it was quickly apparent that judgments on the central issues of content and format required a thorough understanding of the institutional setting of federal label regulation. Furthermore, the achievement of some of the Committee's goals, such as broadened coverage and uniformity of nutrition labeling, may depend on which agency exercises authority in this field.

FDA and USDA Uniformity

The Committee believes that different approaches to providing nutrition information on food labels diminish the utility of labels to consumers and impede efforts to increase nutritional literacy. Although no single label format is perfect and debate over the components that should be required (or allowed) in nutrition labeling is to be expected, it is essential that one format be established and that a single list of mandatory components be prescribed by federal law. Therefore, the Committee was concerned about reports that FDA and USDA often differ in what they require or allow on food labels and that they have sometimes embraced conflicting positions on identical issues, such as the criteria for approving reduced-fat claims on food labels. A detailed comparison of FDA and USDA labeling requirements was not undertaken, but it was the Committee's impression that the charges of inconsistency are exaggerated. They are not, however, groundless.

Federal requirements for food labels should be uniform, and the Committee recommends that legislation should mandate uniformity, subject to narrow exceptions. There may be instances in which the marketing context, the character of a food, or the use of a food may justify different approaches even on common questions. Thus, legislation should not demand uniformity without exception;

it should require that either agency provide for the record justifications for distinctive approaches for labeling specific foods, justification couched in terms that are relevant to the goals of nutrition labeling (e.g., consumer health and understanding).

The Committee also believes that requirements for nutrition labeling should be spelled out in regulations and not left to case-by-case decisionmaking. Legislation should require both FDA and USDA to adopt implementing regulations by a fixed date.

Consolidation of Labeling Authority

From time to time, individuals familiar with federal food labeling control have suggested that the authority to regulate labeling for all foods should be placed in a single federal agency, either FDA or USDA. The Committee did not closely study the implications of placing federal labeling authority exclusively in FDA or USDA, although the case for doing so is not obvious. The Committee also concluded that any recommendation made on this subject would entirely obscure the central objective: to improve nutrition labeling expeditiously.

Choice of Regulatory Mode

The Committee gave greater attention to the different modes of implementing labeling requirements by FDA and USDA. USDA requires approval in advance for all labels of meat and poultry products. FDA, by contrast, establishes labeling requirements by regulation and attempts to secure compliance through a combination of advice giving, publicity, and periodic enforcement proceedings. The latter type of system is obviously more vulnerable to budgetary constraints and personnel cutbacks, which slow the issuance of new regulations and diminish private expectations of enforcement. In the USDA context, resource cutbacks chiefly produce delays in label approval. In the USDA system, since no label may be used until it has been approved, marketplace behavior and official prescription, at least in theory, always coincide.

These significant differences prompted the Committee to reflect on whether FDA should be empowered to require advance approval of all labels used on foods within its jurisdiction. (It would seem imprudent for USDA to relinquish the kind of control it is able to exert over the labels of foods within its jurisdiction.) Practicality, however, prompted the Committee to refrain from recommending such a scheme. Its implications for FDA's budget would be dramatic and, thus, would surely be unsustainable as a political matter. The Committee therefore assumed that FDA will continue to regulate nutrition labeling in the mode it now employs, a mode that almost inevitably results in some gap between the requirements of the law and regulations and the labeling practices that actually occur. It is critical, however, that FDA have the resources it needs to effect a high level of compliance with its labeling requirements.

National Uniformity

National uniformity of food labeling is a controversial issue, one on which views are strongly held and fiercely defended. Resolution of the issue will affect the achievement of the Committee's goals of improved nutrition labeling and increased nutrition literacy.

The Committee believes that uniform federal requirements for nutrition labeling should apply nationwide and that state and local governments presumably should not be able to require different or additional nutrition information on food labels or in nutrition labeling. Legislation should include language that would accomplish this goal.

The Committee's position does not include or imply support for, or for that matter opposition to, proposals to preempt labeling requirements by states whose purpose is to warn consumers about the health risks thought to be associated with individual foods. It does mean that no state should ordinarily be able to require that food labels include nutrient information that is not mandated by FDA or USDA regulations. Nor should a state be able to adopt a different definition of any descriptor whose meaning has been established by federal statute regulation. In principle, the Committee believes that any food that bears nutrition labeling meeting federal requirements should be marketable in every state.

The Committee acknowledges, however, that there may conceivably be circumstances in which local needs might justify some compromise of this principle. To allow for that possibility, legislation could permit a state to seek FDA approval for requiring specific additional nutrition information on specific foods sold within its borders. The sort of provision visualized by the Committee is similar to one that Congress included in the 1976 Medical Devices Amendments to the FD&C Act, and could direct FDA to consider both the scientific basis of a state's claim and the impact of its recognition on the interstate movement and cost of food. No proposal that would prevent the sale of complying foods in other states would be approvable; a state should not be allowed to require label information that another state forbids, thereby forcing sellers to adopt two different labels.

This recommendation is made with the awareness that two of the three key federal food labeling statutes—the FMI Act and the PPI Act—currently provide, without qualification, for preemption of state and local labeling requirements. By contrast, the FD&C Act does not displace state labeling requirements; only if there is a clear conflict with federal requirements or if FDA determines that a specific requirement should be exclusive are state regulations displaced. The Committee could discern no sound justification for this disparity. However, pragmatism leads the Committee to refrain from recommending any change in the USDA-administered statutes.

State Participation in Setting Federal Labeling Standards

The recommendation described above reflects a judgment that national label uniformity and easy movement of foods throughout the United States are important goals. The Committee also recognizes, however, the strong interests of state and local public health officials in ensuring that their citizens are well informed about the nutrient content of foods. Furthermore, the Committee recognizes that federal agencies must often depend on the assistance of state officials to enforce federal requirements. Two steps would strengthen state-federal cooperation in this area.

A formal mechanism such as a national food labeling committee that would include representatives of state governments that would advise FDA and USDA on the design of nutrition labeling requirements could increase the willingness of states to collaborate in enforcement and, perhaps, persuade federal authorities to fashion their requirements to reflect states' interests. Such a committee could be established without new legislation, but a legislative mandate to FDA and USDA to form such a committee would ensure implementation of this inexpensive proposal.

The second step would be more controversial because it would have financial resource implications. If state and local regulatory officials are going to be needed as partners in enforcing requirements to improve the content and broaden the coverage of nutrition labeling, as would surely be true if the Committee's recommendations for labeling produce, fresh and frozen meats, poultry, and seafood, and some foods sold in restaurants were implemented, federal financial assistance to states and localities may be essential. Congress should consider this suggestion either as part of new labeling legislation or in conjunction with other proposals for federal aid to local public health programs.

Timing of Implementation

Several current bills to expand federal authority to regulate food labeling provide for a specific date by which, except for administrative approval of exceptions, new labeling regulations must be complied with. The Committee is eager to see its recommendations or other sound recommendations for improving the nutrition information on food labels implemented quickly. It is more important, however, to set deadlines for the administrative development of new labeling regulations than to fix the date by which all foods must be in compliance. It would be appropriate for new legislation to fix dates for action by the two agencies. The Committee is less confident that a statutory schedule for private-sector compliance that allows for administrative exceptions would expedite implementation of new labeling rules.

Other Legislative Changes

Ingredient Labeling

The Committee recommends two changes in the current rules governing ingredient labeling for foods. First, all sugars in a food should be aggregated—and named individually, albeit perhaps in the alternative—for purposes of listing in order of predominance. Implementation of this recommendation would not require legislation.

Second, manufacturers of all foods covered by FDA standards of identity should be required to list ingredients in the same manner as other FDA-regulated foods. This will require Congress to amend sections 403(g) and 403(i) of the FD&C Act to eliminate the current language, which indicates that only those optional ingredients specified by the standard need to be listed. Ingredients of meat and poultry products for which USDA has adopted standards of identity are generally already required to be listed.

Procedure for Adopting and Amending FDA Standards of Identity

A more careful study of the nutrition implications of FDA standards of identity might lead to the conclusion that the current system of standards should be substantially revised or even abandoned. One need not have arrived at firm judgments about the current appropriateness of food standards, however, to be confident that the current procedures for adopting and amending standards should be changed. The arguments for such change were presented above. Accordingly, the Committee recommends that Congress repeal section 701(e) of the FD&C Act (and other requirements for formal rulemaking). Alternatively, it should amend this provision to exclude the reference to standards of identity adopted pursuant to section 401 of the Act. Either form of amendment would leave FDA, in adopting, amending, or repealing standards of identity, subject to the conventional rulemaking procedures of the Administrative Procedure Act (5 USC § 553).

Implementing Reform if Congress Fails To Act

The Committee believes that the advantages of new legislation outweigh the disadvantages, which are not negligible. It is possible, however, that Congress may fail to act in the near future to clarify the authority of FDA and USDA to reform and broaden their nutrition labeling requirements. It is also possible that one or both agencies may decide to proceed with reforms without, or while awaiting, new legislation. These interrelated scenarios raise several questions, two of which the Committee addressed.

FDA Action in the Absence of New Legislation

The nutrition labeling legislation currently pending in Congress addresses the authority and obligations of FDA. There are probably greater uncertainties about FDA's than USDA's authority to implement the Committee's recommendations for reform. Nonetheless, FDA and DHHS have already initiated rulemaking to revise and expand current nutrition labeling requirements for foods within FDA's jurisdiction. FDA's notice of proposed rulemaking asserts that the proposed reforms can all be supported by its current statutory authority.

Although the Committee is not as confident as FDA that its assertions of authority will be sustained, the chances are likely enough that the agency should proceed with its rulemaking even in the absence of confirmatory or clarifying legislation.

This statement should not be understood to mean that the Committee endorses all substantive features of FDA's proposals. Some are essentially congruent with the Committee's recommendations; some are compatible with the Committee's views. Others, however, reflect different judgments about the information to be included, how information should be expressed, and the foods to be covered. With respect to these differences the Committee stands by the conclusions and recommendations set forth in this report.

USDA Action in the Absence of New Legislation

USDA does not appear to confront the same uncertainties about either legal authority or likely congressional action that FDA currently faces. Nor has USDA yet shown the same interest in broadening the coverage or reforming the content of its requirements for nutrition labeling of meat and poultry products.

The Committee believes that, whether or not Congress acts to clarify and direct FDA's authority to reform nutrition labeling, USDA should promptly initiate administrative proceedings to implement the recommendations set forth in this report. The Committee is satisfied that USDA currently has adequate legal authority to adopt all, or surely most, of these recommendations. Moreover, the Committee regards USDA action in this arena as essential for accomplishment of the desired long-term nutrition goals set forth in the reports of the Surgeon General (DHHS, 1988) and NRC (1989). Indeed, the most serious common deficiency of the bills pending in Congress for broadening nutrition labeling is their failure to cover the foods regulated by USDA. The reasons for this omission may be understandable in political terms, but it remains a deficiency nonetheless. The Committee urges USDA to join with FDA in leading the overdue effort to enhance and expand the information that U.S. consumers are provided about the nutritional quality of the foods they consume.

REFERENCES

DHEW/USDA/FTC (U.S. Department of Health, Education, and Welfare, U.S. Department of Agriculture, and Federal Trade Commission). 1979. Food Labeling Background Papers. Government Printing Office, Washington, D.C. 124 pp.

DHHS (U.S. Department of Health and Human Services). 1988. The Surgeon General's Report on Nutrition and Health. Government Printing Office, Washington, D.C. 727 pp.

GMA (Grocery Manufacturers of America). 1989. Statement by Sherwin Gardner, Vice President, Science and Technology, Grocery Manufacturers of America, Inc., to the Committee on the Nutrition Components of Food Labeling, Food and Nutrition Board, Institute of Medicine, Washington, D.C., December 4, 1989.

Hutt, P.B. 1989. Regulating the misbranding of food. Food Technol. 43(9):288.

Hutt, P.B., and R.A. Merrill. 1990. Food and Drug Law: Cases and Materials. The Foundation Press, Mineola, N.Y. In press.

Kushner, G.J., R.S. Silverman, S.B. Steinborn, and R.A. Johnson. 1990. A Guide To Federal Food Labeling Requirements. Prepared for the U.S. Department of Health and Human Services and the U.S. Department of Agriculture. Government Printing Office, Washington, D.C. 37 pp.

Merrill, R.A., and P.B. Hutt. 1980. Food and Drug Law: Cases and Materials. The Foundation Press, Mineola, N.Y. 959 pp.

NRC (National Research Council). 1989. Diet and Health: Implications for Reducing Chronic Disease Risk. Report of the Committee on Diet and Health, Food and Nutrition Board, Commission on Life Sciences. National Academy Press, Washington, D.C. 750 pp.

Young, F. 1989. Testimony before the Subcommittee on Health and the Environment, Committee on Energy and Commerce, U.S. House of Representatives, Washington, D.C., August 3, 1989.

APPENDIXES

A

Participants at the Public Meeting Held by the Committee on the Nutrition Components of Food Labeling December 4, 1989

SANDRA BARTHOLOMEY, Manager, Nutrition Laboratory, Gerber Products Company

SUSAN BRAVERMAN, Director-at-Large, The American Dietetic Association

J.B. CORDARO, President, Council for Responsible Nutrition

SHERWIN GARDNER, Vice President of Science and Technology, Grocery Manufacturers of America

HILARIE HOTING, Vice President for Nutrition, American Meat Institute

MICHAEL JACOBSON, Executive Director, Center for Science in the Public Interest

JAMES MARSDEN, Vice President for Science and Technical Affairs, American Meat Institute

ALLEN MATTHYS, Director, Technical and Regulatory Affairs, National Food Processors Association

ELAINE McLAUGHLIN, Nutritionist, United Fresh Fruit and Vegetable Association

MONICA OLSEN, Nutrition Scientist, National Dairy Council

CLAIRE REGAN, Research Manager, National Restaurant Association

SARAH SETTON, Vice President of Public Affairs, The Sugar Association, Inc.

ANN WINSLOW, Director of Nutrition, National Cattlemen's Association

B

Participants at Workshops Conducted by the Committee on the Nutrition Components of Food Labeling

Workshop on Label Content
February 7, 1990

DAVID KRITCHEVSKY, Associate Director, Wistar Institute
JUDY MARLETT, Professor, Department of Nutrition Science, University of Wisconsin–Madison
DONALD McCORMICK, Professor and Chair, Department of Biochemistry, School of Medicine, Emory University
WALTER MERTZ, Director, Human Nutrition Research Center, Agricultural Research Service, U.S. Department of Agriculture
LEON PROSKY, Deputy Chief, Experimental Nutrition Branch, Division of Nutrition, Center for Food Safety and Applied Nutrition, Food and Drug Administration, U.S. Department of Health and Human Services
JANET TENNEY, Manager of Nutrition Programs, Giant Food, Inc.

Workshop on Legal Issues Surrounding Food Labeling
February 16, 1990

EDWARD DUNKLEBURGER, Covington and Burling
RICHARD FRANK, Olsson, Frank and Weeda
THOMAS SCARLETT, Hyman, Phelps and McNamara

WILLIAM SCHULTZ, Counsel, Subcommittee on Health and the Environment, Committee on Energy and Commerce, U.S. House of Representatives

BRUCE SILVERGLADE, Director of Legal Affairs, Center for Science in the Public Interest

MICHAEL TAYLOR, King and Spaulding

Workshop on Consumer Understanding and Use of Food Labels
March 13, 1990

CHERYL ACHTERBERG, Assistant Professor, Department of Nutrition, College of Health and Human Development, Pennsylvania State University

ROBERT GOULD, Vice President, Director of Research, Porter Novelli

JAMES HEIMBACH, Deputy Administrator, Human Nutrition Information Service, U.S. Department of Agriculture

JAMES HEISLER, Senior Vice President, Opinion Research Corporation

ALAN LEVY, Head, Research Staff, Division of Consumer Studies, Center for Food Safety and Applied Nutrition, Food and Drug Administration, U.S. Department of Health and Human Services

VICKIE PETERS, Manager, Marketing Research, American Heart Association

Workshop on Label Formats
April 25, 1990

MICHAEL AUDETTE, Marketing Manager, New Ventures, Stouffer Foods

JOHN BLAIR, Vice President, Marketing Research, The Quaker Oats Company

MICHAEL GOLDERMAN, Product Group Manager, ConAgra Frozen Foods

MICHAEL JACOBSON, Executive Director, Center for Science in the Public Interest

PAT KUNTZE, Deputy Associate Commissioner for Consumer Affairs, Office of Consumer Affairs, Food and Drug Administration, U.S. Department of Health and Human Services

GRAHAM MOLITER, President, Public Policy Forecasting, Inc.

RAY SCHUCKER, Director, Division of Consumer Studies, Center for Food Safety and Applied Nutrition, Food and Drug Administration, U.S. Department of Health and Human Services

CAROLE SUGARMAN, Staff Writer, *The Washington Post*

**Workshop on the Impact of Nutrition Labeling Options on Food
Package Design, Marketing, and Advertising
May 2, 1990**

MARGUERITE COPEL, Manager, Nutrition Communications, Simplesse
    Group, The NutraSweet Company

MAURICE COX, Director of Public Affairs, Pepsi-Cola Company

ROBBI RICE DIETRICH, Director, Government Affairs, Frito-Lay, Inc.

HAROLD J. HANDLEY, Vice President and General Manager, McCormick/
    Schilling Division, McCormick & Company, Inc.

ARTHUR W. HARCKHAM, Associate, Dixon & Parcels Associates

DORIS LENNON-THOMPSON, Manager, Consumer Nutrition Affairs, Con-
    sumer Center, Kraft General Foods

KELLY LEWIS, Brand Manager, Edible Oil Products Division, The Procter &
    Gamble Company

CHARLES F. MARTIN III, Vice President, Marketing Services, Kraft General
    Foods

CRAIG SHULSTAD, Director, Public Relations, General Mills

ROBERT K. WHERMANN, Senior Marketing Director, Kellogg Company

C

International Food Labeling

The Committee was cognizant of the larger environment in which U.S. food labeling reform was being considered. Sensitivity to the trends and developments in other countries is important in a world where trade and national economies depend on the ability of companies to sell goods on the international market. This Appendix briefly discusses the current guidelines of the European Community, the Codex Alimentarius Commission, and the results of an informal survey conducted to better understand the situation in specific countries.

EUROPEAN COMMUNITY

The efforts to create a single market by the end of 1992 for the 12 nations of the European Community (EC) will have an enormous impact on the composition of food products and on their labels. Many companies have already created and started advertising "Eurobrands," single brand names for products sold throughout Europe (Prokesch, 1990). In anticipation of this unified market, the Council of the European Community (the Council) recently adopted the *Directive on Nutrition Labeling for Foodstuffs* (the directive), which is a common position on nutrition labeling of food products that is a prelude to the establishment of a standardized format that will apply in all EC countries (CEC, 1990). The Council was inspired by the same concerns that are driving U.S. food labeling policies: the growing public interest in the relationship between nutrition and long-term health, the need for nutrition education of the public, and the need to improve diet to improve health. In its preamble to the directive, the Council noted that to appeal to the average consumer, "given the current low level of knowledge on the subject of nutrition, the information provided should be simple and easily understood" (CEC, 1990, p. 3).

The directive creates guidelines for voluntary nutrition labeling. Labeling would be mandatory only when a nutrition claim appears on a food package or in an advertisement for the product. Nutrition claims (descriptors) would be restricted to those related to calories, protein, carbohydrates, fat, fiber, and 18 vitamins and minerals. The directive applies to foodstuffs to be delivered ultimately to consumers and to products intended for mass caterers, such as restaurants and hospitals. Natural mineral or other waters intended for human consumption and diet integrators/food supplements are exempted. Nonpackaged foodstuffs sold ultimately to consumers or mass caterers and food products packaged at the request of the purchaser or prepackaged with a view to immediate consumption are to be covered by the laws of individual EC countries until the eventual adoption of measures for the EC as a whole.

Two formats for nutrition information are outlined in the directive, either of which may be used when nutrition labeling is voluntary or required. The first format includes only calories and protein, carbohydrate, and fat (in grams). The second adds sugars, saturated fats, fiber, and sodium. If a nutrition claim is made for sugars, saturated fatty acids, fiber, or sodium, the label must include the expanded format. In addition, a manufacturer may include information on starch, polyols, monounsaturated and polyunsaturated fatty acids, cholesterol, and any of the 18 vitamins or minerals, for which there are RDAs, that are present in significant amounts. A nutrition claim may be made for a nutrient only if the food provides 15 percent of the RDA. If the label lists polyunsaturated and/or monounsaturated fatty acids or cholesterol, it must also list the amount of saturated fatty acids.

Calories are to be described in a numeric format, expressed per 100 g, per 100 mg, or per 100 ml. The directive also allows the use of graphic formats in addition to the numerical listing, if permitted by the member country. In declaring sugars, polyols, or starch, the following format must be used:

- carbohydrate (g), of which:
  - sugar (g)
  - polyols (g)
  - starch (g)

Assessment of the amount or type of fatty acid or cholesterol must immediately follow the declaration of total fats, in the following format:

- fat (g), of which:
  - saturates (g)
  - monounsaturates (g)
  - polyunsaturates (g)
  - cholesterol (mg)

Declared values must be based on averages, as calculated from the (1) manufacturer's analysis of the food, (2) the known or actual average values of the ingredients used, or (3) generally established and accepted data.

The directive gives ample time for compliance by member countries. Within 18 months of final adoption of the directive, trade in complying products will be permitted. Three years after adoption, products that are not in compliance with the directive will be prohibited from trade. However, the requirements for labeling of sugars, saturated fatty acids, fiber, and sodium will not take effect for 5 years (CEC, 1990b). The directive also addresses the powers of individual countries to add to its requirements: "Member states shall refrain from laying down requirements more detailed than those already contained in this directive concerning nutrition labeling" (CEC, 1990a, p. 14).

CODEX ALIMENTARIUS COMMISSION

The Food and Agriculture Organization of the World Health Organization (FAO/WHO) established the FAO/WHO Codex Alimentarius Commission in 1962 (hereinafter referred to as Codex) to implement the Joint FAO/WHO Food Standards Program. As of June 1986, the Codex had 129 member countries. Codex guidelines for food labeling are outlined in the *Codex Alimentarius* (FAO/WHO, 1987). The announced purposes of these guidelines are to provide consumers with information so they can make wise food choices, to encourage improved formulation of foods, and to prevent deceptive nutrition labeling (FAO/WHO, 1987).

Codex guidelines contain advisory criteria and standards for the nutrition labeling of foods. The guidelines state that nutrient declarations should be mandatory on any food for which a nutrition claim is made (Codex sections 3.1–5.1), but voluntary for all other foods. When provided, energy value and amount of protein, available carbohydrate (not fiber), fat, and any other nutrient for which a nutrition claim is made should be declared. A carbohydrate claim also triggers the disclosure of total sugars. If a fatty acid claim is made, then saturated and polyunsaturated fatty acids should be declared. Vitamins and minerals present in significant amounts, defined as 5 percent of the recommended intake, should be declared only for those for which there are recommended intakes or those that are of nutritional importance to individuals in a particular country.

Nutrient content is to be presented in a numeric format, but additional depictions, such as graphics, are not prohibited. Information should be expressed per 100 g, 100 ml, or per package if it contains a single serving. Information may be provided per serving if the total number of servings is stated. Vitamin and mineral information may be expressed in metric units and/or as a percentage of the Recommended Dietary Intake (RDI) per 100 g, per 100 ml, or per package if it contains a single serving.

The guidelines prescribe a specific format for carbohydrate disclosure:

- Carbohydrate (g)
- x (g)
  - of which sugars (g)

Total carbohydrate may be followed by x (g), where x represents the specific name of any other carbohydrate constituent. For fatty acids the specified format is as follows:

- Fat (g)
  - of which polyunsaturated (g)
  - and saturated (g)

The Codex guidelines include provisions for supplementary information to be given in addition to the nutrient declaration mentioned above. Recognizing that there are individuals in the population who are illiterate and/or have little knowledge of nutrition, the guidelines suggest food group symbols or other pictorial or color presentations. Consumer education programs are urged to enhance nutrition labeling. Also recommended is a periodic review of nutrition labeling to keep pace with health information.

SURVEY OF FOOD LABELING IN OTHER COUNTRIES

In 1990, the Committee sent a questionnaire (see box) on two occasions to 32 respondents in 27 countries. Twenty-one replies to the first questionnaire were received from 18 countries and 10 replies to the second questionnaire were received from 10 countries. The countries included Belgium, Bulgaria, Canada, Denmark, Finland, the Federal Republic of Germany, Israel, Japan, Luxembourg, Monaco, The Netherlands, Norway, Portugal, Spain, Sweden, the United Kingdom, and the USSR; a reply was also received from the Council of the European Community. Eight respondents were members of the EC and, as such, they reported using the labeling provisions expected to be adopted in the near future. A brief summary of all responses is found in the survey summary box.

OBSERVATIONS ON INTERNATIONAL FOOD LABELING

As a result of this review, it is clear that there is a great deal of interest and activity in nutrition labeling in other industrialized nations. Most of this activity is inspired by the same concerns about diet and long-term health that led to the formation of the Institute of Medicine committee and to the interest in nutrition labeling by U.S. federal agencies and the U.S. Congress.

Even in nations with comparable standards of living, however, food produc-

Questionnaire Sent to Officials Working in
the Field of Food and Nutrition in 27 Countries
To Determine International Food Labeling Practices

1. Does your country have any regulations or guidelines concerning labeling at all?

    Yes   No   Do Not Know

2. Whose responsibility is it to inform users (i.e., those who decide on the design of labels) about these regulations or guidelines? (Name and address of responsible institution)

3. Please list the main groups of foods/commodities covered by labeling requirements, and indicate whether these are mandatory or voluntary.

4. What is the scope of the labeling regulation/guidelines?

    Do they cover ingredient listing?

    Yes   No   Do Not Know

    Do they cover nutrient presentation?

    Yes   No   Do Not Know

    Do they cover claims on foods or descriptions of foods?

    Yes   No   Do Not Know

5. What do the regulations/guidelines say about presentation of labeling concerning:

    Use of graphics or symbols

    Use of numbers (percentages, relative numbers, servings, other)

6. What are the reasons for choosing one mode of presentation over another?

7. Which nutrients are included in the presentation and why?

8. Does your country have an "officially" endorsed set of dietary guidelines?

    Yes   No   Do Not Know

9. Have labeling requirements been designed to correspond with the message in the dietary guidelines?

    Yes   No   Do Not Know

10. Do you have available any studies of how consumers perceive and use labeling?

    Yes   No   Do Not Know

If the answer is yes, could you please let the nutrition unit of the WHO Regional Office for Europe have a copy?

Summary of Responses to the 1990 Survey Sent to 27 Countries

Purposes of Labeling

The countries that responded to the questionnaires indicated that the purposes of nutrition labeling are to convey information to consumers to enable them to improve their diets, allow consumers to compare products and choose the better alternative, provide information for general health promotion purposes, avoid misleading information, standardize messages, and provide general information without further specification.

Responsibility for Labeling Regulations

Institutional responsibility for labeling regulations among the countries that responded to the questionnaire varied and included ministries of health, trade, or agriculture; consumers; and the national food agency. In most countries, however, ministries of health are responsible for nutrition labeling. Announcements of nutrition labeling requirements are generally made through some type of official gazette.

Food Supply Coverage

All countries reported that they have some form of food labeling regulation or guidelines. Ingredient labeling is mandatory and covers either all foods or all prepackaged foods. Ingredients that are required to be listed on food labels are specified. Nutrition labeling is voluntary in most of the responding countries except when nutrient-related claims are made, in which case it is mandatory. Several countries limit the types of claims that are allowed. A few countries have plans to implement mandatory nutrition labeling.

Relation to Dietary Guidelines

Six countries responded that they have publicly approved national dietary guidelines and that nutrition labeling requirements are designed to correspond with those guidelines. However, several countries did not explicitly state that national dietary recommendations and regulation of nutrition labeling are connected.

Presentation of Labeling

All European respondents use the metric system or percentages in nutrition labeling. Only Canada recently changed to using "per serving" as a basis for nutrition labeling. Three countries and the EC permit the use of per serving as a basis for nutrition labeling, but they also allow metric units.

Nutrients Covered

Most countries reported inclusion of the following items when nutrition labeling is used: energy, fat, protein, and carbohydrate. Few countries require vitamins or minerals in nutrition labeling, and in most countries, listing of vitamins and minerals is optional.

Consumer Studies

Studies on consumer perception of labeling were reported to have been conducted in half of the countries that responded to the questionnaires. Those studies were conducted in conjunction with the adoption or revision of nutrition labeling regulations.

tion and sales data display different dimensions. Mass catering has a larger role in Europe, where many workers are fed on the job. Sales of food at limited-menu restaurants are nowhere as significant a part of food sales as they are in the United States. Europeans are literate with regard to the metric system, whereas the U.S. population is resistant to changing from the English system. Advertising of foods is more prevalent and perhaps less controlled in the United States than it is elsewhere. Food variety is probably greater in the United States.

Foods must bear labels that meet local legal requirements. Foods produced in Europe for sale in the United States must bear labels that meet U.S. regulations and vice versa. Very few foods bear precisely the same label worldwide, and this is likely to remain true for the balance of the twentieth century. Thus, the United States needs its own system. The U.S. system, however, should be designed keeping in mind the interesting innovations that have been tried in other countries, to the extent that such innovations are consistent with domestic requirements, consumer desires, and dietary recommendations.

REFERENCES

CEC (Council of the European Communities). 1990a. Common Position Adopted by the Council of European Communities 1990 with a View to the Adoption of a Directive on Nutrition Labeling for Foodstuffs. European Council, Brussels. 17 pp.

CEC (Council of the European Communities). 1990b. Reexamined proposal for a Council Directive on nutrition labeling of foodstuffs. European Council, Brussels. 6 pp.

FAO/WHO (Food and Agriculture Organization of the United Nations, World Health Organization). 1987. Codex Alimentarius, vol. VI, 2nd ed. Food and Agriculture Organization of the United Nations, World Health Organization, Rome.

Prokesch, S. May 31, 1990. Eurosell Pervades the Continent. The New York Times. p. D1.

D

Food Standards and the Quest
for Healthier Foods

Alvin J. Lorman*

INTRODUCTION AND SUMMARY

In 1938, in order to protect the American public from what it perceived to be increasing debasement of the traditional food supply, Congress enacted legislation that authorized the Food and Drug Administration (FDA) to create legally binding "standards of identity"—or recipes—for foods. FDA took up this challenge with enthusiasm, and by 1950 about half of the consumer food dollar was spent on foods that were governed by food standards (or standardized). But in dictating the level of "valuable" ingredients that should be in specific foods, FDA understandably reflected the thinking of the country at that time. Thus, whereas today many Americans seek to reduce their intake of fat, saturated fat, and cholesterol, 30 years ago FDA adopted food standards that assured that manufacturers did not cheat consumers by providing lower levels of those ingredients. In short, ingredients considered valuable in a food 30 years ago may be considered that food's nutritional liability today.

With increased knowledge of the relationship between diet and health, it is fair to ask whether a government program originally adopted in 1938 to promote

*Alvin J. Lorman is a partner of the law firm Baker & Hostetler in Washington, D.C.

one set of nutritional values has successfully evolved so that it promotes the nutritional values of the 1990s.

This paper first reviews the history of FDA's implementation of its food standards authority and then examines the impact of food standards on the availability and the consumer acceptance of new and "healthier" versions of standardized foods.

For many decades, FDA enforced its food standards authority so as to impede the development of alternatives to standardized foods. At least since the 1970s, however, FDA has evidenced no hostility to the existence of modified standardized foods, but only to the use of the standardized name as part of the name of the substitute food. On the issue of nomenclature, however, FDA has tended to act in an ad hoc fashion and create confusion as to what the applicable rules are and has been unable to articulate a defensible rationale for whatever policy exists.

Several alternatives can remedy the current situation. First, the procedures for adopting and amending food standards could be relaxed by Congress so that procedural requirements do not serve to discourage the modification of standards. Second, FDA could adopt procedural regulations to streamline the cumbersome statutory process, as it has done when faced with similar statutory mandates, such as for withdrawing approval of new drugs. Third, a general rule could be adopted to permit the accurate use of defined descriptors, such as low-fat, with any food name, whether standardized or nonstandardized. Fourth, if altered versions of standardized foods are to be treated differently than altered versions of nonstandardized foods, as appears to be the current rule, FDA should, through public rulemaking, articulate a coherent distinction (if one exists) for the disparate treatment. Finally, Congress could abolish food standards entirely (or FDA could revoke them) on the grounds that informative labeling and an educated public obviate the need for standards that, no matter how liberally applied, inevitably have anticompetitive impacts and costs.

HISTORY OF FOOD STANDARDS

The Legislative Mandate

The Pure Food and Drug Act of 1906[1] was the first attempt at a comprehensive federal statute governing both the safety and the quality of food. Under the Act, which prohibited the adulteration or misbranding of food products,[2] the government had little trouble bringing adulteration cases against those who engaged in such traditional forms of economic cheating as diluting milk with water. More sophisticated forms of economic adulteration, however, often proved beyond the scope of the statute. Thus, when the government tried to condemn a product that was labeled as "Bred Spread," a fruit spread containing less fruit than jam would normally contain, the court held that the product was not adulterated jam, but a truthfully labeled unique product that contained less fruit than jam.[3]

Debasement of processed foods was sufficiently common that in 1930, at the behest of the canning industry, Congress authorized FDA to establish so-called standards of quality for canned foods.[4] These standards established the minimum quality necessary to employ a particular name without declaring the product to be "substandard."

Congress sought to comprehensively remedy the defects of the 1906 Act when it enacted the Federal Food, Drug, and Cosmetic Act of 1938.[5] In a dramatic departure from the 1906 Act, section 401 of the 1938 Act authorized FDA to promulgate definitions and standards of identity for foods.[6] The statutory mandate provides that:

> Whenever in the judgment of [FDA] such action will promote honesty and a fair dealing in the interest of consumers, [it] shall promulgate regulations fixing and establishing for any food, under its common or usual name so far as practicable, a reasonable definition and standard of identity . . . . In prescribing a definition and standard of identity for any food or class of food in which optional ingredients are permitted, [FDA] shall, for the purpose of promoting honesty and fair dealing in the interest of consumers, designate the optional ingredients which shall be named on the label . . . .[7]

Having thus concluded that FDA should be empowered to establish standards for foods, Congress also gave it the authority to enforce any standards it adopted. Congress provided that a food would be deemed to be misbranded:

> If it purports to be or is represented as a food for which a definition and standard of identity has been prescribed by regulations as provided by section 401, unless (1) it conforms to such definition and standard, and (2) its label bears the name of the food specified in the definition and standard . . . .[8]

A food that is not subject to a standard of identity is required to disclose its common or usual name, if there is one, and its ingredients, if it contains more than one.[9] Congress also continued the ban, found in the 1906 Act, against imitation foods, declaring a food misbranded "[i]f it is an imitation of another food, unless its label bears . . . the word 'imitation' and, immediately thereafter, the name of the food imitated."[10]

Procedural Requirements

Although Congress empowered FDA to issue food standards whenever in its "judgment" to do so would promote "honesty and fair dealing in the interest of consumers," it afforded FDA little leeway in the procedures to be followed to adopt a standard.[11] Congress enacted the Federal Food, Drug, and Cosmetic Act 8 years before the Administrative Procedure Act was adopted.[12] Thus, the concept of notice and comment rulemaking was essentially alien to Congress in 1938. Accordingly, Congress mandated, in section 701(e) of the Act, that food standards be adopted by formal rulemaking on a record, a process that combines elements of both rulemaking and adjudication.[13] The first step in this process is a proposal to create a standard, issued either by FDA on its initiative or by petition of any interested party to FDA. Interested parties may comment on the proposal orally or in writing. After receiving comments, FDA issues an order establishing the standard. Any person who disagrees with the standard may, within 30 days after entry of the order, file objections, stating the grounds therefore, and request a public hearing. The filing of the objections automatically stays the operation of the standard. At a public hearing, both FDA and those opposed to the standard introduce evidence and testimony, and witnesses are subject to cross-examination. At the conclusion of the hearing, FDA must issue an order, "based only on substantial evidence of record at such hearing . . . ." A person who disagrees with this final order can challenge it in the court of appeals. Even setting aside cases of notorious food standard proceedings, such as the one to define peanut butter,[14] the standard-setting process has proved more and more bothersome to FDA over time.

FDA IMPLEMENTATION OF FOOD STANDARDS

The Traditional Approach

Food standards are a potent force in the marketplace. The 1989 edition of Title 21 of the *Code of Federal Regulations* contains 257 discrete food standards regulations, some of which cover many foods. (For example, 21 CFR § 155.200 establishes a definition and standard of identity for "certain other canned vegetables." In fact, it is a generic standard covering 34 named canned vegetables.) At one time it was estimated that standardized foods account for approximately half of the supermarket bill of the American consumer.[15] There are 19 categories of food standards, although two categories alone—milk and cream, and cheese and cheese products—account for 104 discrete standards.

The largest single category of food standards is cheese and cheese products, totaling 73 discrete foods. The large number of standards in this category is probably a reflection of both the dairy industry's traditional belief in the use of standards to prevent imitations and competition as well as the facility with which large cheese companies managed to create new standards for their new products in the past.

For most of the past 52 years, FDA has enforced the food standards provision of the 1938 Act so as to serve as a disincentive, or at least a discouragement, to product innovation. For much of this period, it has probably done so intentionally, for the "innovation" of 30 years ago was often considered debasement rather than improvement. New products have evolved, however, sometimes by creating new standards and sometimes by adopting new common or unusual names acceptable to FDA. But, there is general agreement (if not evidence) that, until the 1970s, FDA stood in the way of product innovation. More recent standards have tended to be more broadly drawn, characterizing many ingredients as "optional," thus affording some flexibility in formulation and invoking the statutory requirement that optional ingredients be listed on the label.[16]

In examining the history of FDA implementation of food standards and related provisions, it is important to remember that the outcome was not mandated by statute nor was it necessarily suggested by public policy. Much of the history of food standards is guided by a narrow enforcement philosophy and by untested assumptions about how consumers will react to product labels. FDA's traditional protectiveness of the use of a standardized name as part of the name of a nonstandardized food seems to be based, in part, on the theory that the latter would be confused with the former, when it is the very difference between the two that industry is trying to promote. Yet, the early rigidity of food standards was amply supported by the congressional intent. The failure of the 1906 Act to effectively prevent the adulteration of food for economic reasons led to the passage of the food standards provisions in the 1938 Act. According to Congress, the evil to be remedied was that under the 1906 Act, "[t]he Government has had difficulty in holding such articles as commercial jams and preserves and many other foods to the time-honored standards employed by housewives and reputable manufacturers."[17] Accordingly, the early standards of identity adopted a "recipe" approach. The term "recipe" is used here in a very formal way: the right of a person to vary a recipe to either decrease the quantity of one ingredient and increase the quantity of another, or to substitute for an ingredient temporarily absent from the cupboard, was not provided to food manufacturers.

> Two objectives explain the FDA's prolonged adherence to its original recipe format: (1) a desire to preclude any modifications of basic food formulas that could contribute to consumer deception, and (2) a concern to restrain the growing use in food production of chemical additives if safety had not been demonstrated.[18]

The importance of food standards in the marketplace went far beyond the food being standardized. FDA broadly interpreted the prohibition against "purporting to be" a standardized food. Although a literal reading of "purports to be" might imply an attempt to "pass off" the substitute as the real thing, FDA took the position that any food, no matter how truthfully labeled, which looked like or tasted like a standardized food "purported to be" that food. Thus, establishment of a standard essentially outlawed foods similar to the product defined in the standard. In 1941, when FDA established standards for farina products and enriched farina products,[19] it outlawed the sale of a product that had been on the market for over 20 years: farina with vitamin D.[20] Since the product did not contain all of the vitamins specified in the enriched farina standard and the plain farina standard did not permit the addition of any vitamins, FDA argued that the product could not be sold at all. Because avoidance of consumer confusion is one of the goals of the food standards program, the court upheld this claim, stating that "the statutory purpose to fix a definition of identity of an article of food sold under its common or usual name would be defeated if producers were free to add ingredients, however wholesome, which are not within the definition."[21] This extraordinarily strict reading of the statutory provisions can most likely be explained by an inherent distrust on the part of FDA of the ability of consumers to detect differences in food products based on their labeling and by the agency's desire to have a simple black and white test for whether or not a product "purported to be" a standardized food.

The statutory ban against imitating another food product without disclosing that fact prominently was another tactic FDA used to protect the traditional ingredients of foods. Interestingly, because the penalty for purporting to be a standardized food is that the food cannot be marketed at all, the first litigated case involving the imitation prohibition involved an attempt to use it as a sword rather than as a shield. In *62 Cases of Jam v. United States,*[22] FDA argued that a product labeled as "imitation jam" could not be sold because it "purported" to be jam, a standardized food. "Delicious Brand Imitation Jam" contained only 25 percent fruit, rather than the 45 percent required by the applicable standard of identity.[23] The product was sold principally to institutional buyers rather than to consumers. FDA argued that the product "purported to be" jam, and was not, and thus could not be sold. Although the appellate court agreed, the Supreme Court did not. The court declined FDA's invitation to read "purports to be" and "imitation" as coextensive.

> Section 403(g) [which bans foods that purport to be standardized foods] was designed to protect the public from inferior foods resembling standard products but marketed under distinctive names . . . . Congress may well have supposed that similar confusion would not result from the marketing of a product candidly and flagrantly labeled as an "imitation" food.[24]

The imitation jam case thus permitted manufacturers to label a food as "imitation" and thus deviate from an applicable standard of identity while still using, in part, the standardized name. Because it has been generally believed by industry that the word "imitation" would be the kiss of death in the marketplace, imitation foods have succeeded, if at all, only in institutional settings where consumers do not make the purchase choice and do not see the product label.[25] Although FDA "lost" the imitation jam case, it was a Pyrrhic victory for industry. A conjunction of the readings of "purports to be" and "imitation" led to the following situation: A food that resembled a standardized food could not be sold, regardless of how informative its labeling, unless it called itself "imitation," a form of labeling that told the consumer only what the product was not, and which largely guaranteed that the product would not reach supermarket shelves.

FDA's war against "imitation" foods continued to erupt episodically. In 1953, FDA sought to brand as "imitation ice cream" a nondairy product that resembled ice cream in taste, color, texture, and melting properties.[26] The product, called Chil-Zert, was conspicuously labeled "not an ice cream" on all four sides of the carton, immediately below the product name. On two sides there appeared the disclaimer "contains no milk or milk fat!" The court agreed with FDA's assertion that Chil-Zert was an imitation ice cream, even though there was no evidence whatsoever that any misleading statements about the product had been made or that consumers would in any way be misled. Indeed, at the time, ice cream was not a standardized food.[27]

In 1966, FDA sought unsuccessfully to condemn a product labeled as "imitation margarine" which contained less fat than the level required for standardized margarine.[28] FDA's argument, that *all* products made in semblance of butter must be called margarine, was rejected by the court.

At the same time that the agency was enforcing its expansive view against using standardized names for substitute foods, it was also enshrining substitutes in standards of their own. Perhaps the best-known example of a standardized substitute food is margarine. In the cheese area, for example, there is pasteurized blended cheese, pasteurized processed cheese, pasteurized processed cheese food, pasteurized cheese spread, pasteurized processed cheese spread, and a host of similar products. Presumably, the same agency that believes that consumers would be confused by "nonfat" versions of standardized cheeses expects consumers to know the subtle distinctions between cheese and cheese food or between blended cheese and processed cheese. More obviously, FDA has defined ice cream, ice milk (ice cream with less milk fat), and mellorine (the ice cream–like product that may legally contain nondairy fats).

FDA's Policy Evolves

Two separate developments helped push FDA into resolving the conflicts created by its interpretation of food standards and substitutes for standardized foods. First, improvements in technology and an increased reliance upon processed foods by consumers made possible the development of a greater variety of foods which had not been traditionally part of the American diet. Second, starting in the late 1950s and accelerating through the 1960s, there was an increasing recognition of the role played by diet in development of certain chronic diseases, especially heart disease.[29] The 1970 report of the White House Conference on Food, Nutrition, and Health, which summarized the new learning and which criticized FDA's efforts to stigmatize as imitation many new and healthful substitute foods, helped push FDA to attempt to resolve the simmering conflict.[30]

In the 1970s, FDA began a concerted effort to ensure that foods were informatively labeled, rather than labeled with terms that revealed what the food was not. In a regulation announcing the agency's policy on common or usual names, FDA both announced the principles it would use in establishing common or usual names for food products (and which industry could use for the same purpose) and sought a way to impose regulatory standards on food products without the elaborate procedures and the commitment of agency resources required in a section 701(e) rulemaking.[31]

Similarly, in a regulation adopted in 1973, FDA for the first time defined the term "imitation" so that alternative or substitute foods could be formulated in such a way as to avoid the use of that stigmatized term.[32] The regulation provides that a food that is a substitute for and resembles another food would be considered an imitation only if it is nutritionally inferior to the food for which it substitutes and resembles. Nutritional inferiority was defined as a reduction in the content of an essential nutrient present at a level of 2 percent or more. Reflecting current thinking, however, a reduction in the caloric or fat content of the food did not signify nutritional inferiority. This regulation permitted manufacturers to produce variants of standardized foods and know that they could do so without running the risk of being branded an imitation. The regulation was upheld against challenge by consumers.[33]

Having defined objective criteria for avoidance of the term imitation, the agency attempted to apply nomenclature standards evenhandedly to substitutes for both standardized and nonstandardized foods. As one of the participants has described the change:

> In the early 1970's, FDA made the decision to apply the same policy in common and usual names to standardized and nonstandardized foods. Previously the Agency had taken a position that any new substitute for a standardized food was required to be labeled as an imitation but a new substitute for a nonstandardized food was not required to be so labeled. Dressings for salad illustrate the impact of this policy. FDA had promulgated a standard for French dressing, 21 C.F.R. § 169.115, but not for Italian or Russian dressing. Under its traditional policy a reduced calorie version of French dressing had to be labeled as imitation French dressing, but a reduced calorie version of Italian or Russian dressing could be described as "reduced calorie" Italian or Russian dressing. Under its new policy FDA took the position that the common or usual name for a nonstandardized food could *include* the name of the standardized food, as long as the difference between the products was made clear . . . . This new policy was intended to prevent standards of identity from operating as barriers to the development of new food products, especially new versions of traditional [foods] with micronutrient composition modified to meet national nutritional goals. Food

producers responded by developing dozens of new products with a reduced content of calories, sodium, cholesterol, and fat.[34]

By the mid-1970s, FDA's policy had changed so dramatically it was affirmatively stating that "tomato juice enriched with vitamin C" does not purport to be standardized tomato juice,[35] that enriched macaroni fortified with protein does not purport to be standardized enriched macaroni,[36] and that raisin bread, a standardized food, made with appropriately fortified flour could be sold as nonstandardized "enriched raisin bread."[37]

FDA's Current Policy

Many individuals thought that with the decisions and regulations cited above, the then-40-year-old dispute on naming nonstandardized versions of standardized foods had ended, but that assumption was wrong. Whether as a result of a conscious change in policy or simply regulation on an ad hoc basis without a written or explicit policy, FDA has once again asserted that the name of a new or modified food depends upon whether it is intended to substitute for a standardized or a nonstandardized food. (Indeed, the current director of the Center for Food Safety and Applied Nutrition said he is not aware that the unified naming policy had *ever* been FDA policy.[38]) For example, in a regulatory letter issued on May 1, 1986, FDA argued that a low-fat yogurt sweetened with concentrated fruit juice could not be called "yogurt" because fruit juice was not an acceptable sweetener under the standard of identity.[39] Other than the use of a nonrecognized sweetener, the product complied with the standard for low-fat yogurt. FDA recommended that the product be called "low fat yogurt substitute" or "flavor-cultured dairy dessert." To confuse the issue, on November 23, 1988, the agency stated in a letter that it was acceptable to call a food "lowfat yogurt with aspartame sweetener."[40] While inconsistent with its position 2 years earlier, this opinion appears to be consistent with FDA's current position (see p. 331).

The principal disputes today and in the near future over the use of standardized names in nonstandardized food products will involve reduced-calorie and reduced-fat versions of standardized foods. With over 100 food standards governing products with milk fat as a mandatory ingredient and at mandatory levels, "reduced-fat" labeling of standardized foods will continue to occupy a major portion of industry's efforts and FDA's objections. It is important to note that FDA does not object philosophically to all low-fat versions or reduced-fat versions of standardized foods that use the standardized name. Indeed, the agency has standardized many such foods itself. One of the more recent standards of identity is that for yogurt, low-fat yogurt, and nonfat yogurt. Most consumers are familiar with nonfat milk, low-fat milk, and milk, each a standardized food. It is only when a manufacturer on his attempts to apply the "low-fat" or "nonfat" terminology to a nonstandardized version of a standardized food and use the standardized name that FDA objects. FDA's position seems to be that consumers would be misled by a nonstandardized, low-fat version of a standardized dairy product such as sour cream, but that they are not misled when FDA itself determines the identity of yogurt and low-fat yogurt, for example. The assumption implicit in this distinction seems to be that consumers know which foods are standardized and which are not, and that that somehow makes a difference.

Industry's Views

The recent round of FDA hearings on food labeling issues demonstrated that there is no unified industry view on the role of food standards in today's marketplace. Understandably, attitudes appear to reflect the competitive position of the commentator as much as any deep philosophical position. For example, the dairy industry, whose products appear to be most under attack today because of the fat content of those products, takes the most inflexible approach. The recently completed *Report and Recommendations* of the National Commission on Dairy Policy, an organization of dairy producers created by Congress, proposed that FDA enforce existing food standards "to protect the consumer from fraud and deception" and more strictly enforce the misbranding provisions of the Act, "particularly with regard to non-standardized foods which purport to resemble foods for which standards of identity or common or usual names have been established."[41] The Commission took issue with FDA's definition of "imitation" as being based solely on nutritional inferiority and asked Congress to define the term imitation "to be applied to any food product that simulates a standardized food."[42]

Cheese makers are bearing the brunt of the consumer's changing attitude toward the value of fat in foods. Unlike the National Commission on Dairy Policy, however, the United States Cheese Makers Association has supported the adoption of a system to name fat-modified cheeses by using qualified versions of the standardized name.[43] Using a Wisconsin regulation as a model, the Association urged the creation of a general standard for versions of standardized cheeses with reduced milk fat content. That standard would require that the reduced-fat version of the standardized cheese have "the same or substantially same flavor, texture, and body characteristics" as the standardized product, limit the increase in moisture content to 25 percent above that allowed in the standardized cheese, and require a one-third reduction in milk fat content. The cheese makers also noted:

> If it is to be the Government's policy to encourage Americans to consume less fat, edible products containing less fat must be available to them. A 50 percent or more milk fat reduction requirement makes that virtually impossible in the cheese industry and denies consumers the ability to reduce fat intake and still enjoy and get the nutrition cheese provides.[44]

Without specifying the reduction that should be required, others agreed with the suggestion that "low-fat" or "reduced-fat" cheeses should be available. For example, Quaker Oats Company noted that FDA

> should countenance formulation and labeling, for example, of "low-fat cheddar cheese" with a reduced milk fat content, but with the organoleptic properties of "cheddar cheese." Standards of identity should not stand as a disincentive to production of more healthful foods and ingredients (*e.g.*, soy-based dairy alternatives). Moreover, these new innovative products should not be saddled with pejorative names such as "substitute," so long as they are nutritionally equivalent to the products which they resemble.[45]

The Quaker Oats comment is interesting because it, in some ways, reflects some of the confusion surrounding this issue. Regardless of its past attitudes, FDA has, for at least 15 years, "countenanced" formulation of low-fat cheeses and has not used standards as a disincentive to production of, for example, soy-based dairy alternatives. It is only the last sentence of the quoted comment that addresses the real issue: What are these modified or substitute foods to be called, and what impact will these names have on their acceptability to the consumers the companies are trying to serve?

Kraft General Foods (KGF) also endorsed the use of appropriate modifiers with standardized names to describe altered versions of standardized foods. KGF asked: "What clearer or more concise method could be used to describe a 'low fat cheddar cheese' except by those very terms? It describes a product with the physical and organoleptic characteristics of cheddar cheese except that it is low in fat."[46] The company stated that it supported the existence of food standards, which serve as a benchmark upon which to build modified products, but urged FDA to use sufficient regulatory flexibility to use those standards in a manner that encouraged the development of new, healthier modified products "marketed in terms which will clearly describe the new products in relation to the familiar existing benchmarks."[47]

Consumer groups, as well, supported those segments of industry that charge that the current system discourages the development of more healthful foods. The Center for Science in the Public Interest (CSPI) charged both that a standardized food name was misleading and that modified products should not be required to bear "unfamiliar or pejorative names."[48] CSPI stated that "the current law poses obstacles to updating nutritionally-obsolete standards and to marketing new, more healthful products. FDA should take steps to encourage the food industry to reformulate and name foods more consistently with current nutritional goals, without violating consumers' expectations about the quality of such foods."[49] CSPI also urged FDA to first review the names of standardized foods that include nutritional terms and revise those that no longer reflect contemporary thinking. For example, CSPI objected to the standardized name "low-fat milk," which allows for 2 percent fat, a 50 percent reduction from that in regular milk. Two percent milk still derives 38 percent of its calories from fat.

CSPI also argued that:

> FDA should make it more possible for truly low or reduced in fat, sodium, or low-sugar alternatives to standardized foods to bear attractive names. Health authorities and consumers alike would appreciate a wider selection of lower-fat and lower-sodium dairy products, lower-sodium canned vegetables and juices, and lower-sugar canned fruits, fruit juices, jams, and jellies, named as such. FDA, however, has prohibited names such as "low-fat cheddar cheese" by concluding perhaps too readily that such names cause foods to "purport to be" or be "represented as" standardized foods. As a result, new, more healthful foods must often bear unfamiliar or pejorative names.[50]

Similar support for modifying existing standards to establish subgroups of standardized foods, using criteria for lowered fat, sugar, or sodium, came from the American Public Health Association, which argued that those foods meeting the established criteria should be allowed to be labeled as, for example, "low-fat" cheese or "low-fat" ice cream.[51]

Even those segments of industry that support the continued use of food standards agree that changes to the procedures for adopting standards and modifying existing standards should be considered. In joint comments to FDA, both the Chocolate Manufacturers Association and the National Confectioners Association stated that they would

> strongly support a change which would permit the adoption of standards and their alteration by notice and comment rulemaking rather than by the far more cumbersome and time-consuming formal evidentiary hearings procedure. There should be no automatic stays of the effective date of a standard simply because an objection has been filed.[52]

The proposed change, however, would require Congress to amend the Act. The Milk Industry Foundation and the International Ice Cream Association similarly criticized the cumbersome procedure for amending standards. These associations urged FDA to "appoint a blue ribbon committee of qualified individuals from FDA, the states, the food industry, and consumer organizations to develop a mechanism by which the process for amending existing standards and establishing necessary new standards can be improved."[53]

Examination of industry's comments demonstrates that there is some confusion concerning exactly what FDA's policy is on the use of standardized names in nonstandardized foods. A March 13, 1990, letter to KGF spells out that policy as clearly as it has been spelled out in recent years.[54] In response to a request from KGF that the agency state that Kraft's "nonfat ice cream" is being lawfully marketed, or, alternatively, that FDA has not yet formulated an institutional position concerning that name, the Director of the Center for Food

Safety and Applied Nutrition, Fred R. Shank, laid out the agency's views on the use of standardized names.

> FDA has allowed the name of a standardized food in the name of a nonstandardized food when ingredients have been added to the standardized food to make a new food. For example, FDA has countenanced the marketing of "yogurt sweetened with aspartame," "calcium fortified orange juice," and "tomato juice with added vitamin C." In each instance, the standardized portion of the new food (e.g., the tomato juice "tomato juice with added vitamin C") has complied with the applicable standard.[55]

When a manufacturer chooses to subtract ingredients from the standardized food, thus no longer meeting the standard, FDA's position is that the standardized name cannot be used with the simple qualification of "nonfat" or "low-fat."[56]

Shank also stated that the existence of standards for yogurt, low-fat yogurt, and nonfat yogurt do not support KGF's position. The use of those modifiers, he noted, is a direct crossover from the standards for milk. Thus, low-fat yogurt is made with low-fat milk. In addition, Shank noted that in standardizing the three yogurts, the agency was simply standardizing the names industry itself had been calling various foods prior to the standard's enactment.

Although FDA's position does not seem to satisfy industry today because of the desire to delete or reduce ingredients such as fat from standardized foods, it must be recognized that it in fact represents a substantial departure from the agency's traditional interpretation. There is little question that a court following the *Quaker Oats* precedent would hold calcium-fortified or vitamin C-fortified tomato juice or enriched raisin bread to be illegal as foods that purport to be the standardized food but that do not meet the standard. Similarly, FDA has not receded at all, despite considerable pressure from some quarters, from its position that nutritional inferiority, and nutritional inferiority alone, is the standard to determine whether a food is an "imitation." Thus, for all practical purposes the issue of imitation foods has been buried and not revisited. It is, as suggested earlier and as recognized by the agency, only in the nomenclature of foods that disputes still exist.

Interviews with FDA officials responsible for food labeling decisions reveal that the public confusion and dispute are mirrored by internal disagreement. Just as some dairy producers believe that the standards of identity should be enforced as they were in the 1940s, some agency officials believe that any use of the standardized name in a food from which standardized ingredients have been removed is both illegal and wrong. Others recognize that, by and large, the issue is really one of the removal of fat from dairy products and are genuinely struggling to reach an agreement as to how modified products should be named.

One FDA official, for example, stated that it would be a "violation of the English language" to permit the sale of a product called "nonfat ice cream" because fat is the component that makes milk cream and to produce a "creamless" ice cream was perceived by this official as not only violating the English language but also debasing the Act. Another senior official, however, said that he had no problem with redefining the English language so long as the result yielded a level playing field. He noted that simply permitting the use of the term "reduced fat" with a name of a standardized food set no standards as to how that reduction in fat could be achieved. When fat is removed from many dairy products, something must be put in its place. The ingredients used to replace the fat can have a substantial impact on the nutritional and organoleptic characteristics of the resulting product.

When asked whether the use of defined descriptors such as reduced-fat or low-fat would make it easier to use standardized names, there was again disagreement. Shank stated that since the agency would probably require a 50 percent reduction in fat to qualify for the reduced-fat modifier, he did not believe that that would be a practical alternative for most dairy products. (The cheese makers agreed with him on this point. See the discussion on p. 329.) On the other hand, when asked whether he would object to the sale of a product called reduced-fat cheddar cheese if that product shared the organoleptic properties of standardized cheddar cheese and achieved the agency's expected 50 percent reduction in fat, he said he would be hard-pressed not to accept it. Another FDA official, however, flatly refused to countenance the use of such a name, although he could provide no reasoned explanation for his position.

The agency officials interviewed were unable to articulate a principled distinction between applying descriptors to nonstandardized names and applying them to standardized names. It may be that there are some products, such as ice cream, for which the public perception is so inextricably tied up with the traditional ingredients that descriptive distinctions ultimately fail. Yet, whether or not consumers would be misled by a product called "nonfat ice cream" may depend in part on consumers' expectations when they buy ice cream. If consumers in fact expect to receive flavored cream that is frozen while stirring, "nonfat ice cream" probably would be misleading. If, on the other hand, consumers expect to receive a frozen dairy dessert with the organoleptic properties of ice cream, then they may not be disappointed by a product with those properties but with no fat. Similarly, one would probably get different results if one asked consumers whether they would buy ice cream without any cream in it, or ice cream without any fat in it.

It is also important to consider whether use of the standardized name as part of a modified food has policy implications or is merely an attempt to "pass off" an inferior product by using the name of a superior product. After all, some venerable substitute products, such as margarine, have developed an identity of their own and are now the object of modified versions themselves. If one believes that consumers will try more readily a modified standardized food that promises health benefits if it looks like, tastes like, and is named after that food, then requiring cumbersome names probably does have a marketplace and health impact. (The marketplace impact may simply be the added costs of advertising and promotion to establish the franchise for the food; see p. 335.)

Despite the agency's firmly entrenched attitude against sanctioning the use of reduced-fat or nonfat as part of the name of a nonstandardized version of a standardized food, it has, in fact, not always taken vigorous action to prohibit that use. The agency has stated that it does not like the name "reduced-calorie mayonnaise," but that product remains on the market. One company is selling a "French nonfat dressing," a name that appears to violate current agency policy, and another company is selling cheddar reduced-fat cheese.

Finally, the state of flux in which the agency finds itself on this issue is perhaps best reflected by the fact that it is apparently quite willing to issue temporary marketing permits for the manufacture and sale of altered versions of standardized foods. The agency has issued three temporary marketing permits for "light ice cream," a product whose label declares it to contain "reduced calories" and "reduced fat."[57] Similarly, in 1989 the agency issued six temporary marketing permits for "light" sour cream. The Director of the Center for Food Safety and Applied Nutrition said that the agency is perfectly willing to use temporary marketing permits as a method to bring altered products to the market using the standardized name until such time as a new policy is developed. How the existence of a temporary marketing permit means that "light sour cream" is not confusing to consumers when that same name would be, in FDA's view, in the absence of the permit is not apparent.

Shank also stated that the agency is seriously considering asking Congress to amend the Federal Food, Drug, and Cosmetic Act to abolish the requirement that food standards be adopted and amended by using section 701(e) formal rulemaking procedures. He said the agency would be willing to make more changes to food standards if it could do so using notice and comment rulemaking.

THE MARKET IMPACT OF FOOD STANDARDS

In view of the vast array of foods available in the supermarket today, it is fair to ask whether FDA's attitudes and enforcement priorities have, in fact, hindered the development of new and potentially more healthful food products. Industry observers suggest that in the 1960s, the trade literature contained numerous articles concerning the hindrance to new product development caused by FDA's enforcement attitudes. There is no real evidence that these products could not actually be sold, yet the strongly held belief that a conservative FDA stifled innovation may, in fact, have contributed to stifling innovation. With the changes in the available products brought about by changes in FDA's attitudes in the 1970s, it is clear that companies felt that the law provided more leeway for product innovation and that innovation took place. Promulgation in 1978 of FDA's rule on labeling of reduced-calorie and low-calorie foods established rules that could help support the naming of altered versions of standardized foods. The availability of products such as low-sugar apricot preserves, low-sugar orange marmalade, and reduced-calorie salad dressing are ample testimony to the perceived consumer market for such products.

There is, however, a persistent belief that FDA policy stifles innovation. The clear message of many companies during the food labeling hearings was that FDA's attitude toward the naming of nonstandardized versions of standardized foods was hindering innovation. FDA's Shank believes that "standards have not kept manufacturers from developing more healthful foods. If they can achieve the organoleptic properties [that consumers want], they've been able to come up with names that adequately position the products."[58] Shank believes that technological problems in making modified foods are the primary forces that either drive or hinder new foods. "Problems of formulating an acceptable food are a bigger issue than what you call it."

Shank's assessment is supported by the development of products such as Simplesse®, a new substitute for dairy fat. Within weeks after its approval, it appeared on the market, replacing the fat in a fat-free ice-cream-like frozen dessert product which reportedly looks and tastes like premium ice cream. Its manufacturer is promoting it by its brand name, Simple Pleasures®, and has satisfied the statutory requirement that it bear a common or usual name by calling it "frozen dairy dessert." Of course, with a large enough advertising budget for the first product of its type, it may be that the product would sell, regardless of its name.

One of the consequences of limiting the use of standardized names in modified standardized products is that trademarks assume a greater role and enhanced advertising budgets are required. If the common or usual name of the food cannot easily disclose to consumers the alteration that has been accomplished to the standardized food and do so in a manner that is not thought to be counterproductive from a commercial standpoint, it is necessary to create or use trademarks and to advertise them heavily to create a market for the product. The expenditure necessary to create brand recognition means that smaller companies with smaller advertising budgets are less likely to be able to introduce innovative products and that lower-cost generic products are not likely to be created at all. For example, many supermarket chains sell house-brand cream cheese. If such a chain wanted to sell a reduced-fat version of cream cheese in response to perceived consumer demand for lower-fat food, it could not legally call the product House-Brand Reduced-Fat Cream Cheese, although that is a name that provides a good idea of what the food is and is not. Without a large advertising budget, it is unlikely that this supermarket chain would try to market the same product as House-Brand Reduced-Fat Spreadable Cheese Product.

The use of trademarks and money to circumvent common or usual name requirements can create new problems. Philadelphia brand cream cheese is probably one of the best-known trademarks in the marketplace. Capitalizing upon that franchise, there are now two Philadelphia Light products in the marketplace. One Philadelphia Light is a foil-wrapped cheese packaged to resemble Philadelphia brand cream cheese. Upon superficial examination, most consumers will probably assume that Philadelphia Light is a low-fat or low-calorie version of Philadelphia brand cream cheese. In fact, it is and it is not. Upon closer examination, one can see that Philadelphia Light bears the common or usual name of neufchatel cheese, a standardized cheese whose principal difference from cream cheese is its fat content.[59] Once popular in the United States, it has fallen into disfavor in recent years. But the manufacturer, by being able to trade on its well-known Philadelphia trademark, is able to convey the accurate message that this is a reduced-calorie or reduced-fat version of cream cheese without running afoul of the Act. (Generic neufchatel cheese, however, would not have that advantage, and most consumers would not recognize that neufchatel cheese is, in fact, a standardized version of reduced-fat cream cheese.)

Further shopping in the supermarket cheese department would reveal another Philadelphia Light cheese, this one resembling whipped cream cheese in a plastic tub. This Philadelphia Light, however, is called pasteurized process cheese food product and contains cream cheese and low-fat cottage cheese.

Where, as here, the brand name intentionally overpowers the common or usual name of the food, one might question whether the need to avoid the use of standardized names in nonstandardized products serves to protect or to mislead consumers.

USING FOOD STANDARDS TO IMPROVE THE NUTRITIONAL QUALITY OF FOOD

A reduction in the levels of ingredients that are thought to be undesirable is only one way of adapting foods, including standardized foods, to promote a healthier population. Food standards can also be used to encourage the consumption of more healthful ingredients, either by mandating their presence or by providing labeling rules that permit the use of the standardized name in an altered version.

In fact, the earliest food standards were emphatically used to help promote nutrition of Americans by encouraging and requiring the addition of vitamins and minerals. In 1940, FDA proposed to establish a standard of identity for flour. Partly in response to the American Medical Association's 1938 recommendation encouraging the fortification of milk, butter, and grain products, FDA developed an enriched-flour standard. Industry's voluntary use of enriched flour became widespread, and during World War II it was required. Although these changes sought to correct diseases due to deficiencies, not diseases of affluence, they provide ample precedent of the use of standards of identity to attempt to improve the health of Americans.

Assuming the existence of widespread agreement that fortification with a particular nutrient is desirable, one is still faced with the question of how to achieve it in a standardized food. Taking fiber as an example and macaroni and noodle products as the vehicle, one could encourage the consumption of more fiber by amending the standards of identity for various noodle products to require the addition of a specified level of an identified fiber. Alternatively, one could determine that a specified percentage increase in the fiber content of macaroni would entitle that standardized food to be called "high-fiber macaroni" or, perhaps less attractively, "macaroni with X percent added fiber." Since FDA's current policy permits the use of standardized names in nonstandardized foods if one is adding something to a food that otherwise meets the standard, the addition to standardized foods of nutritional components such as fiber is presumably permitted without further regulatory action (assuming, of course, that the fortification did not displace a required level of a mandatory nutrient, such as protein).

Food standards could also be used to promote the public health by reducing or eliminating the intake of ingredients thought to be unhealthful. Salt, for example, is an optional ingredient in many canned vegetables and a risk factor for hypertension. As an optional ingredient, its presence is declared (in small type) in the ingredient statement. A strongly proactive health policy might prohibit the addition of salt to standardized foods on the (untested) assumption that, left to their own choosing, consumers would use less salt. Similarly, the minimum fat levels of cheeses could be reduced to the lowest level capable of maintaining the general characteristics of the product.

Prohibiting or reducing ingredient levels in standardized foods is likely to arouse considerably more opposition than permitting or encouraging fortification would. And, as discussed below, until procedures to adopt or amend food standards are changed, the commitment of resources that such an approach would require make it unlikely that it will be attempted.

OPTIONS FOR CHANGE

The inconsistencies of FDA's behavior in recent years demonstrate that it has not articulated a coherent and principled body of rules to determine when the name of a standardized food may or may not be used in the name of an altered version of that food. Until such rules exist, it seems likely that decisionmaking will continue to be varied and ad hoc. Also, the agency's apparent abandonment of the view in the 1970s that the rules for naming foods should be the same whether those foods were standardized or nonstandardized should once again be enforced. It is not apparent why the names "low-sodium cheddar cheese" (a standardized food) and "low-sodium havarti" (a nonstandardized food) are nonmisleading to consumers, while "low-sodium swiss cheese" (a modified version of a standardized food) is misleading.

Yet, FDA's concern for the consumers' expectations for a standardized food can be appropriately recognized as well. A regulation to define reduced-fat and low-fat products would go a long way toward making the use of the descriptor appropriate in connection with the name of the standardized food. For example, if reduced-fat always means a one-third reduction in fat, it seems entirely appropriate and nonmisleading to suggest that ice cream made with one-third less fat than that called for in the standard could reasonably be called "reduced-fat ice cream," so long as its organoleptic properties and nutritional content were essentially the same as that of standardized ice cream. (If they were not, the product could be called reduced-fat frozen dessert.)

Similarly, a standardized product such as jam that contains one-third less sugar could appropriately be called reduced-sugar jam without being misleading to the concept of jam. As consumers become more sophisticated and as the agency looks to appropriate descriptors, it may be that the current regulation permitting the use of "reduced-calorie" in connection with the names of nonstandardized foods and, perhaps, some standardized foods should be reexamined. A reduction in calories can be accomplished in a number of ways, usually by reducing fat or carbohydrates, and it may be that the price that industry will have to pay for using standardized names should be disclosure of how the reduction in caloric content took place.

One alternative would be to permit the use of the descriptors "low" and "non" in connection with a standardized name only when fat, for example, has been removed but not replaced with other ingredients. This is how the various forms of milk are named. Similarly, there seems to be little chance of consumer deception when a totally different characterizing ingredient is used— and disclosed—to make an otherwise complying version of a standardized food. For example, the nonstandardized food "goat's milk yogurt" is unlikely to be confused with regular yogurt, which is made with cow's milk. (On the other hand, there is a standard for goat's milk ice cream.) The most difficult problem to resolve is the nomenclature of foods from which both some ingredient has been removed and another has been added to replace it.

Also needed are changes in the procedures used to adopt and amend standards. The formal adjudicatory hearing represents what Congress thought was necessary in 1938 to protect the rights of interested parties. For better or worse, today Congress routinely grants regulatory agencies the power to adopt equally important regulations by the less formal notice and comment procedure. It is difficult to explain why adopting and amending food standards should require a more formal and legalistic procedure than, for example, setting the mortgage interest rate on government-insured loans.[60]

Although formal adjudication is a useful tool to test the validity of rules based on determinable and contested fact, the findings involved in setting food standards are more like policy decisions than objectively verifiable facts. The procedures used to establish and amend food standards should assure that all policy and factual predicates are recognized, all differing views are acknowledged and responded to, and all decisions are explained adequately. This approach, plus meaningful judicial review, should more than adequately protect the public and private interests at stake.

Absent congressional revision of the food standards procedures, FDA could adopt regulations that have the effect of sharply limiting an objector's right to a hearing and thus streamline the procedure administratively. Similar regulations have been issued, and upheld, in the drug withdrawal area,[61] and other agencies as well have successfully adopted regulations limiting what otherwise appeared to be an absolute right to a hearing.[62]

Lest adopting and amending food standards by informal rulemaking be considered a panacea, it should be remembered that recent regulatory reform initiatives and declining budgets have made the issuance of any kind of rule difficult and time-consuming. If informal rulemaking is not the answer, then Congress should consider simply abolishing the food standards provisions of the Act and rely instead upon fully informative labeling and a better educated public to achieve the same consumer protection goals Congress had in mind in 1938.

Whatever policy its internal debates ultimately yield, FDA must resolve this issue and test its conclusion in a public forum. Ad hoc decisionmaking is as dangerous to progress as an intentionally negative rule is. The issues raised by the question of the use of standardized names in nonstandardized foods create enough controversy and implicate enough different values that fairness dictates that it be adopted in a public setting conducive to airing and responding to all conflicting views.

Finally, FDA needs sufficient resources to enforce whatever naming scheme is ultimately adopted. Consumers are probably most frequently confused when an absence of FDA rules and FDA enforcement leaves manufacturers to their own devices.[63]

NOTES

1. Act of June 30, 1906, ch. 3915, 34 Stat. 768, *repealed by* 52 Stat. 1059 (1938).

2. *Id.* §§ 7 & 8, 34 Stat. 769.

3. *See United States v. Ten Cases Bred Spred,* 49 F.2d 87 (8th Cir. 1931). *See generally* R. Merrill & E. Collier, "'Like Mother Used to Make': An Analysis of FDA Food Standards of Identity," 74 Colum. L. Rev. 561, 565 (1974) (hereinafter cited as "Merrill & Collier").

4. Act of July 8, 1930, ch. 874, 46 Stat. 1019. *See* H.T. Austern, "The F-O-R-M-U-L-A-T-I-O-N of Mandatory Food Standards," Food Drug Cosm. L.Q. 559 (December 1947).

5. Act of June 25, 1938, ch. 675, 52 Stat. 1040. It is customary to refer to provisions of the Act by their original section number with a parallel citation to Title 21 of the *United States Code,* and that practice will be followed here.

6. The Federal Food, Drug, and Cosmetic Act actually authorizes "the Secretary" to enforce its provisions. Since 1938, "the Secretary" has been, variously, the Secretary of Agriculture, the Federal Security Administrator, the Secretary of Health, Education and Welfare, and the Secretary of Health and Human Services. FDA is a nonstatutory agency, a part of the U.S. Department of Agriculture first, then the Federal Security Administration, then the U.S. Department of Health, Education, and Welfare, and now the U.S. Department of Health and Human Services. For simplicity, this paper uses the term "FDA" in place of "the Secretary" and as if it had existed since 1938.

7. Section 401, 21 USC § 341. Section 401 also authorized FDA to continue to adopt standards of quality and empowered it to adopt standards of fill of container as well.

8. Section 402(g), 21 USC § 342(g).

9. Section 403(l), 21 USC § 343(i).

10. Section 402(c), 21 USC § 342(c).

11. Section 701(e), 21 USC § 371(e).

12. Codified at 5 USC § 551 *et seq.*

13. FDA also received from Congress the authority to adopt rules by a different, less onerous process. Contained in section 701(a) of the Act, this authority was originally thought to permit the agency simply to issue the kinds of housekeeping rules required to operate any organization, such as the hours it would be open for business, the number of copies of documents to be submitted, and similar matters. With the passage of time, this general grant of housekeeping rulemaking has in fact been interpreted by the agency, with the support of the courts, to be a general grant of notice and comment rulemaking authority.

14. FDA and the food industry argued for 11 years to adopt a standard of identity for peanut butter, with much of that time devoted to the question of whether the food should contain 87 or 90 percent peanuts. FDA prevailed, and peanut butter contains 90 percent peanuts. *See generally* Merrill & Collier, 74 Colum. L. Rev. at 585–591.

15. *Id.* at 561.

16. Section 401, 21 USC § 341, authorizes FDA to "designate the optional ingredient which shall be named on the label." This has been read to mean that mandatory ingredients need not be listed on the label.

17. H.R. Rep. No. 2139, 75th Cong. 3d Sess. 5 (1938).

18. Merrill & Collier, 74 Colum. L. Rev. at 568.

19. Now codified at 21 CFR §§ 139.110 and 139.115 (1989), respectively.

20. *Federal Security Administrator v. Quaker Oats Co.,* 318 U.S. 218 (1943).

21. *Id.* at 232.

22. 340 U.S. 593 (1951).

23. Now codified at 21 CFR § 150.160 (1989).

24. 340 U.S. at 600.

25. It is interesting to speculate whether the fact that consumers never saw the imitation jam label was part of FDA's motivation in attempting to outlaw the product.

26. *United States v. 651 Cases . . . Chocolate Chil-Zert,* 114 F. Supp. 430 (N.D.N.Y. 1953).

27. The prohibition against imitating a food without prominently labeling it as imitation applies to all foods, not just standardized foods.

28.   *United States v. 856 Cases . . . "Demi,"* 254 F. Supp 57 (N.D.N.Y. 1966).

29.   *See, e.g.,* National Academy of Sciences, *The Role of Dietary Fat in Human Health* (1958); American Heart Association, Dietary Fat and Its Relation to Heart Attacks and Strokes, 23 *Circulation* 133 (January 1961); American Medical Association, The Regulation of Dietary Fat, 181 *JAMA* 411 (Aug. 4, 1962).

30.   White House Conference on Food, Nutrition, and Health, Final Report, Report of Panel III-2 at 120 (1970).

31.   Now codified at 21 CFR § 102.5 (1989).

32.   Now codified at 21 CFR § 101.3(e) (1989).

33.   *Federation of Homemakers v. Schmidt,* 539 F.2d 740 (D.C. Cir. 1976).

34.   R. Merrill & P. Hutt, *Cases and Materials on Food and Drug Law* at 126 (2d ed.) (in press). Peter Barton Hutt served as Chief Counsel of FDA from 1971 to 1975.

35.   39 Fed. Reg. 31,898 (Sept. 3, 1974).

36.   43 Fed. Reg. 11,695 (Mar. 21, 1978).

37.   43 Fed. Reg. 43,456 (Sept. 26, 1978).

38.   Interview with Fred R. Shank, Director, Center for Food Safety and Applied Nutrition, Food and Drug Administration (Mar. 23, 1990).

39.   FDA Regulatory Letter No. SEA-86-11, to Parker Hentage (May 1, 1986).

40.   Letter from L. Robert Lake, Director, Office of Compliance, Center for Food Safety and Applied Nutrition, FDA, to Stuart Pape (Nov. 23, 1988). The author of this letter conceded in a telephone interview that when he wrote the second letter, he recognized that the underlying product—yogurt—conformed to the standard of identity.

41.   National Commission on Dairy Policy, *Report and Recommendations* at 88 (1989).

42.   *Id.*

43.   Comments of the United States Cheese Makers Association, FDA Docket No. 89N-0226 (Dec. 13, 1989).

44.   *Id.* at 5.

45.   Comments of the Quaker Oats Company at 12, FDA Docket No. 89N-0226 (Jan. 5, 1990).

46.   Comments of Kraft General Foods at D-2, FDA Docket No. 89N-0226 (Jan. 5, 1990).

47.   *Id.*

48.   Comments of the Center for Science in the Public Interest at 39, FDA Docket No. 89N-0026 (Jan. 5, 1990).

49.   *Id.* at 38.

50.   *Id.* at 39.

51.   Comments of the American Public Health Association at 6, FDA Docket No. 89N-0026 (Jan. 5, 1990).

52.   Comments of the Chocolate Manufacturers Association and the National Confectioners Association at 16, FDA Docket No. 89N-0026 (Jan. 5, 1990).

53.   Comments of the Milk Industry Foundation and the International Ice Cream Association at 3, FDA Docket No. 89N-0026 (Nov. 1, 1990).

54.   Letter from Fred R. Shank, Director, Center for Food Safety and Applied Nutrition, Food and Drug Administration, to Merrill S. Thompson (Mar. 13, 1990).

55.   *Id.*

56. KGF changed the name of the food in question after receiving this letter.

57. The most recent temporary market permit was noticed at 55 Fed. Reg. 12,736 (Apr. 5, 1990). *See also* 55 Fed. Reg. 3772 (Feb. 5, 1990).

58. Interview with Fred R. Shank, Director, Center for Food Safety and Applied Nutrition, Food and Drug Administration (Mar. 23, 1990).

59. Now codified at 21 CFR § 133.162 (1989).

60. *See, e.g.*, 38 USC § 1803 (setting of interest rates for Veterans Administration loans).

61. The regulations themselves were upheld in *Pharmaceutical Manufacturers Ass'n v. Finch*, 318 F. Supp. 301 (D. Del. 1970), and their application in a series of Supreme Court cases, *USV Pharmaceutical Corp. v. Weinberger*, 412 U.S. 655 (1973); *Weinberger v. Bentex Pharmaceuticals, Inc.*, 412 U.S. 645 (1973); *Ciba Corp. v. Weinberger*, 412 U.S. 640 (1973); and *Weinberger v. Hynson, Westcott & Dunning, Inc.*, 412 U.S. 609 (1973).

62. *See, e.g., United States v. Florida East Coast R. Co.*, 410 U.S. 224 (1973).

63. One author has suggested that FDA use its "enforcement discretion" and establish "action levels" for "selected 'lite' standardized foods." J. Agar, "Generally Recognized as Sour Cream: Treating Standards of Food Identity as a Success," 44 Food Drug Cosm. L. Rev. 237, 248 (1989). He argues that the Act contains sufficient discretion that the agency can permit the sale of modified standardized foods that are somehow not legal: "The analysis suggested in this article does not suggest that honestly labeled modifications of standardized foods *must* in all cases be within the law." It is hard to imagine how the statute could be interpreted in such a way that a truthful and nonmisleading food name would be unexceptional from an enforcement standpoint but illegal nonetheless. A policy that cannot be articulated in the *Federal Register* and defended successfully in court should not govern the future of modified standardized foods.

Index

descriptor definitions, 14–16, 18–21,
    24, 171, 176, 179, 181, 185,
    199
dietary fiber information, 18, 178–179
education of consumers, 30, 269
exemptions from mandatory
    requirements, 12, 132, 179
fat information, 16–17, 171
fatty acid information, 16, 17, 171
food analysis, 11
format of labels, 13, 29, 142, 171,
    259, 261, 264
fresh foods, 12–13, 142–143
ingredient listing, 17–18, 25, 171,
    176, 227
institutional packages, 12, 134
iron information, 21, 199
mandatory nutrition labeling
    requirements, 132
meat, 12–13, 142–143
micronutrient information, 199
noncommercial food service
    operations, 14, 154
placement and prominence of food
    components, 28, 259
point-of-purchase information, 12–13,
    14, 142
potassium information, 20, 186–187
poultry, 12–13, 142–143
"as prepared" nutrient declaration, 259
produce (fruits and vegetables),
    12–13, 142–143
protein information, 19, 181
restaurant foods, 13–14, 150–151
seafood, 12–13, 142–143
serving size, 22–23, 28, 214–216, 259
sodium information, 19, 185
source definitions, 24, 199, 224
standards of identity, 231
testing of label formats, 25, 29, 261,
    264
units of measurement, 28, 259
U.S. RDAs, 24, 224
voluntary nutrition labeling, 14, 154
Recommended Dietary Allowances
    (RDAs)

as basis for U.S. RDAs, 5, 23, 45, 58,
    68, 216
comparison with U.S. RDAs, 218
nutrients in standard serving of food
    ranked by, 222–223
Reforms, see Food labeling reforms;
    Recommendations
Regulation of food labeling
authority to expand nutrition labeling,
    280–289; see also FDA
    regulation of nutrition labeling;
    USDA regulation of nutrition
    labeling
in commercial food service industry,
    147–150
enforcement issues, 142
overlap in FDA and USDA
    jurisdictions, 53–54
overview of U.S. system, 1–2, 3–6,
    39–40, 51–55
statutory authorities, see Federal
    Food, Drug, and Cosmetic Act;
    Federal Meat Inspection Act;
    Poultry Products Inspection Act
uniformity in, 54, 64
see also Deficiencies in food label
    requirements; Legislative
    reforms; Mandatory nutrition
    labeling
Restaurant foods
attention to dietary recommendations,
    13, 144–147
computation of nutrient information,
    13, 146–147
costs of labeling, 273–274
dissemination of nutrition and
    ingredient information by food
    chain operators, 147
eating trends and attitudes of
    consumers, 144–145
FDA regulatory authority over, 60–61,
    285–287
industry characteristics, 13, 143–144
ingredient labeling of, 147–148, 286
legislation on labeling, 294